Ontogeny

of

IMMUNITY

Ontogeny
of
IMMUNITY

Edited by

RICHARD T. SMITH
ROBERT A. GOOD
PETER A. MIESCHER

University of Florida Press ⅃ Gainesville ⅃ 1967

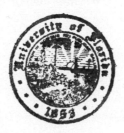

Proceedings of the second Developmental Immunology Workshop held February 6, 7, 8, 1966, at Sanibel Island, Florida, under the sponsorship of the National Institute of Child Health and Human Development

A University of Florida Press Book

Published with Assistance from the National Institute of Child Health and Human Development

Library of Congress Catalog Card Number: 66-29457

PRINTED BY THE H. & W. B. DREW COMPANY, JACKSONVILLE, FLORIDA
BOUND BY UNIVERSAL-DIXIE BINDERY, INC., JACKSONVILLE, FLORIDA

The
Editors'
Preface

● ●

● ●

THIS VOLUME summarizes and formalizes the proceedings of the second of a series of developmental immunology workshops. These workshops came about originally as a result of the interest of Drs. Robert Aldrich and Dwain Walcher of the National Institute of Child Health and Human Development in fostering more rapid and effective communication among the investigators concerned with the time-linked aspects of immune mechanisms. It is patterned after the highly successful antibody workshops which have served as an informal arena for exchange of ideas and data for immunologists in the recent past.

Sanibel Island proved again to be ideal for the workshops because of ease of access by air transportation, but sufficient remoteness to insure an atmosphere conducive to exchange. The proceedings of the first workshop have appeared in the volume "Phylogeny of Immunity," published in early 1966. This companion volume is published because no comprehensive resource material was available concerning the ontogenetic aspects of immunity. Accordingly, the participants agreed to prepare formal manuscripts, and the discussions were recorded and edited. It is hoped that the body data represented and discussion collected in this volume will be helpful to investigators concerned with developmental biology as well as to immunologists who see in the ontogenetic approach an engaging opportunity to gain new understanding of immune mechanisms. A third workshop will be held in 1967, on the subject of "The Immunologic Deficiency Diseases in Man." Under joint sponsorship with the National Foundation, the proceedings of that conference will also be published.

This volume would not have been possible without the adroit editorial and administrative assistance of Sondra Smith, Jean Curry, and Rosemary Welch, for which the editors and participants are deeply grateful. The workshop and the preparation of the book have been supported by grants from the National Institute of Child Health and Human Development (HD-1124-02) and the Department of Pediatrics, University of Florida.

RICHARD T. SMITH
ROBERT A. GOOD
PETER A. MIESCHER

Participants

William H. Adler, III, M.D.
Research Fellow, Department of Pediatrics, University of Florida, Gainesville, Florida

William A. Altemeier, M.D.
Instructor, Department of Pediatrics, University of Florida, Gainesville, Florida

Robert A. Auerbach, Ph.D.
Professor of Zoology, Department of Zoology, University of Wisconsin, Madison, Wisconsin

Matthew Block, Ph.D., M.D.
Professor of Medicine and *Chief of Hematology Service,* University of Colorado Medical Center, Denver, Colorado

Werner Braun, Ph.D.
Professor, Institute of Microbiology, Rutgers University, New Brunswick, New Jersey

John J. Cebra, Ph.D.
Associate Professor of Microbiology, University of Florida, Gainesville, Florida

Edwin L. Cooper, Ph.D.
Assistant Professor, Department of Anatomy, University of California, Los Angeles, California

Max D. Cooper, M.D.
Instructor, Department of Pediatrics, University of Minnesota Medical School, Minneapolis, Minnesota

James D. Ebert, Ph.D.
Director, Department of Embryology, Carnegie Institution of Washington, Baltimore, Maryland

Michael Feldman, Ph.D.
Head, Section of Cell Biology, Weizmann Institute of Science, Rehovoth, Israel

Joanne Finstad, M.S.
Research Fellow, Departments of Pediatrics and Microbiology, University of Minnesota, Minneapolis, Minnesota

Marvin Fishman, Ph.D.
Associate Member, Public Health Research Institute of the City of New York, Inc., New York

Robert A. Good, M.D., Ph.D.
American Legion Memorial Heart Research Professor of Pediatrics and Microbiology, University of Minnesota Medical School, Minneapolis, Minnesota

William H. Hildemann, Ph.D.
Associate Professor of Immunology, Department of Microbiology and Immunology, University of California, Los Angeles, California

Kurt Hirschhorn, M.D.
Associate Professor of Medicine, New York University School of Medicine, New York

Arthur G. Johnson, Ph.D.
Associate Professor, Department of Microbiology, University of Michigan, Ann Arbor, Michigan

Charles B. Kimmel, B.A.
Student, Department of Biology, Johns Hopkins University, Baltimore, Maryland; Department of Embryology, Carnegie Institution of Washington, Baltimore, Maryland

PARTICIPANTS

Irwin R. Konigsberg, Ph.D.
Staff Member, Department of Embryology,
Carnegie Institution of Washington,
Baltimore, Maryland

Rose G. Mage, Ph.D.
Staff Member, Immunochemistry Section,
Laboratory of Immunology, NIAID,
National Institutes of Health,
Bethesda, Maryland

Peter A. Miescher, M.D.
Professor of Medicine, Department of
Medicine, New York University School of
Medicine, Bellevue Medical Center,
New York, New York

N. A. Mitchison, D. Phil.
Medical Research Council Staff, National
Institute for Medical Research, Mill Hill,
London, England

John Papaconstantinou, Ph.D.
Staff Member, The Oak Ridge National
Laboratory, Biology Division,
Oak Ridge, Tennessee

Raymond D. A. Peterson, M.D.
Established Investigator, American Heart
Association; *Visiting Investigator,* Univer-
sity of Uppsala, Uppsala, Sweden

Robert T. Schimke, M.D.
Chief, Section on Biochemical Regulation,
NIAMD, National Institutes of Health,
Bethesda, Maryland

Howard A. Schneiderman, Ph.D.
Director, Developmental Biology Center,
Western Reserve University,
Cleveland, Ohio

Martin L. Schulkind, M.D.
Instructor, Department of Pediatrics,
University of Florida, Gainesville, Florida

Arthur M. Silverstein, Ph.D.
Associate Professor, The Wilmer Institute,
Johns Hopkins University School of
Medicine, Baltimore, Maryland

Richard T. Smith, M.D.
Professor and *Chairman,* Department of
Pediatrics, University of Florida,
Gainesville, Florida

Arthur J. L. Strauss, M.D.
Head, Section on Autoimmunity,
Laboratory of Immunology, National In-
stitute of Allergy and Infectious Diseases,
National Institutes of Health,
Bethesda, Maryland

G. Jeanette Thorbecke, M.D.
Assistant Professor of Pathology, Depart-
ment of Pathology, New York University
School of Medicine, New York

Ralph van Furth, M.D.
Department of Microbial Diseases, Leiden;
Guest Investigator, Rockefeller University,
New York, N. Y.

Introduction

THE LYMPHORETICULAR SYSTEM shares with the hematopoeietic system the characteristic that, continuously throughout the life-span, the processes of cell differentiation from primitive precursors is critical to the function of the system. It is not surprising, therefore, that the mechanisms which control the differentiation of cells and tissues that lead to immunological recognition or antibody formation share in principle the characteristics of differentiation in more general systems which have been studied by developmental biologists.

Accordingly, immunological development can be described in terms of the same levels of ontogeny which have been used to describe the general cases of development by Grobstein.

Immunological function may be examined at the level of genetic control over transcription processes leading to the formation of antibody proteins. At a second level of ontogeny, the form, function, and organization of the individual cells involved in this translation process can be investigated, and the lymphocytes and plasma cells characterized in terms of the relation of organization to cell products characteristic of the immune response. At another level, interactions between cells—particularly cells of epithelial and mesenchymal origin—which direct differentiation are particularly characteristic of the lymphoreticular system. The process of induction is active in the formation of the primitive thymus in higher mammals, and possibly other contexts. At a higher degree of organization, the ontogeny of organs and the interactions of the cells and cell systems within these organs during early development can be manipulated experimentally, and the effects of initial and continuing contact with the microbiologic and antigenic components of the environment can be evaluated.

The ontogeny of immunity has been considered in this book roughly in terms of these levels, as a basis for continuity of the presentations and discussions. This operational division did not inhibit vertical integration in terms of mechanisms applicable at several levels of ontogeny. Where whole organ or whole organism events might be explained in terms of processes occurring at the molecular level, this was attempted.

The common interest between cell biologists concerned with the general and the immunological cases of differentiation has been such as to make this delineation of the current state of the art an easy task, and it has stimulated definition of major and unexplored problems. This volume is the outcome of discourse between such individuals in a developmental immunology workshop.

RICHARD T. SMITH

Contents

CONTENTS

PART III

Embryonic Development of Form and Function of the Lymphoreticular System

EDITOR: ROBERT AUERBACH

PART IV

Pre- and Postnatal Function of the Lymphoreticular System

EDITOR: ARTHUR SILVERSTEIN

CONTENTS

Synthesis and Speculation

**EDITORS: R. T. SMITH, R. A. GOOD,
and P. A. MIESCHER**

PART I

DIFFERENTIATION AND GENETIC CONTROL OF DIFFERENTIATION: GENERAL ASPECTS PERTINENT TO THE LYMPHORETICULAR SYSTEM

Editor: James D. Ebert

I

JAMES D. EBERT

Developmental interactions at cellular and molecular levels

THE CONTRIBUTORS were charged with presenting a brief, but clear, overview of current thought on mechanisms of cellular differentiation and regulation of protein synthesis to serve as a background for more specific discussions of the differentiation of immunologically competent cells and the synthesis of antibodies. Attention was to be centered on cell differentiation, deliberately excluding problems of morphogenesis. Contributors were asked to bear in mind the two principal components in antibody formation: intrinsic and extrinsic— genetic limitations and antigenic stimuli. It followed naturally, therefore, that attention was paid on the one hand to the mechanisms underlying the synthesis of tissue-specific proteins in relation to the stage of cellular maturation, and, on the other, to the interplay of genetic and environmental or physiological factors controlling protein synthesis in tissues of adult animals.

A second consideration to which contributors were asked to address themselves was the following: Do any of the techniques now employed by students of development need to be exploited by those whose efforts are directed largely toward problems of immunogenesis? This question evoked discussions of, at first, the effectiveness and limitations of clonal techniques in studying differentiation, a subject which appears to have obvious importance to immunologists; and, subsequently, the importance of cell interactions.

The statements of the four principal con-

tributors are presented separately, without editorial change or comment. The very fact that this is possible attests to the care taken by each contributor to assure that his presentation fitted the framework, and matched the mood, of the Workshop.

One of the questions which courses through and underlies not only the first session, but the Workshop as a whole, concerns the requirement for rapid cell division, or at least for DNA synthesis, prior to differentiation. It has long been known that the beginning of *overt* cellular differentiation, at least, and the synthesis of tissue-specific proteins, occurs after DNA synthesis has ceased. Recent evidence from several laboratories re-enforces this argument: *cellular* DNA synthesis appears to be essential for the fixation of the transformed state when cells are transformed by tumor viruses. Cell growth is essential for the transformation of fibroblasts of line 3T3 by SV40 virus (1). Cellular DNA synthesis has been observed in cultures infected by polyoma virus (2, 3, 4). Bader (5) has advanced evidence that the transformation of fibroblasts by Rous sarcoma virus (RSV) fails when cellular DNA synthesis is inhibited.

Todaro and Green have presented an excellent summary of the evidence supporting the essentiality of DNA synthesis for transformation: (a) organs containing cells with a high growth rate are usually among those more susceptible to neoplastic change; (b) cells which never divide in adults do not give

3

rise to neoplasms; and (c) young animals are more susceptible than adults to viral onco-genesis. In our own laboratory we have been exploring the interaction of RSV with differ-entiating muscle cells, using the cloning tech-niques of Konigsberg (6) and Hauschka and Konigsberg (7). From these studies, carried out in collaboration with M. E. Kaighn, H. H. Lee, and P. M. Stott (8, 9), it is clear that RSV will infect and transform myoblasts, which are capable of division; however, al-though the virus is detected in multinucleated myotubes, the myotubes are not transformed.

Is there an example of "differentiation with-out DNA synthesis"? Brachet (10) showed that "differentiation without cleavage" (11) did involve DNA synthesis. Is the question meaningful? Possibly we will be able to decide only when we know more about the stability of DNA-like RNAs.

The extent to which these questions are pertinent to our discussion of antibody forma-tion will be revealed in the pages that follow.

REFERENCES

1. Todaro, C. G., and Green, H. (1966): Cell growth and the initiation of transformation by SV40. Proc. Nat. Acad. Sci., U.S. *55*, 302.
2. Dulbecco, R., Hartwell, L. H., and Vogt, M. (1965): Induction of cellular DNA synthesis by polyoma virus. Proc. Nat. Acad. Sci., U.S. *53*, 403.
3. Weil, R., Michel, M. R., and Ruschmann, G. K. (1965): Induction of cellular DNA synthesis by polyoma virus. Proc. Nat. Acad. Sci., U.S. *53*, 1468.
4. Gershon, D., Hausen, P., Sachs, L., and Wino-cour, E. (1965): On the mechanism of polyoma virus-induced synthesis of cellular DNA. Proc. Nat. Acad. Sci., U.S. *54*, 1584.
5. Bader, J. P. (1965): Transformation by Rous sarcoma virus: a requirement for DNA synthesis. Science *149*, 757.
6. Konigsberg, I. R. (1963): Clonal analysis of myogenesis. Science *140*, 1273.
7. Hauschka, S., and Konigsberg, I. R. (1966): The influence of collagen on the development of muscle clones. Proc. Nat. Acad. Sci., U.S. *55*, 119.
8. Kaighn, M. E., Ebert, J. D., and Stott, P. M. (1965): Animal viruses and embryos. Carnegie Inst. of Washington Year Book *64*, 483.
9. Lee, H. H., Kaighn, M. E., and Ebert, J. D. (1966): Carnegie Inst. of Washington Year Book *65*, in press.
10. Brachet, J. (1957): Biochemical Cytology. New York, Academic Press, p. 191.
11. Lillie, F. R. (1902): Differentiation without cleavage in the egg of the annelid *Chaetopterus pergamentaceus*. Wilhelm Roux Arch. Entwick-lungsmechanik *14*, 477.

2

HOWARD A. SCHNEIDERMAN

Control systems in developing insects

IT HAS BEEN a fruitful custom to bring various experimental biologists together to provide a counterpoint for discussions of immunological mechanisms. An entomologist is appropriate because insects have begun to provide some interesting clues to the nature of the control systems that regulate the development of multicellular organisms.

The following points will be covered: (a) Possible sites of regulation, (b) Insect hormones as agents which control differentiation, (c) Possible site of action of these hormones, and (d) The reversibility of differentiation.

A central problem of development is what determines the career of a cell in a developing organism. The cells of an organism carry identical genomes, but in different tissues and in different stages of development they have very different protein compositions and engage in very different biochemical activity. For many years it was assumed that such differences were brought about by regulatory processes operating in the cytoplasm. For example, students of development conceived of metabolic cycles and chain reactions which could, once set into motion, perpetuate themselves. These cycles were thought to be regulated by only a few specific factors such as hormones and inducers. The role of the nucleus was recognized as a central one but most of the "action" was in the cytoplasm.

This view is no longer possible. Today the search for mechanisms of regulating cell metabolism in general and cell differentiation in particular focuses more and more on the genome. It is widely held that a great deal of metabolic regulation occurs at the level of the gene and that much of differentiation can be understood in terms of the management of genetic information.

One formulation goes as follows: During the course of the cell life different parts of the genome express themselves at different times and the cell makes different sorts and amounts of specific proteins. By determining the rate of synthesis of specific proteins differentiation of the cell is controlled. How are these rates of specific synthesis controlled in the cells of multicellular organisms? Quite frankly, nobody knows. But we have learned a good deal about control mechanisms in microorganisms, and there is good reason to suppose that many of these ideas are relevant to multicellular organisms. To simplify subsequent discussions allow me to summarize a few bits of the familiar dogma and pinpoint some possible sites and mechanisms of regulation.

The genome is a large collection of separate units of information. Transcription of information from the genome into messenger RNA is usually blocked by repressors. Only when the genome is unblocked can the cell make specific messenger RNAs. To unblock a specific part of the genome the cell has to inactivate a specific repressor. This can be done by specific control substances—inducers—which combine with the repressor to activate it. By this means the organism can derepress or acti-

5

vate specific genes in a cell and the cell is enabled to synthesize specific mRNA molecules. Once a mRNA is produced, other sorts of regulation are possible. Now each mRNA must combine with ribosomes (in the nucleus or cytoplasm) to form clusters of ribosomes or polysomes which serve as sites of nuclear or cytoplasmic protein synthesis. The rate at which specific mRNAs combine with ribosomes is a process that could be subject to both extrinsic and intrinsic regulation. The rate at which a particular mRNA is read and a particular protein synthesized is a process that can be regulated. The lifetime of a specific mRNA is something that could be regulated either intrinsically in terms of the particular sequence of bases in the mRNA or extrinsically.

Thus, rates of protein synthesis may be regulated by synthesizing new messenger RNAs (as in *E. coli*) or activating previously synthesized messenger RNAs (as in fertilized eggs or adult liver cells).

There are doubtless also other sites of regulation besides the nucleus and the polysomes. These become apparent when one looks at an electron micrograph of a cell. Surely cellular and intracellular membranes play a central role in the regulation of specific syntheses.

What is the chemical nature of the controlling substances and from where do they originate? Some control substances like repressors originate within the cell itself. Others originate in the environment of the cell as products of other cells. It is the controlling substances that originate outside of target cells themselves that I wish to deal with in this discussion; in particular, with certain hormones that control the development of insects. The principal interest of my laboratory has been the chemical nature of these hormones and the mechanism of their action in development.

As a text for my discussion I shall use various wild silkworms of the family Saturniidae such as *Cecropia, Cynthia, Polyphemus,* and others. These wild silkworms are familiar creatures common to much of North America and their life cycle is familiar to you. The caterpillar hatches from its egg and periodically it molts. This molting is a distinguishing feature of insect growth. Now the epidermis of an insect is bound to an outer layer of cuticle and cannot grow unless it detaches

from the cuticle. Periodically the epidermal cells of immature insects detach from their cuticle, grow by cell division or cell enlargement or both, and secrete a new and extensible cuticle with folds. When this cuticle is nearly complete the epidermal cells produce and release enzymes which digest the inner layers of the old cuticle which they then absorb. Thereupon the epidermal cells waterproof the new cuticle and the old cuticle is shed. In the *Cecropia* silkworm there are four larval molts, a larval-pupal molt and a pupal-adult molt.

The periodic cell multiplication and molting of *Cecropia* and other immature insects is brought about by two hormones, one produced by secretory cells in the insect's brain and the other by glands on the prothorax, the prothoracic glands. The "brain hormone" acts by stimulating the prothoracic glands. The prothoracic glands respond to this stimulus by releasing prothoracic gland hormone—called ecdysone—which in turn acts on various cells of the insect and causes them to grow. In the case of the epidermal cells of the insect, ecdysone causes them to deposit a new cuticle and to molt.

A third hormone, the juvenile hormone, is secreted by the corpora allata, endocrine glands located near the brain of the insect. More than thirty years ago V. B. Wigglesworth showed that this hormone promotes larval development but prevents metamorphosis. Its presence in the immature insect insures that when the larva molts it will retain its larval characters and not differentiate into an adult. The juvenile hormone is a remarkable agent which permits growth but prevents maturation.

When larval cells are stimulated to grow and molt by the prothoracic gland hormone, the presence of a high concentration of juvenile hormone causes them to use their synthetic machinery to secrete larval cuticle. In the presence of juvenile hormone, the cells secrete pupal cuticle; in the absence of juvenile hormone, these cells may secrete adult cuticle directly and by-pass the pupal molt. By regulating the release of brain hormone molting is controlled; by regulating the release of juvenile hormone maturation is controlled. In simplest terms, in some way ecdysone stimulates the synthetic activity necessary for growth and molting. Juvenile hormone influences the kind of synthetic activities that occur.

Let us consider the chemical nature and mode of action of the molting hormone ecdysone. To bio-assay for ecdysone one takes an isolated abdomen of an insect and injects the extract to be tested. If the isolated abdomen molts, then the extract contained ecdysone. Peter Karlson and Adolph Butenandt began work on ecdysone twenty-four years ago. They crystallized it eleven years ago and Karlson has recently announced its structure. From an analysis of 250 mg of crystals isolated from 1,000 kg of pupae of the commercial silkworm Karlson and his coworkers have found ecdysone to be a steroid closely resembling cholesterol with the empirical formula $C_{27}H_{44}O_6$. Its identification marks the culmination of twenty-four years of painstaking work. It appears to act on all arthropods—insects, crustacea, etc. It is the first steroid hormone identified in an invertebrate. Shortly after their announcement of the structure of this insect hormone, the isolation and structural identification of the corresponding hormone in the crustacea was announced. This hormone, called crustecdysone, differs from ecdysone only in having an extra hydroxyl group. The fact that ecdysone and its relatives are steroids indicates that steroid hormones are not a recent innovation of the vertebrates.

The discovery that ecdysone is a steroid is of uncommon interest, but equally remarkable are some recent reports on its mode of action which appear to have important consequences for students of growth and suggest that this hormone may act on the nucleus, perhaps on the genes themselves or on the nuclear membrane and bring about the elaboration of specific RNA molecules that are destined to participate personally in the cytoplasmic syntheses that characterize growth and molting. Principal support for this conjecture comes from experiments of Ulrich Clever and Peter Karlson on the puffing pattern of giant chromosomes of the midge *Chironomus*. In *Chironomus* as in most Diptera the daughter chromatids do not separate following replication. Instead, they line up side by side to form giant chromosomes consisting of hundreds of sister chromatids paired gene for gene. Chromosomal puffs indicate a local loosening of the bundles of threads. Clever and Karlson have

shown that injections of pure ecdysone into *Chironomus* larvae cause prompt and characteristic changes in the puffing pattern of the chromosomes, changes identical to those that occur during pupation. These changes begin within fifteen minutes of injection and the size of the puffs is proportional to the dose. As little as 10^{-5} micrograms is effective. One particular puff in one chromosome seems to be affected before all the others. These puffs are regions of high RNA synthesis and Clever and Karlson equate puffing of a chromosome region with gene activation. They interpret these experiments to mean that ecdysone acts on the chromosomes and activates particular gene loci to bring about the syntheses that culminate in molting.

Experiments of this sort have led to the hypothesis that steroid hormones and perhaps several other hormones of vertebrates directly regulate gene activity. How they act is not yet known. Are they inducers, corepressors? Do they combine with DNA, with histones, with the nuclear membrane? Or notwithstanding the attractiveness of the hypothesis, must we look for sites of steroid action in the cytoplasm rather than in the nucleus? Do these hormones cause cytoplasmic derepression of some sort or act on the cellular and intracellular membranes?

The last matter I wish to discuss is the reversibility of differentiation with particular reference to insects. Is differentiation of insect cells reversible? If insect cells can dedifferentiate, is DNA synthesis an obligatory step in this process? Answers to these questions have been revealed by a number of simple experiments. If one injects a pupa of a moth with juvenile hormone, the pupal epidermal cells do not secrete adult cuticle. Instead, they secrete a new pupal cuticle. This is clearly not a reversal of differentiation but the prevention of progress in differentiation. Juvenile hormone prevents the pupa from using adult instructions. Indeed, reversing the differentiation of a whole insect has so far proved impossible and no one has succeeded in causing a moth to molt into a caterpillar. However, it is possible to reverse differentiation in a fragment of an insect. This was accomplished by Hans Piepho who implanted a fragment of skin of an adult wax moth into a young larval host (which contains a high concentration of juvenile hormone) and discovered that the adult epidermis in a few instances dedifferentiated and secreted larval cuticle. Invariably several molts were required before the implanted fragment of adult integument secreted larval cuticle. Apparently, prolonged exposure to juvenile hormone and repeated molts enabled the cells to reuse larval instructions and synthesize larval cuticle.

From these experiments it appears that cytodifferentiation of insect cells is not irreversible. Nor can it be argued that the adult epidermal cells that form the new larval cuticle were "reserve" cells which did not participate in the formation of the adult cuticle. So far as we can ascertain, the epidermis of insects is but a single cell layer in thickness, and each cell is responsible for secreting the cuticle that overlies itself.

The experiments also emphasize a special interest of the juvenile hormone from the viewpoint of developmental biology. It is an agent which permits the larval part of the genome to express itself. In the absence of juvenile hormone the adult part of the genome expresses itself and adult development is accompanied by a variety of syntheses which do not occur in larval life or occur at very different rates.

Two further features of these experiments are noteworthy. First, is the fact that it took several molts and some time before the adult epidermal cells "retooled" for the task of making larval cuticle. This period of retooling probably involved both the degradation (or excretion) of enzyme molecules specifically associated with adult syntheses as well as the reprogramming of the genome. The second feature is that in these experiments with fragments considerable regeneration occurred and most, and perhaps all, of the cells in the implanted fragment were the products of regeneration-induced mitosis. In short, DNA replication occurred in the adult epidermal cells before they began to secrete larval cuticle. Is this DNA synthesis necessary? May it be that a genome which is functioning in a particular way cannot switch to a new kind of function without replication? Perhaps DNA replication erases some earlier applied biases for particular functions and enables the genome to be reprogrammed. There is considerable evidence that in insects DNA replication is prerequisite for reprogramming of the genome. For example, epidermal cells around a wound synthesize DNA and are many times more sensitive to reprogramming by juvenile hormone than epidermal cells in an uninjured area. If you prevent DNA replication with an inhibitor of DNA synthesis such as mitomycin C, then the cells in the injured area lose their sensitivity to juvenile hormone and behave like other epidermal cells.

Much more work needs to be done, but the evidence at hand favors the view that in many insects reversibility of differentiation depends upon DNA replication. If this turns out to be generally true, it implies that dedifferentiation involves primarily changes in the control of transcription (mRNA synthesis) rather than of translation (protein synthesis).

In this brief discussion I have attempted to demonstrate ways in which insects can be used to answer a number of basic questions about development. Because of their short generation time which permits extensive genetic studies, a wealth of information about their genetics, desirable cytological features like giant chromosomes, an extensive literature on their physiology, and their great convenience as laboratory organisms, it appears likely that in the future insects will become principal objects for the study of developmental problems in multicellular organisms.

BIBLIOGRAPHY

Clever, U. (1966): Gene activity patterns and cellular differentiation. Amer. Zool. 6, 33.

Krishnakumaran, A., and Schneiderman, H. A. (1964): Developmental capacities of the cells of an adult moth. J. Exp. Zool. 157, 293.

Krishnakumaran, A., Oberlander, H., and Schneiderman, H. A. (1965): Rates of DNA and RNA synthesis in various tissues during larval moult cycle of Samia cynthis ricini (Lepidoptera). Nature 205, 1131.

Meyer, A. S., Schneiderman, H. A., and Gilbert, L. I. (1965): A highly purified preparation of juvenile hormone from the silk moth *Hyalophora cecropia L.* Nature *206,* 272.

Oberlander, H., Berry, S., Krishnakumaran, A., and Schneiderman, H. A. (1965): RNA and DNA synthesis during activation and secretion of the prothoracic glands of saturniid moths. J. Exp. Zool. *159,* 15.

Schneiderman, H. A., and Gilbert, L. I. (1964): Control of growth and development in insects. Science *143,* 325.

Wigglesworth, V. B. (1964): The hormonal regulation of growth and reproduction in insects. Adv. in Insect Physiol. *2,* 247.

DISCUSSION

EBERT: Does ecdysone stimulate cell division?

SCHNEIDERMAN: Not in general. In these insects, there is little cell division in most larval cells, except for the imaginal discs. The larvae grow by cell enlargement. DNA is replicated, but there is no cell division.

Let me restate your question. "Is one of the primary actions of ecdysone to stimulate the synthesis of DNA and is this synthesis prerequisite for further differentiative events?" Or, "If one blocks DNA synthesis in epidermal cells, will they differentiate?" Now the answer is straightforward: if one prevents epidermal cells from making DNA, they will not differentiate. It appears as if DNA synthesis were an obligatory first step before certain cells can undergo further developmental change.

PETERSON: It is clear that RNA is being formed in the puffs. Has it not also been said that DNA is disproportionately replicated in these sites?

SCHNEIDERMAN: The literature on DNA synthesis in puffs is confused; I do not know of a critical experiment. In a recent article Kroeger [H. Kroeger and M. Lezzi (1966): Regulation of gene action in insect development. Ann. Rev. Ent. *11,* 1] reviewed the literature on puffing of chromosomes. He points out that in the giant chromosomes of sciarids there is often some local DNA synthesis in certain regions after puffing, but the phenomenon is not general and the function of this locally synthesized DNA is not known.

PETERSON: It is a critical question. Does DNA have to be replicated? Is it replicated in specific sites and not throughout the whole chromosome?

SCHNEIDERMAN: There clearly are many puffs in which DNA synthesis has not been demonstrated. Moreover, there is no evidence I know of that DNA synthesis occurs in *parts* of a chromosome after ecdysone treatment and not in the whole chromosome. A selective DNA synthesis in which multiple copies of a particular part of the genome would be produced would be an interesting kind of regulation.

MITCHISON: Could you give us some indication of the number of genes activated in these puffs?

SCHNEIDERMAN: May I rephrase your question and ask "After ecdysone is added, are there any loci that puff before all the others?" The answer is clear. In *Chironomus tentans,* Ulrich Clever has shown that there are two puffs that are more sensitive than any others to ecdysone. Moreover, the size of these puffs is proportional to the dose of ecdysone injected, and the amounts that are required to produce these puffs are extremely small.

FELDMAN: The induction of puffing by ecdysone indicated that the hormone acts as a specific inducer of specific genes of *Chironomus.* Could you then comment on findings published a few years ago which led to the conclusion that ecdysone could induce protein synthesis in mammalian liver cells *in vitro?*

SCHNEIDERMAN: So far as I am aware, those experiments have not yet been confirmed. The data initially presented did not permit an assessment of their possible significance. There is no question but that the hormone preparations that were used were good. The experiments are interesting, but I don't think that the results presented thus far would enable one to draw any conclusions.

FELDMAN: You mentioned histones as possible repressors in multicellular organisms. Yet recent studies have indicated that the blocking effect of histones on DNA may be attributed simply to the fact that DNA-histone complexes in the test tube are non-soluble and therefore do not manifest polymerization of RNA, unlike unmasked DNA. In this respect the effect of histone is non-specific.

JOHN PAPACONSTANTINOU

Tissue-specific protein synthesis and cellular maturation in the vertebrate lens

IN THE COURSE of cellular differentiation, interacting cells are induced to initiate the synthesis of a new protein or series of proteins. Similarly, during the terminal stages of cellular differentiation, or during the process of cellular maturation, the synthesis of highly specialized proteins (structural proteins or enzymes) is initiated. Some examples of tissue-specific protein synthesis associated with cellular maturation are seen in the maturation of the erythrocyte (1) or the differentiation of the lens fiber cell (2). In both of these cases morphological changes are accompanied by the initiation of synthesis of tissue-specific proteins.

The initiation of tissue-specific protein synthesis is a problem of differential gene action and, as shall be shown below, the continued synthesis of these proteins is a problem of regulation of protein synthesis, but not necessarily at the level of the gene. Since the initiation and early regulation of tissue-specific protein synthesis is inhibited by actinomycin treatment, these observations indicate that the initial regulation of protein synthesis may be on the transcriptional level (3, 4). Furthermore, as the cells mature, the synthesis of these same proteins becomes insensitive to actinomycin D and the regulation of their synthesis is on the translational level (3-6). The transition from an actinomycin-sensitive to an actinomycin-insensitive status of protein synthesis has been shown to occur in the differentiation of the lens epithelial cell to fiber cell (5, 7). In all of the cases where this pattern of variation of actinomycin sensitivity is observed, the synthesis of the mRNA is turned off and the existent RNA is stabilized or "long-lived." One of the important factors, therefore, in describing the molecular mechanisms of cellular differentiation is the mechanism of stabilization of mRNA.

Antibody synthesis has often been referred to as a model system for cellular differentiation. In view of the fact that the antibody-synthesizing cells are highly differentiated and their proteins, the immunoglobulins, are tissue-specific, this system may fall into the same category as those I have mentioned above, i.e., the terminal cellular maturation systems. Thus, the questions which are of interest in problems of cellular maturation may be pertinent to the antibody-synthesizing system. Some of the questions which are of interest to us with respect to lens cell differentiation might be asked, therefore, of the antibody-synthesizing cells. These are as follows:

(a) Is the regulation of immunoglobulin synthesis on the transcriptional level at all times?

(b) Does the synthesis of antibodies go through an actinomycin-sensitive—actinomycin-insensitive period? Does antibody synthesis occur, at any time, on stable RNA templates?

These are just a limited number of questions of interest to the developmental biologist. Our data on the maturation of the lens cell involve the initiation of synthesis of a new, specific group of proteins, the γ-crystallins. It also involves the stabilization of mRNA. It is possible that some of our observations may be of interest to those working along the same lines in immunoglobulin synthesis.

MORPHOLOGICAL CHANGES IN FIBER CELL DIFFERENTIATION

The structure of the lens.—The lens is an avascular tissue composed of the following distinct cell types: (a) an outer single layer of epithelial cells; (b) a zone of cellular elongation, composed of cells which are in the process of developing into fiber cells; and (c) the inner fiber cells (Fig. 1). Initiation of the differentiation of epithelial cells to fiber cells occurs at the peripheral or equatorial zone of the lens. It is in this region where the gross morphological changes associated with fiber cell differentiation occur, i.e., the transition from a cuboidal lens epithelial cell to the elongated fiber cell. After the embryonic lens has been formed, fiber cells are continuously laid down throughout the prenatal and postnatal life of the animal. The bulk of the lens is composed of layer upon layer of these fiber cells, and this continuous formation of fiber cells accounts for the growth of this tissue. It can be seen, therefore, that (a) fiber cell formation represents the final stage of lens cell differentiation and (b) in the adult lens the fiber cells formed during embryonic growth compose the central or nucleus region while the newly formed fiber cells are found in the peripheral or cortex region.

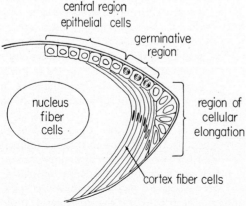

FIG. 1. A diagrammatic presentation of the structure of the vertebrate lens, and the relationship of the lens epithelial cells to the lens fiber cells.

Cytological and cytochemical observations on the process of fiber cell formation.—The lens epithelial cells are characterized by their cuboidal shape, their basophilic staining properties, and their ability to replicate (8). In the zone of elongation (Fig. 2), where the epi-

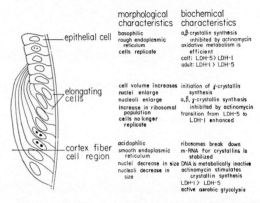

FIG. 2. A diagrammatic presentation of the area of cellular elongation in the vertebrate lens. The morphological and biochemical alterations which occur during lens fiber cell differentiation are also listed.

thelial cells begin the process of fiber cell formation, the following changes occur in the intracellular structures: (a) the cell sends out cytoplasmic processes anteriorly and posteriorly beneath the cuboidal epithelial cell layer to form the fiber cell; (b) the nucleus and nucleoli enlarge (9); (c) the ribosomal population increases significantly, especially in the cytoplasm adjacent to the enlarged nucleus (10, 11).

In the completed fiber cell, (a) the cytoplasm loses its basophilic properties and takes on acidophilic properties; (b) the nucleus and nucleoli reduce in size and the endoplasmic reticulum, which has a granular appearance in the epithelial cell, takes on a smoother appearance in the fiber cell; (c) through electron microscope studies it has been shown that a significant decrease in the ribosomal population occurs in the differentiated fiber cell (10, 11). These differences in staining properties and changes in intracellular structure indicate that significant macromolecular changes are associated with fiber cell differentiation. The enlargement of the nucleus and nucleoli, for example, as well as the increase in ribosomal population are an indication of increased nucleic acid and protein synthesis during elonga-

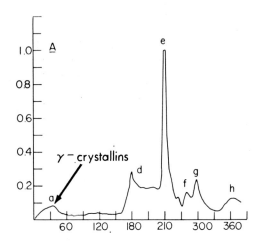

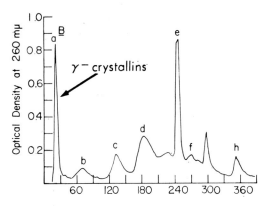

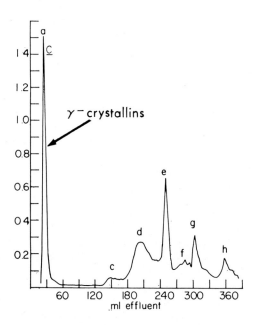

tion. These structural changes are probably the result of a series of biochemical events which are associated with fiber cell formation.

PROTEIN AND NUCLEIC ACID CHANGES ASSOCIATED WITH FIBER CELL FORMATION

The association of γ-crystallin synthesis with fiber cell differentiation.—There are three major groups of proteins synthesized by lens fiber cells: the α-crystallins, the β-crystallins, and the γ-crystallins. These proteins can be separated into the three main groups by DEAE-cellulose chromatography (12). Typical patterns showing a stepwise elution of the crystallins from DEAE-cellulose columns are shown in Fig. 3. The pattern in Fig. 3A shows that the epithelial cells from calf lenses contain only traces of γ-crystallins in comparison to the amounts found in the cortex and nucleus fiber cells (Figs. 3B and 3C). These data indicate that the γ-crystallins are proteins which are characteristic of the fiber cell. The small amounts of γ-crystallins that are detected in the epithelial cell patterns are due to the adherence of the elongating cells, which are unavoidably mixed with the epithelial cells when they are removed for homogenization.

Since lens fiber cell formation is analogous to cellular maturation and is associated with the synthesis of a tissue-specific protein, the question I would like to consider is whether the γ-crystallins are synthesized initially on "long-lived" stable templates or whether there is a progressive transition from a relatively short-lived mRNA with a rapid turnover to a long-lived stable mRNA with a very slow turnover. To answer this question we studied the effect of actinomycin D on protein and nucleic acid synthesis in calf lens epithelial and fiber cells (2, 13). Since small amounts of γ-crystallins are detectable in epithelial cell homogenates by fractionation on DEAE-cellulose, this procedure was used to determine whether actinomycin D could differentially affect the synthesis of this protein. Radioactive crystallins synthesized by actinomycin treated and control epithelial and fiber cells were frac-

FIG. 3. The fractionation of α-, β-, and γ- crystallins by DEAE-cellulose chromatography. A. Calf lens epithelial cell crystallins. B. Calf cortex fiber cell crystallins. C. Calf nucleus fiber cell crystallins.

13

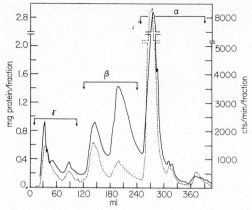

FIG. 4. The fractionation of calf lens epithelial cell crystallins after a 2-hour incubation in C^{14}-amino acid algal hydrolysate.

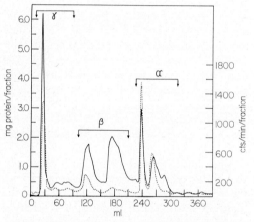

FIG. 5. The fractionation of calf lens epithelial cell crystallins after a 2-hour incubation in C^{14}-algal hydrolysate plus actinomycin D (10 μg/ml).

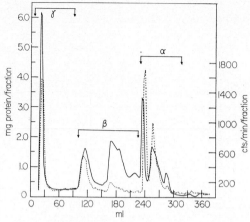

FIG. 6. The fractionation of calf lens cortex fiber cell crystallins after a 2-hour incubation in C^{14}-amino acid algal hydrolysate.

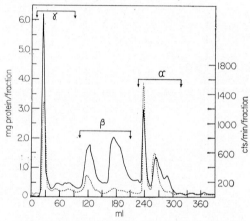

FIG. 7. The fractionation of calf lens cortex fiber cell crystallins after a 2-hour incubation in C^{14}-amino acid algal hydrolysate plus actinomycin D (10 μg/ml).

tionated on DEAE-cellulose, and each fraction was counted. The patterns in Figs. 4 and 5 show the effect of actinomycin D on lens protein synthesis in epithelial cells. It can be seen that the γ-crystallins (as well as the α- and β-crystallins) are strongly inhibited by actinomycin D. A similar series of experiments is shown in Figs. 6 and 7 for the fiber cells. These data show that γ-crystallin synthesis in the fiber cells is stimulated by actinomycin D. Thus these proteins, whose synthesis is initiated in the region of cellular elongation, are inhibited by actinomycin at the time of their initial synthesis. In addition, the data indicate that the synthesis of γ-crystallins occurs initially via an actinomycin-sensitive mechanism and progresses, with the differentiation of

the epithelial cell to the fiber cell, to an actinomycin-"insensitive" mechanism. One explanation for this is that the crystallins are synthesized on stable templates in the fiber cell and that this stabilization occurs at some time after the initiation of fiber cell formation.

mRNA in epithelial cells and fiber cells.— The data on protein synthesis indicate that mRNA in the fiber cell is long-lived. These data are in agreement with the autoradiographic studies which show that protein synthesis in the fiber cells is insensitive to actinomycin D (7). In addition, the autoradiography experiments show the occurrence of a sharp decrease in the incorporation of uridine by fiber cells. It appears, therefore, that the turnover of RNA in the fiber cells is significantly slowed down and that the protein synthesis that does occur in the fiber cells occurs on stable templates.

Both epithelial cell and fiber cell phenol extracted RNA have been analyzed by sucrose density gradient centrifugation (13). The gradients showed that RNA synthesis in the epithelial cells is significantly greater than that of the fiber cells; i.e., that there is a natural slowing down of RNA synthesis in the fiber cell. In the presence of actinomycin D, RNA synthesis is almost completely inhibited in both epithelial and fiber cells. Under these conditions, protein synthesis is significantly inhibited in the epithelial cells (Fig. 5), but stimulated in the fiber cells. Thus, the synthesis of proteins in the fiber cells proceeds in the absence of RNA synthesis and must be presumed to occur on stable templates. (The stimulatory effect is due to the control of protein synthesis by the epithelial cells, over the fiber cells. Removal of the epithelial cells results in neither an inhibition nor stimulation of γ-crystallin synthesis.)

In view of the active turnover of RNA in the epithelial cells, attempts were made to pulse label these cells with radioactive uridine and to isolate mRNA by methylated albumin columns (MAK). Similar experiments were carried out with fiber cell RNA. The MAK column patterns (Fig. 8) show a highly radioactive portion of the ribosomal peak which is significantly staggered. This fraction was found to have a high percentage of hybridizability (25-30%) with calf thymus DNA, thus indicating that this is DNA-like RNA. In addition, it should be noted that there is a very significant decrease in the incorporation of

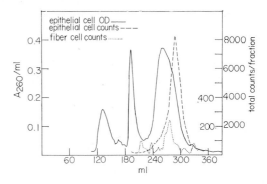

Fig. 8. Pulse labelled calf lens epithelial cell and cortex fiber cell RNA. C^{14}-uridine was used as an RNA precursor. The RNA was phenol extracted and fractionated on a methylated albumin kieselguhr column. Epithelial cell RNA counts – – – – ; fiber cell RNA counts ....; OD_{260}————.

uridine into this same RNA fraction in the fiber cells. This gives some indication of the sharp decrease in mRNA turnover in these fiber cells.

In summary, therefore, I would like to point out that during cellular maturation, which involved fiber cell formation in the lens, the synthesis of a new group of proteins, the γ-crystallins, is initiated. The synthesis of these proteins is initially sensitive to actinomycin D, and this sensitivity is lost in the fiber cell. This differential sensitivity to a potent inhibitor of mRNA synthesis is due to the rapid turnover of mRNA in the epithelial cells and the stabilization and slowing down of mRNA synthesis in the fiber cells. Antibody synthesis also involves the synthesis of a highly specific protein. It would be of interest to know whether there is a differential rate of mRNA turnover in the antibody-synthesizing cells and whether this is a function of the control of the synthesis of these protein molecules.

REFERENCES

1. Bessis, M. (1965): Cytology of the Blood and Blood-Forming Organs. New York, Gruen and Stratton, p. 232.
2. Papaconstantinou, J. (1965): Biochemistry of bovine lens proteins. II. The γ-crystallins of adult bovine, calf and embryonic lenses. Biochim. Biophys. Acta 107, 81.
3. Wilt, F. H. (1965): Regulation of the initiation of chick embryo hemoglobin synthesis. J. Molec. Biol. 12, 331.

4. Garren, L. D., Howell, R. R., Tomkins, G. M., and Crocco, R. M. (1964): A paradoxical effect of actinomycin D: The mechanism of regulation of enzyme synthesis by hydrocortisone. Proc. Nat. Acad. Sci., U.S. 52, 1121.
5. Papaconstantinou, J., Stewart, J. A., and Koehn, P. V. (1965): A localized stimulation of lens synthesis by actinomycin D. Biochim. Biophys. Acta 114, 428.
6. Scott, R. B., and Bell, E. (1965): Messenger

RNA utilization during development of chick embryo lens. Science *147*, 405.

7. Reeder, R., and Bell, E. (1965): Short- and long-lived messenger RNA in embryonic chick lens. Science *150*, 71.

8. Cogan, D. C. (1962): Anatomy of lens and pathology of cataracts. Exp. Eye Res. *1*, 291.

9. Hertl, M. (1955): Kernvolumen und Nukleolarapparat wachsender Linsenzellen. (Cell nucleus volume and the nucleolar apparatus of growing lens cells.) Z. Zellforsch. Mikroskop. Anat. *43*, 228.

10. Eguchi, G. (1964): Electron microscope studies on lens regeneration. II. Formation and growth of lens vesicle and differentiation of lens fibers. Embryologia *8*, 247.

11. Karasaki, S. (1964): An electron microscopic study of Wolffian lens regeneration in the adult newt. J. Ultrastruct. Res. *11*, 246.

12. Papaconstantinou, J., Resnik, R. A., and Saito, E. (1962): Biochemistry of bovine lens proteins. I. Isolation and characterization of adult α-crystallins. Biochim. Biophys. Acta *60*, 205.

13. Stewart, J. A., and Papaconstantinou, J.: Unpublished observations.

DISCUSSION

HIRSCHHORN: After injury of the reversibly stationary epithelial cell, it turns into a replicating cell. What is known about RNA metabolism during this process? Is there breakdown and synthesis of ribosomes?

PAPACONSTANTINOU: As far as I am aware, evidence on breakdown of ribosomes under those conditions has not been presented. The synthesis of ribosomes has been described.

KIMMEL: Can you visualize any particular economy to the cell in the specific way in which ribosomes are being broken down? May this relate to the preservation of mRNA in the 40S particle?

PAPACONSTANTINOU: We need a better grasp of the mechanisms involved before we attempt to draw conclusions.

MIESCHER: Do cortical fiber cells synthesize proteins?

PAPACONSTANTINOU: α- and γ-crystallins, but only in the presence of epithelial cells.

MIESCHER: How do you explain the influence of epithelial cells in protein synthesis in fiber cells?

PAPACONSTANTINOU: We suggest that the epithelial cells regulate what goes into fiber cells. It appears likely that they control the amino acid pool. Moreover, it is possible that they regulate the energy available to fiber cells by providing, say, ATP.

BLOCK: Are there cells in the lens which completely lose their endoplasmic reticulum and are therefore unable to synthesize protein thereafter and so became "mature" in the sense that red cells are mature?

PAPACONSTANTINOU: You are correct.

These cells do "mature" in the sense that erythrocytes do in that they lose their nucleus. But we have been able to show that they incorporate amino acids into protein.

SCHNEIDERMAN: Your assertion that protein synthesis continues in living cells in the fiber nucleus has a number of interesting implications. The cells have no nucleus. Your data indicate that they have no DNA. You argue that they are alive and that in an old cow they may be years old. Followed to its logical conclusion one must conclude that stabilized messengers for all of the constitutive enzymes plus some of the lens proteins persist for months and years in these cells. I find this hard to believe. Are you certain that these cells in the fiber nucleus are very old? Are you certain they really make protein? Have you ruled out non-specific binding of labelled amino acids? Could programmed ribosomes from younger cells or proteins made in younger cells diffuse to the cells of the fiber nucleus?

PAPACONSTANTINOU: With respect to the age of the nucleus fiber cells we have biochemical data which indicate that these are the original cells laid down and that they are not replaced. This evidence is based on our observation that there are chromatographic (DEAE) and electrophoretic differences in embryonic and adult γ-crystallins. Since the embryonic fibers may be found in the nucleus region of the adult lens we looked at the γ-crystallins from this region and found that they have the properties of the embryonic γ-crystallins, not the adult γ-crystallins.

With respect to the ability of nucleus fiber

cells to incorporate amino acids into protein, we have found a small but significant amount of radioactive protein in the nucleus region of calf lenses. These calves are 3-6 months old.

Your question of whether protein can be transferred from younger cells to the older cells is very interesting and I have thought about this recently. It may be possible that protein synthesized in the epithelial cells is transferred to fiber cells. This will be very difficult to prove. We are planning a series of experiments to try to answer this question.

4

ROBERT T. SCHIMKE

On the control of protein synthesis in animal tissues

UNDERSTANDING of the control of protein synthesis has been based largely on studies with microorganisms, where the availability of multiple types of mutants has allowed for use of experimental approaches not readily possible with animal tissues. These studies have led to the now familiar model for control of protein synthesis of Jacob and Monod in which the synthesis of a protein is controlled at the DNA, or genetic, level by the rate at which a specific messenger RNA is synthesized (1). This model has dominated most current thinking on the control of protein synthesis in animal tissues and has led to much fruitful research and speculation. Nevertheless, a number of recent studies have suggested that such a model is not adequate to explain all events in the control of protein synthesis in animal tissues. The following remarks, then, are made in a spirit of questioning and speculation, with the hope that this may lead to new approaches to an understanding of the control of protein synthesis in animal tissues.

As a basis for this discussion we might consider Fig. 1, which gives a highly simplified representation of the major known events of protein synthesis, starting at the level of DNA and ending with the secretion and/or degradation of the final product (2). Thus at the DNA level, there is the synthesis of three classes of RNA, i.e., messenger, transfer (soluble), and ribosomal. The specific messenger RNA subsequently interacts with assembled ribosomes to form polysomes, on which protein

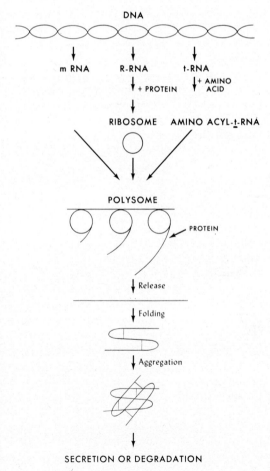

Fig. 1. Steps in protein synthesis.

synthesis actually occurs. The messenger RNA determines the ordered stepwise attachment of different amino acyl-RNAs on the ribosome, with the subsequent formation of peptide bonds between the amino acids, thereby allowing for the synthesis of a growing peptide chain. The peptide chain then must be released from the ribosome and undergo folding into a specific configuration. Such a protein may then undergo aggregation with like or dissimilar proteins to form more complex, active enzymes or structural units. A protein may then be secreted, and/or may undergo degradation within the cell.

Inasmuch as each of the events of protein synthesis and metabolism may be catalyzed by multiple enzymes and may occur in different cellular compartments, or even in different cells, control of protein synthesis could be exerted at potentially multiple sites or levels. In *Escherichia coli* the control of protein synthesis is exerted primarily at the genetic level. Thus the synthesis of a given protein is dependent on the presence of specific messenger RNA, whose synthesis is controlled by the interaction of small molecules such as amino acids and sugars, with genetically determined aporepressors (1). Messenger RNA is highly labile, having a half-life of only 2 to 3 minutes (3). Thus the ability to make specific proteins can be rapidly changed every several minutes by altering of complement of messenger RNA species. Such a control mechanism is well suited to an opportunistic, rapidly growing, unicellular organism, which is accustomed to rapid adaptation to a wide variety of nutritional conditions. This organism, however, should be contrasted with an individual cell in a multicellular organism. Such a cell is often not growing rapidly, may carry out a highly specialized function, and is associated with similar and dissimilar cells into tissues and organs. Each cell exerts influence on other cells by direct cell-cell interaction as well as by humoral or nervous control. Thus the types of control mechanisms suited for bacteria may not be entirely adequate for control of protein synthesis in multicellular organisms.

Let us then look at some examples of investigations in animal systems to illustrate the following major points: (a) the complexities of the events of protein synthesis and metabolism which may be separated in time in the cell, as well as occurring in different cellular compartments, (b) the potential, if not actual, control of protein synthesis at multiple levels in animal tissues, (c) the lack of fundamental knowledge concerning certain events of protein synthesis.

SEPARATION OF EVENTS OF PROTEIN SYNTHESIS IN TIME AND SPACE

Time.—There are a number of studies which show that the effect of a specific hormone, or the initiation of a developmental process, can be divided into two distinct time periods: an early period in which a subsequent effect can be prevented by administration of actinomycin D, and a later period during which this antibiotic has no effect. The actinomycin D-sensitive period can be of variable duration, being 1 to 2 hours in the case of hydrocortisone induction of tyrosine transaminase and tryptophan pyrrolase of rat liver (4), or 4 to 6 hours for diethylstibestrol induction of phosphoprotein synthesis in livers of male chickens (5). Similar observations have been made in a number of developmental systems, including embryonic pancreas (6), hemoglobin synthesis in chick embryo (7), and embryonic skin and lens (8), as well as the development of spores in *B. subtilis* (9). Since actinomycin D inhibits RNA synthesis (10), such findings suggest that the early, actinomycin D-sensitive event is associated with the synthesis of specific messenger RNA, which becomes active for protein synthesis only at some later time. Such a time may reflect the time-dependent steps involved in the assemblage of the active protein-synthesizing unit (polysome), or result from the potentially active polysomal unit being regulated at a subsequent step in protein synthesis, a process which is not dependent on RNA synthesis.

Space.—An animal cell is highly organized into multiple compartments and organelles, in each of which various of the events of protein synthesis may be taking place independently, as indicated by the following examples. For instance, Perry (11) and Girard *et al.* (12) have demonstrated that ribosomal precursors are synthesized in the nucleus and are subsequently assembled and transferred to the cytoplasm. In addition, the place within the cell where a specific protein may be synthesized can vary. Thus, although the bulk of protein synthesis occurs in cytoplasm of the animal cell, hemoglobin synthesis in the duck erythrocyte occurs in the nucleus (13). Another type of compartmentalization involves the synthesis of carbamyl phosphate synthetase subunits and their subsequent assemblage into enzymatically and immunologically active forms within mitochondrial particles (14). Pancreatic enzymes, synthesized on rough endoplasmic reticulum, are initially collected in organelles (Golgi apparatus), following which they are secreted into the intestinal lumen (15). Although little is known about the physiological process(es) of protein degradation, in various animal tissues, the presence of organelles containing a variety of hydrolytic enzymes, i.e., lysozymes, in multiple cell types (16), suggests a separation of this function within a cell.

Not only may events of protein synthesis occur in different portions of the same cell, as indicated above, they also may occur in differing cell types. The results of Amos et al. (17) and Segal et al. (18), which indicate that the addition of exogeneous RNA can direct specific protein synthesis in cultured cells and ovary respectively, suggest the potential of cell-cell interaction involving transfer of RNA or other compounds. The passage of essential factors for one cell type to another has been observed in a number of differentiating systems (6, 19, 20, 21).

MULTIPLE LEVELS FOR THE CONTROL OF
PROTEIN SYNTHESIS AND METABOLISM

DNA (genetic) level.—It is obvious that, ultimately, control of specific protein synthesis is dependent on the activation of specific DNA segments (genes) to allow for the synthesis of appropriate RNA species. The mechanism whereby such a DNA segment is activated is one of the central problems of molecular and developmental biology, irrespective of whether the system under study be microbial or a higher animal.

The best available evidence for the control of specific protein synthesis at the level of DNA in animal tissues comes from studies with hormones. Most dramatic are those studies described by Schneiderman (this volume) on the effects of the steroid insect hormone, ecdysone, on chromosomal "puffing" (21, 22). Such direct observations of hormonal effects on chromosomal behavior and the known ability of actinomycin D to prevent hormone effects in mammalian tissues have led to the suggestion that many hormones act at the DNA level by stimulating the synthesis of specific messenger RNA (23). Thus Karlson (24) and Bonner (25) have suggested that hormones may interact with histones to release inhibition of specific DNA segments, thereby allowing for RNA synthesis to proceed. Such interpretations are, of course, beclouded by lack of knowledge of the functions of histones, by lack of knowledge of the potentially varied physiological and biochemical effects of actinomycin D, as well as by the fact that the observed chromosomal behavior may represent a second or third order response to the hormone.

Ribosomal level.—In contrast to the very short half-life of messenger RNA in bacteria, that of messenger RNA in animal systems would appear in general to be far longer (26). This, of course, would be in keeping with the previously cited studies indicating a time during which appearance of a specific protein is not dependent on continued RNA synthesis (4-9). The presence of a long-lived messenger RNA, then, provides the possibility that control of specific protein synthesis can occur at the so-called "translational level," that is, by how rapidly a previously coded polysome synthesizes a given protein. Indeed, there are now a number of studies indicating that various types of control of protein synthesis exist at the ribosomal level. In the case of feather development, Bell et al. (27) have shown that ribosomes destined for specific protein synthesis exist in an inactive four-membered aggregate, which opens when protein synthesis commences. In addition, Monroy et al. (28) have found that inactive ribosomes of the unfertilized sea urchin egg can be activated by brief treatment with proteolytic enzymes. They suggest that such a mechanism is involved in the initiation of protein synthesis after fertilization.

Studies on hemoglobin synthesis have suggested another type of mechanism for the acceleration of ribosomal protein synthesis. Thus it has been known for some time that the rate of synthesis of B chains of hemoglobin increases as the chain length increases (29). More recently it has been found that the addition of iron (30), or of hemin (31), to a ribosomal preparation from reticulocytes markedly increases the rate of hemoglobin synthesis. A somewhat analogous example in the intact animal involves the stimulation of ferritin biosynthesis in rat liver following administration of ferrous iron (32), a process that is insensitive to actinomycin D (33). Such observations, taken together, suggest that the rate of synthesis of a protein may be dependent on the conformation of the growing peptide chain, a conformation that may be affected by prosthetic groups such as hemin or iron. A prosthetic group might also function to actually pull a preformed protein off of a ribosome. There are a number of reports of specific proteins bound to ribosomes, including triose phosphate dehydrogenase in yeast (34), tryptophan synthetase (35) and β-galactosidase in *E. coli* (36), and albumin in rat liver (37). One could therefore postulate that an agent, such as a substrate, cofactor, or protein subunit, might act to alter the conformation of a ribosomal bound protein to affect its release, and thereby allow continued enzyme synthesis. Such an explanation has been advanced for the mechanism for the substrate (tryptophan) induction of tryptophan pyrrolase of rat liver (38).

Other support for the regulation of protein synthesis at the ribosomal level comes from studies of an effect of actinomycin D in actually increasing the appearance of a specific protein when actinomycin D is given some time after an induction process has been initiated. Thus Garren *et al.* have found that actinomycin D given 5 to 6 hours after hydrocortisone actually increases the levels of rat liver tryptophan pyrrolase and tyrosine transaminase, whereas it totally prevents the induction of these enzymes when given at the same time as the hydrocortisone (4). They postulated that the secondary effect of actinomycin D resulted from an inhibition of synthesis of a species of RNA that acts as a repressor at the ribosomal level. Rosen *et al.*, on the other hand, have shown that this actinomycin D effect can be mimicked by administration of casein hydrolysate and have suggested that the effect is due to replenishing a depleted amino acid pool (39). Kenney has indicated that the synthesis of rat liver tyrosine transaminase is under control of several

hormones, at least some of which occurs at the ribosomal level (40). Korner has also suggested that growth hormone acts at some step at the ribosomal level in facilitating protein synthesis (41).

Peptide folding and aggregation.—The process of the folding of a peptide into its appropriate conformational state and the subsequent aggregation can be sites for control of protein synthesis. Thus Anfinsen and his collaborators have isolated an enzyme from the microsomal fraction of a variety of rat tissues that catalyzes disulfide interchanges (42). This enzyme can increase the rate at which unfolded peptides assume a proper conformation for biological activity when that conformation requires disulfide bonds. In addition the entire spectrum of effects of substrates, cofactors, and products to affect the conformation or aggregational state and activities of enzymes (43) may be considered as control of the terminal stages of synthesis of biologically active proteins.

Protein degradation.—The process of protein degradation can be under various types of control. Schimke (44) and Segal (45) have emphasized the significance of continual protein turnover, i.e., both synthesis and degradation, in the control of enzyme levels in animal tissues. Schimke *et al.* (46) have presented evidence indicating that the rate at which rat liver tryptophan pyrrolase is degraded *in vivo* can be markedly affected by administrations of its substrate, tryptophan, presumably by altering the conformation of the enzyme protein structure and thereby making it more resistant to the degradative process.

It is apparent from the above-cited examples that the control of the total metabolism of a specific protein can be highly complex, and that one need not be limited to mechanisms directed only to the DNA (genetic) level. It should be pointed out that many of the concepts concerning sites of control of protein synthesis in animal tissues have been based on effects of actinomycin D, as indicated above. Although this drug inhibits RNA synthesis, it is becoming increasingly clear that it also has other actions, including disruption of the ribosomal relationship to endoplasmic reticulum (47) and interference with respiration and anaerobic glycolysis (48), all occurring in the dose ranges used in the above-cited studies. Therefore conclusions based on the assumption that the observed effects of actinomycin D result only from inhibition of RNA synthesis may not be entirely justified.

Another problem that arises in determining the site of action of a given agent in affecting protein synthesis concerns the possibility that the events of protein synthesis are highly coupled, such that each reactant, i.e., protein, peptide, ribosomal bound protein, etc., may feed back to inhibit an earlier reaction in the sequence. Thus an agent could increase the rate of protein synthesis by acting at any given site which can be rate limiting. Thus by mass action (49) or by releasing a feed-back inhibition, the rate of enzyme synthesis could be increased. At the extreme such a stimulus could theoretically be that for the secretion of a given protein, which in turn could release the inhibition all the way back to the level of messenger RNA synthesis. Any one or part of the protein synthesis sequence could be involved in such control mechanisms. Indeed Stent has proposed such a mechanism for bacteria whereby an inducer could act at the ribosomal level to initiate the pulling off of a messenger RNA from the DNA such that more messenger could be synthesized (50). Experimental evidence for such a hypothesis has been provided by the studies of Byrne *et al.*, indicating an *in vitro* association of ribosomes with RNA and DNA (51), as well as by the kinetic studies on RNA synthesis of Bremer and Konrad (52).

Areas in which knowledge of protein synthesis is lacking.—Formulations of possible regulatory mechanisms are obviously limited by knowledge of the events of protein synthesis. One area of current interest is the relationship of DNA replication to protein synthesis. Thus in yeast (53) and in *B. subtilis* (54) the synthesis of a specific enzyme occurs only during a definite time of the replication cycle, suggesting that replication and the ability to synthesize specific messenger RNA are related processes. The extent to which chromosomal replication and the synthesis of specific messenger RNAs and protein are coupled events in animal tissues will be an area of future interest. Another area in which a better understanding of the process of protein synthesis will be important involves the role of membranes in the synthesis of protein. Thus both in bacteria and in animal tissue the bulk of protein synthesis occurs on ribosomes associated with membranes.

What are the functions of such membranes, and does the interaction of membranes and polysomes play a regulatory function, as suggested by Pitot (55)? Finally, as emphasized by Hendler (56), since only 1 to 5% of the protein-synthesizing ability of the intact cell can be recovered in broken cell preparations, is it correct to assume that this small percentage is representative of the remaining protein-synthesizing ability of the cell? Hendler's recent studies indicating the potential importance of lipo-amino acid complexes in the synthesis of protein in hen oviduct homogenates (56) suggest that some re-evaluation of the events of protein synthesis may be necessary.

CONCLUSION

The objective of this presentation is to indicate by example the great number of ways in which the synthesis and metabolism of a protein can be regulated in animal cells. Although these remarks have not been directed at the specific problem of antibody synthesis, it is clear that the events of antibody synthesis and subsequent metabolism are similar to those of other proteins in animal cells, and therefore, presumably, are potentially subject to the same multiplicity of regulatory mechanisms. It is apparent that knowledge of certain aspects of protein synthesis is quite limited, and therefore the ability for formulate concepts of regulatory mechanisms is also limited. In attempting to understand the complex process of antibody formation, a completely open mind is suggested as to the many possibilities of regulatory phenomena which might be important in the individual model.

REFERENCES

1. Jacob, F., and Monod, J. (1961): Genetic regulatory mechanisms in the synthesis of proteins. J. Molec. Biol. *3*, 318.
2. Schweet, R., and Bishop, J. (1963): Protein synthesis in relation to gene action, in: Taylor, J. H., ed.: Molecular Genetics, Part 1. New York, Academic Press, p. 353.
3. Leive, L. (1965): RNA degradation and the assembly of ribosomes in actinomycin treated *Escherichia coli.* J. Molec. Biol. *13*, 862.
4. Garren, L. D., Howell, R. R., Tomkins, G. M., and Crocco, R. M. (1964): A paradoxical effect of actinomycin D: The mechanisms of regulation of enzyme synthesis by hydrocortisone. Proc. Nat. Acad. Sci. *52*, 1121.
5. Greengard, O., Gordon, M., Smith, M. A., and Acs, G. (1964): Studies on the mechanisms of diethylstibesterol-induced formation of phosphoprotein in male chickens. J. Biol. Chem. *239*, 2079.
6. Grobstein, C. (1964): Cytodifferentiation and its controls. Science *143*, 643.
7. Wilt, F. (1965): Regulation of the initiation of chick embryo hemoglobin synthesis. J. Molec. Biol. *12*, 321.
8. Scott, R. B., and Bell, E. (1964): Protein synthesis during development. Control through messenger RNA. Science *145*, 711.
9. Aronson, A., and del Valle, M. R. (1964): RNA and protein synthesis required for bacterial spore formation. Biochim. Biophys. Acta *87*, 267.
10. Reich, E., and Goldberg, I. H. (1964): Actinomycin and nucleic acid formation, in: Davidson, J. N., and Cohn, W. E., eds.: Progress in Nucleic Acid Research and Molecular Biology, Vol. 3. New York, Academic Press, p. 183.
11. Perry, R. P. (1963): The cellular synthesis of ribosomal and 4S RNA. Proc. Nat. Acad. Sci. *48*, 2179.
12. Girard, M., Latham, H., Penman, S., and Darnell, J. E. (1965): Entrance of newly formed messenger RNA and ribosomes into Hela cell cytoplasm. J. Molec. Biol. *11*, 187.
13. Hammel, C. L., and Bessman, S. P. (1964): Hemoglobin synthesis in avian erythrocytes, J. Biol. Chem. *239*, 2228.
14. Tatibana, M., and Cohen, P. P. (1965): Formation and conversion of macromolecular precursor(s) in the biosynthesis of carbamyl phosphate synthetase. Proc. Nat. Acad. Sci. *53*, 107.
15. Davidson, J. P., and Palade, G. E. (1966): Role of the golgi complex in the intracellular transport of secretory protein. Proc. Nat. Acad. Sci. *55*, 424.
16. DeDuve, C. (1959): Lysosomes, a New Group of Cytoplasmic Particles in Subcellular Particles. Hyaishi, T., ed., New York, The Ronald Press, p. 128.
17. Amos, H., Askonas, B., and Soeiro, R. (1964): Evidence for messenger activity of alien ribonucleic acid in chick cells. J. Nat. Cancer Inst. Monograph *13*, 155.
18. Segal, J. J., Davidson, O. W., and Wada, K. (1965): Role of RNA in the regulatory action of estrogen. Proc. Nat. Acad. Sci. *54*, 782.
19. Cohen, S. (1962): Isolation of a mouse submaxillary gland protein accelerating incisor eruption and eyelid opening in the new-born animal. J. Biol. Chem. *237*, 1555.
20. Lash, J. W., Hammes, F. A., and Zilliken, F. (1962): Induction of cell differentiation. The *in vitro* induction of vertebral cartilage with a low molecular weight tissue component. Biochem. Biophys. Acta *56*, 313.
21. Clever, U., and Karlson, P. (1960): Induktion von Puff-veränderungen in der Speicheldrüsenchromosomen von *Chironomus tentans* durch Ecdyson. Exptl. Cell Research *20*, 623.
22. Clever, H. (1964): Actinomycin and puromycin: Effects on sequential gene activation by ecdysone. Science *146*, 794.
23. Karlson, P. (1963): New concepts on the mode of action of hormones. Perspect. Biol. Med. *6*, 203.
24. Karlson, P. (1965): Biochemical studies of ecdysone control of chromosomal activity. J. Cell. Comp. Physiol. *66, Supp. 1*, 69.
25. Bonner, J. (1965): The template activity of chromatin. J. Cell. Comp. Physiol. *66, Supp. 1*, 77.
26. Revel, M., and Hiatt, H. H. (1964): The stability of liver messenger RNA. Proc. Nat. Acad. Sci. *51*, 810.
27. Bell, E., Humphreys, T., Slayter, H. S., and Hall, C. E. (1965): Configuration of inactive and active polysomes of the developing down feather. Science *148*, 1739.
28. Monroy, A., Maggio, R., and Rinaldi, A. M. (1965): Experimentally induced activation of the ribosomes of the unfertilized sea urchin egg. Proc. Nat. Acad. Sci. *54*, 107.
29. Dintzis, H. M. (1961): Assembly of the peptide chains of hemoglobin. Proc. Nat. Acad. Sci. *47*, 247.
30. Waxman, H. S., and Rabinovitz, M. (1965): Iron supplementation *in vitro* and the state of aggregation and function of reticulocyte ribosomes in hemoglobin synthesis. Biochem. Biophys. Res. Commun. *19*, 538.
31. Bruns, G. P., and London, I. M. (1965): The effect of hemin on the synthesis of globin. Biochem. Biophys. Res. Commun. *19*, 538.
32. Loftfield, R. B., and Harris, A. (1956): Participation of free amino acids in protein synthesis. J. Biol. Chem. *219*, 151.
33. Drysdale, J. W., and Munro, H. N. (1965): Failure of actinomycin D to prevent induction of liver apoferritin after iron administration. Biochim. Biophys. Acta *103*, 185.
34. Warren, W. A., and Goldwaithe, D. A. (1962): The isolation of yeast ribosome associated with triose phosphate dehydrogenase. Proc. Nat. Acad. Sci. *48*, 698.
35. Horibata, K., and Kern, M. (1964): The ribo-

somal association of the dissimilar polypeptide chains of tryptophan synthetase. Proc. Nat. Acad. Sci. *51*, 218.

36. Kiho, Y., and Rich, A. (1964): Induced enzyme formed on bacterial polyribosomes. Proc. Nat. Acad. Sci. *51*, 111.

37. Warren, W., and Peters, T. (1965): Binding of purified antialbumin by rat liver ribosomes. J. Biol. Chem. *240*, 3109.

38. Greengard, O., and Feigelson, P. (1961): The activation and induction of rat liver tryptophan pyrrolase *in vivo* by its substrate. J. Biol. Chem. *236*, 158.

39. Rosen, F., and Milholland, R. J. (1965): Studies on the regulation of enzyme synthesis by cortisol and amino acids. Fed. Proc. *24*, 509.

40. Kenney, F. T., and Albritton, W. L. (1965): Repression of enzyme synthesis at the translational level and its hormonal control. Proc. Nat. Acad. Sci. *54*, 1693.

41. Korner, A. (1965): Growth hormone effects on RNA and protein synthesis in liver. J. Cell. Comp. Physiol. *66, Supp. 1,* 153.

42. Steiner, R. F., Delorenzo, F., and Anfinsen, C. B. (1965): Enzymatically catalyzed disulfide interchange in randomly cross-linked soybean trypsin inhibitor. J. Biol. Chem. *240*, 4648.

43. Monod, J., Changeux, J., and Jacob, F. (1963): Allosteric proteins and cellular control systems. J. Molec. Biol. *6*, 306.

44. Schimke, R. T. (1964): The importance of both synthesis and degradation in the control of arginase levels in rat liver. J. Biol. Chem. *239*, 3808.

45. Segal, H. L., and Kim, Y. S. (1963): Glucocorticord stimulation of the biosynthesis of glutamic-alanine transaminase. Proc. Nat. Acad. Sci. *50*, 912.

46. Schimke, R. T., Sweeney, E. W., and Berlin, C. M. (1965): Studies of the stability *in vivo*

and *in vitro* of rat liver tryptophan pyrrolase. J. Biol. Chem. *240*, 4609.

47. Revel, M., Hiatt, N., and Revel, J. P. (1964): Actinomycin D. An effect on rat liver homogenates unrelated to its action on RNA synthesis. Science *146*, 1311.

48. Laszlo, J., Miller, D. S., McCarty, K. S., and Hochestein, P. (1966): Actinomycin D. Inhibition of respiration and glycolysis. Science *151*, 1007.

49. Mandelstam, J., and Yudkin, J. (1962): Studies in biochemical adaptation. Some aspects of galactozymase production by yeast in relation to the "mass action" theory of enzyme adaptation. Biochem. J. *51*, 693.

50. Stent, G. (1964): The operon on its third anniversary. Science *144*, 816.

51. Byrne, R., Levin, J. G., Bladen, H. A., and Nirenberg, M. W. (1964): The *in vitro* formation of a DNA ribosome complex. Proc. Nat. Acad. Sci. *52*, 140.

52. Bremer, H., and Konrad, M. W. (1964): A complex of enzymatically synthesized RNA and template DNA. Proc. Nat. Acad. Sci. *51*, 801.

53. Halvorson, H., Gorman, J., Tauro, P., Epstein, R., and LaBerge, M. (1964): Control of enzyme synthesis in synchronous cultures of yeast. Fed. Proc. *23*, 1002.

54. Masters, M., and Pardee, A. B. (1965): Sequence of enzyme synthesis and gene replication during the cell cycle of *Bacillus subtilis*. Proc. Nat. Acad. Sci. *54*, 64.

55. Pitot, H., Cho, Y. S., Lamar, C., Jr., and Peraino, C. (1965): The interaction of external and internal controls on enzyme levels in liver and hepatoma. J. Cell. Comp. Phy. 6?, *Supp. 1,* 163.

56. Hendler, R. W. (1965): Lipo-amino acids as precursors in the synthesis of authentic proteins by homogenates of hen oviduct. Proc. Nat. Acad. Sci. *54*, 1233.

DISCUSSION

BRAUN: What one does not know is whether such apparent regulation affects intracellular or intercellular events. It may involve the selective elimination of a cell type rather than the kinds of intracellular regulation that we have been considering thus far.

PAPACONSTANTINOU: Does the antibody-producing system resemble the model shown; i.e., is there an initial actinomycin-sensitive, followed by an actinomycin-insensitive, period of antibody synthesis? If so, does this apply to both γG- and γM-antibodies?

FISHMAN: I will present data showing it does. Moreover, again under conditions similar to those described by Papaconstantinou and others, it can enhance rather than inhibit.

CEBRA: Perhaps the "enhancing effect" of actinomycin D, administered sometime after steroid, on increase of enzyme activity is due to its inhibition of other "irrelevant" messenger RNA synthesis. The irrelevant RNA could compete with messenger for enzyme and for ribosomes and its absence would permit continued, efficient enzyme synthesis.

5

IRWIN R. KONIGSBERG

The application of clonal techniques to problems of cytodifferentiation

THE EXPERIMENTAL APPROACH to be described was developed initially to provide a simple *in vitro* system with which to examine certain problems of the cytodifferentiation of skeletal muscle cells (1, 2, 3). Having developed procedures which provided us with a workable system we became interested in how one of the procedures which we found necessary, indeed essential, operated. Pursuing this question has led to consideration of the role of metabolic interaction between different cell types in the differentiation of muscle cells in culture.

Applying cloning techniques to freshly dissociated embryonic cells has enabled the study of growth and differentiation of colonies of muscle cells from single myoblasts. The source of these myoblasts is the leg musculature of the 12-day chick embryo. Cell suspensions are prepared by controlled trypsinization and small numbers of such cells are inoculated into a 5-cm petri plate containing growth medium. After a two-week incubation period, a macroscopically visible colony can be observed, marking the site where each viable cell had attached to the bottom of the petri plate. Such colonies can be readily observed to constitute two distinct groups. One group can be identified as colonies of muscle cells by virtue of the presence of many long multinucleate cells within which the characteristic pattern of cross-striation can be demonstrated. The other group has a distinctly different colonial morphology, composed of cells which,

by convention, are classified as "fibroblastic" (3).

The ability to form clonal populations in culture which still retain the capacity to express differentiative function is not restricted to the muscle cells. This same phenomenon has been demonstrated recently for embryonic chondrocytes (4) and for embryonic pigmented retinal cells (5).

Not many years ago the prospect of obtaining clones of cells capable of expressing differentiative function was viewed rather pessimistically. The only reliable technique for obtaining differentiation *in vitro* was organ culture—in which a compact mass of embryonic tissue is cultured under conditions which discourage cell migration and consequent thinning of the explant. Cultures of rapidly growing dispersed cells were observed to rapidly lose their capacity to perform the functions characteristic of the differentiated state. Several theoretical explanations have been offered to explain the failure to obtain differentiation in dispersed cell culture—these suffer from being constructed wholly upon negative evidence.

It might be instructive, however, to examine the conditions required by the three cell types which have been successfully cloned in culture —such information should be useful in extending similar studies to other cell types—and more particularly to developing cell systems amenable to the examination of specific questions.

25

For both the chondrocyte and the pigmented retinal cell the decisive factor which permitted successful clonal development was the recognition that the embryo extract which the investigators had been using contained factors which, while permitting proliferation, inhibited differentiation. By using only that fraction of the embryo extract which was retarded on a G-25 Sephadex column the inhibitory fraction could be excluded. In medium prepared with the retarded fraction of the extract, clones of chondrocytes synthesize metachromatic matrix and clones of pigmented retinal cells form pigment. Moreover, cells which are unable to synthesize their differentiated product in the "inhibitory" medium will give rise to differentiated clones when transferred to medium prepared with the retarded fraction. Regardless of the molecular nature of these inhibitory substances, it is clear that a medium which satisfies the requirements for growth does not necessarily permit cellular differentiation.

The conditions required for the development of clones of differentiated muscle cells seem to depend not on the removal of an inhibitor of differentiation but rather on the provision of a macromolecule which in mass culture is provided by a different cell type. Some time ago muscle clones were obtained in high frequency only by using "conditioned" medium (medium recovered from crowded cultures containing both fibroblasts and myoblasts). Colonial morphology was also strikingly different from the muscle clones which developed in unconditioned medium. In conditioned medium muscle colonies are larger, contain many more multinucleated elements, and thus, by virtue of their fibrous, sworling appearance, are readily distinguished by inspection alone from colonies of fibroblastic cells (3).

These observations of the development of muscle clones in conditioned medium suggested that medium exposed to the metabolic activities of large numbers of cells is altered in one or more respects making it more suitable for supporting the development of such colonies. Undoubtedly very many changes occur during conditioning of the medium. However, several observations now suggest that collagen, synthesized by the fibroblasts in the mixed cultures, may be the principal active component in conditioned medium. Studying some of the temporal parameters of the requirement for conditioned medium my student, Stephen Hauschka, and I found first that conditioned medium is required only during the first three days after the cultures are established, and that with certain batches of conditioned medium as short a period as 24 hours was sufficient. After this short initial period the medium could be replaced with unconditioned medium and still yield cultures in no way different from those grown in conditioned medium for the entire period. Secondly, we found that this surprisingly short critical period led to testing the effects of pretreating the petri plate surfaces with conditioned medium before inoculating the cells. Such petri plates, even after several rinses with distilled water, will support muscle cloning even when the liquid overlay is unconditioned medium.

These observations inferred (6) that conditioned medium altered the surface of the petri plate, most probably by the deposition of material upon the surface. Several other pieces of the puzzle now seemed to fit into place suggesting what this material might be.

For example, it was known that medium could be conditioned by mass cultures consisting almost exclusively of fibroblasts. In such fibroblast "farm" cultures what appeared to be atypical collagen fibers could be detected by electron microscopy. By subcloning single colonies, pure populations of muscle cells were found to clone only in conditioned medium. Some fibroblast colonies, however, would clone equally well in both unconditioned and conditioned medium.

We concluded that the fibroblasts were chiefly, if not exclusively, responsible for the conditioning effect. Since collagen is the most characteristic product of the fibroblast and is deposited extracellularly, it seemed reasonable to inquire whether collagen in some form is present in conditioned medium and is deposited on the petri plate surface where it provides a substratum which permits the development of muscle clones.

To test this premise we purified acid-soluble collagen from the tail tendons of the rat. Thin films of precipitated collagen were then deposited on the surfaces of petri plates and cells cultured on such collagen films in unconditioned medium. These cultures were compared to control cultures grown in both conditioned and unconditioned medium in untreated petri plates. The results clearly indicate that the use of a collagen substratum replaces the need for conditioned medium (6,7).

Our working hypothesis is that the development of muscle clones in culture is influenced by the metabolic activities of fibroblasts and that the influence is mediated by collagen or materials associated with collagen.

The necessary condition for the clonal development of the muscle cell would appear to be the provision of a macromolecule produced by another cell type—a cell type with which the myoblast is normally associated *in vivo*. Whether this dependency holds for the development of muscle cells *in vivo* or is manifested only in culture is not known. The paradox, however, is that it is difficult to imagine how such a dependency could be experimentally tested without recourse to cloning procedures since both fibroblast and myoblast are interspersed in muscle tissue.

Interactions between cells of different developmental fates do occur repeatedly in embryogenesis and have been shown to be responsible, in some cases, for directing one or both components into cytodifferentiative pathways that they would not have pursued if the interaction had been blocked. In other cases, particularly those which occur late in embryonic life, such interactions may permit continued differentiation along the same pathway to which a particular group of cells had been committed at some earlier time. The postulated relationship between fibroblast and myoblast in culture would fall in this later category.

It should be noted that the fibroblast participates in a number of tissue interactions involved in the development of a variety of organs. These epitheliomesenchymal interactions occur between the epithelial primordia of a variety of organs and their associated mesenchymal components. In a number of these interactions, mesenchyme from one or more ectopic sites has been shown to substitute for the homologous connective tissue element. This raises the question of whether mesenchyme exerts a similar effect in those situations in which the source of mesenchymal cells is not strictly specified, and in these instances, would the mechanism of interaction involve some universal activity of the fibroblast.

The most extensively studied epitheliomesenchymal system is the developing pancreas. Grobstein and his associates (8, 9, 10) have demonstrated that the pancreatic epithelium, in culture, will form acini, synthesize amylase, and accumulate zymogen granules when cultured in association with mesenchymal cells (of pancreatic origin or from any of the other sources tested). In this system, also, the mesenchyme is required for only a brief period of time (the first 48 hours of culture) (8). After this time, the subsequent course of differentiation is unaltered by the removal of the mesenchyme. During the 48-hour "critical" period when the presence of mesenchyme is required, collagen fibers are deposited at the basal regions of the epithelial cells (11). Radioautographic evidence suggests that soluble collagen is synthesized by the mesenchymal component. It then diffuses across the millipore membrane interposed, in these studies, between the two components and is precipitated into periodic fibers on the epithelial side of the membrane (12). In a similar epitheliomesenchymal interaction which occurs during the development of the salivary gland, such collagen fibers appear to maintain the lobated pattern of the organ and may perhaps also establish physiological differences between basal and apical regions of a single lobule (13).

It is clear that collagen can substitute for conditioned medium. Whether collagen is in fact the "active factor" supplied by conditioned medium is still hypothetical, but testable. The implication of collagen in the development of the pancreas and salivary glands, while not definitive, does warrant consideration of the possibility that this molecule plays some common role in the differentiation of a variety of cell types.

PART I — EDITOR: JAMES D. EBERT

REFERENCES

1. Konigsberg, I. R. (1961): Some aspects of myogenesis *in vitro*. Circulation *24*, 447.
2. Konigsberg, I. R. (1961): Cellular differentiation in colonies derived from single cell platings of freshly isolated chick embryo muscle cells. Proc. Nat. Acad. Sci., U.S. *47*, 1868.
3. Konigsberg, I. R. (1963): Clonal analysis of myogenesis. Science *140*, 1273.
4. Coon, H. G. (1966): Clonal stability and phenotypic expression of chick cartilage cells *in vitro*. Proc. Nat. Acad. Sci., U.S. *55*, 66.
5. Cahn, R. D., and Cahn, M. B. (1966): Heritability of cellular differentiation: clonal growth and expression of differentiation in retinal pigment cells *in vitro*. Proc. Nat. Acad. Sci., U.S. *55*, 106.
6. Konigsberg, I. R., and Hauschka, S. D. (1966): Reproduction: Molecular, Subcellular and Cellular (ed. M. Locke). New York: Academic Press.
7. Hauschka, S. D., and Konigsberg, I. R. (1966): The influence of collagen on the development of muscle clones. Proc. Nat. Acad. Sci., U.S. *55*, 119.
8. Grobstein, C. (1962): Interactive processes in cytodifferentiation. J. Cell. Comp. Physiol. *60*, *Supp. 1*, 35.
9. Grobstein, C. (1964): Cytodifferentiation and its controls. Science *143*, 643.
10. Rutter, W. J., Wessells, N. K., and Grobstein, C. (1964): Metabolic control mechanisms in animal cells. Nat. Cancer Inst. Monogr. *13*, 51.
11. Kallman, F., and Grobstein, C. (1964): Fine structure of differentiating mouse pancreatic exocrine cells in transfilter cultures. J. Cell. Biol. *20*, 399.
12. Kallman, F., and Grobstein, C. (1965): Source of collagen at epitheliomesenchymal interfaces during inductive interaction. Develop. Biol. *11*, 169.
13. Grobstein, C., and Cohen, J. (1965): Collagenase: Effect on the morphogenesis of embryonic salivary epithelium *in vitro*. Science *150*, 626.

DISCUSSION

STRAUSS: In connection with fibroblast-conditioned myoblast cytodifferentiation have you studied such factors as (a) species specificity, i.e., attempts to condition myoblasts of one species with collagen or fibroblasts of another; (b) regional specificity, i.e., the regional source of mesenchyme and its conditioning potential; (c) organ or tissue specificity, i.e., attempts to condition myoblasts with cells other than fibroblasts?

KONIGSBERG: Our conditioned media have been prepared in cultures of embryonic chick cells, including fibroblasts. However, the conditioned medium may be replaced by conventional media provided collagen is present. We have used several collagens, including rat tail tendon and fish swim bladder.

AUERBACH: Collagen may be non-specific but this does not exclude the possibility that specific factors may influence cloning also. Do you have any information on the effects of conditioned media of various tissue origins on differentiation of muscle cells?

KONIGSBERG: We have tried conditioning with medium from liver cell cultures; we did get muscle clones in very small numbers; they were rather "puny" ones. We have tried Hela cells without success. But the development of

protocols for conditioning a medium is quite empirical. One has to work out conditions for each cell type before he can be reasonably sure that it was not effective in conditioning.

VAN FURTH: Does treatment of the conditioned medium or the collagen-treated plates with collagenase prevent the differentiation of muscle?

KONIGSBERG: We have not done this experiment. In theory it is an important one. One of the things we want to do is to study the effects of collagenase on pretreated plates. What discouraged us was the fact that it is difficult to obtain purified collagenase. The other problem is this: since gelatin will substitute for collagen, it would be difficult to interpret results with collagenase treatment.

COOPER: We are familiar with the developmental phenomenon of regeneration in vertebrates. For example, after a salamander limb is amputated there accumulates at the cut surface a blastema which subsequently differentiates into cartilage, muscle, etc. Have you or others cultured blastemal cells in a conditioned medium?

KONIGSBERG: We have not.

COOPER: What about embryonic limb bud cells like those of the chick embryo?

KONIGSBERG: We have cultured limb bud cells and gotten small numbers of rather atypical-looking muscle colonies; at least they are atypical when compared to the colonies that we get from the older tissue.

FELDMAN: Does collagen affect only the incidence of clones which will undergo differentiation, or is the general cloning efficiency also influenced; i.e., the total numbers of clones produced?

KONIGSBERG: No, it doesn't affect cloning efficiency. But it does affect the percentage of colonies which can be scored as muscle. So we assume that it is not simply a matter of enhancing the attachment of single cells.

BLOCK: You have alluded to difficulty in determining whether the effect of collagen in inducing clonal synthesis of striated muscle fibers *in vitro* is also operative *in vivo*.

KONIGSBERG: Heinz Herrmann has presented data that do not answer the question, but do indicate that the rate of accumulation of actomyosin and accumulation of collagen in the skeletal muscle are similar.

EBERT: Cardiac muscle appears to develop in the absence of collagen. The evidence is not crucial, but thus far hydroxyproline has not been detected in the two-day-old chick embryo, at a time when the heart is already beating.

CEBRA: Can you detect myosin in any of the clones grown in unconditioned medium? Perhaps some cells may differentiate with respect to product and not with respect to form.

KONIGSBERG: With techniques that we have used for detecting cross-striated fibrils, we don't see them in the monoculated cells regardless of the medium in which they are grown.

PETERSON: Did you say that neither acid hydrolsates of rat tail tendon collagen nor collagenase-digested collagen will condition the medium?

KONIGSBERG: Yes. Neither equivalent amounts of collagen hydrolsate nor collagenase digest will replace formed collagen.

BRAUN: Can you alter the phenotype of your clones by starting with unconditioned media and then adding conditioned media? The basic problem would appear to be: are you modifying the phenotype or are you possibly selecting another cell type?

KONIGSBERG: We plated cells in unconditioned medium. Then, at intervals—three, six, nine days—we removed the unconditioned medium and added conditioned medium. This procedure greatly increased the number of muscle clones. For example, cells grown exclusively in conditioned medium yield about 60% muscle colonies, whereas in unconditioned medium the yield is about 10%. So we have in a sense "rescued" some of the cells which wouldn't have differentiated into muscle. It appears, therefore, that we are modifying the phenotype.

GOOD: It would seem reasonable to determine whether collagen is affecting more than cell nutrition by testing the responsiveness of myoblasts to the collagen environment by treating the blastic cells with either trypsin or with disaccharidases. Gessner has recently interfered with contact inhibition occurring in the T_3 fibroblast system by treating T_3 fibroblasts with disaccharidases from *Clostridium perfringens*. He has also interfered with recirculation of lymphocytes by treatment of the lymphocytes with disaccharidases. One might inhibit the apparent inducing- or "permitting"-effect of the collagen by altering the surface of the blast cells. The effect of the collagen may require a recognition phenomenon which would be of general significance.

PART II

DIFFERENTIATION OF CELLS OF LYMPHORETICULAR SYSTEM

JOHN CEBRA

ANTIGENIC STIMULATION of an animal causes the differentiation of lymphoid elements and the expression by some of these of specific antibody formation. Antibody-forming cells are usually dedicated to the synthesis of antibody of a single specificity. However, it has now become apparent that antibodies with the same specificity can be resolved into many molecular forms—into classes, types, and allotypes—which differ in their physicochemical and biologic properties. Thus one would like to identify the various cellular changes which precede the appearance of immunoglobulins in the cytoplasm of lymphoid cells and to account for the diversity of these products with respect to both antibody specificity and "gross molecular form." Particularly, one would like to know how closely the control of antibody specificity and molecular form, both presumably aspects of amino acid sequence of the component immunoglobulin chains, were linked. Are individual lymphoid elements precommitted to synthesis of antibodies of a single specificity and molecular form before they express either of these molecular features upon antigenic stimulation? Or, are the lymphoid cells relatively non-differentiated with respect to the specificity and molecular form of their potential product? If so, how does the antigen influence the course of the ensuing differentiation? Finally, is it possible that specificity and molecular form, presently assessed from different parts of the immunoglobulin molecule, may be independently controlled? For instance, is it possible that lymphoid cells are fully differentiated with respect to the molecular form of their potential product, but require additional extracellular stimulation and information, derived from antigen, before the synthesis of complete antibody molecules with a determined specificity can begin?

The following papers will consider different aspects of this general problem—namely, the differentiation of lymphoid elements. Dr. Fishman will consider the differentiation of populations of lymphoid cells stimulated *in vitro* to express antibody specificity in two differentiable molecular forms—γM and γG. Various preparations extracted from macrophage, which have ingested antigen, appear to initiate specific antibody formation. Dr. Feldman will continue by considering the initial phagocytosis of antigen as an essential step for the induction of antibody synthesis *in vivo*. X-irradiated mice which can no longer make an antibody response to antigen can be restored to immunologic competence by administration of macrophage incubated with antigen.

Dr. Hirschhorn will describe a model system in which the events leading to immunoglobulin synthesis may be non-specifically initiated. Phytohemagglutinin, acting on peripheral blood lymphocytes, stimulates transformation to blast cells, preparation for cell division, and the appearance of a variety of immunoglobulin forms in the cytoplasm of individual cells. Dr. van Furth then will deal with the ability of peripheral blood lymphocytes to synthesize immunoglobulins under normal circumstances and with the homogeneity of the molecular forms produced by individual cells. My own paper will endeavor to demonstrate the extreme differentiation of individual lymphoid elements with respect to the class, subclass, type, and allotype of their product immunoglobulin. The proportions of the various immunoglobulins in the blood appear to reflect the relative numbers of cells actively synthesizing these various molecular forms. Finally, Dr. Mage will describe fascinating experiments attempting to alter the normal serum concentrations of different allotypes of immunoglobulins. Specific immunosuppression of the full capacity to produce a particular molecular form (allotype) can result from treating unborn or newborn rabbits.

6

MARVIN FISHMAN and FRANK L. ADLER

The RNA of macrophages in antibody formation

SEVERAL YEARS AGO we reported (4) that macrophages which have been incubated with an antigen (bacteriophage T2) yield a ribonuclease-sensitive material (Macro-T2-RNA) which stimulates lymph node fragments from non-immune animals to produce T2 specific antibodies. More recently similar observations have been published by Askonas (1) and by Friedman (7). Immunogenic material of an apparently related nature had previously been found in the livers of immunized animals (8). It is the purpose of this presentation to summarize some of our more recent findings which indicate that Macro-T2-RNA is heterogeneous, that T2 antigen is demonstrable in some but not all its immunogenic fractions, and that the different fractions evoke antibodies of distinct immunoglobulin classes.

In our earlier phases of these studies (4) we employed minimal doses of antigen (1 PFU of T2 phage per 100 macrophages) and obtained Macro-T2-RNA which contained no demonstrable T2 antigens. Such preparations elicited a short-lived 19S antibody in cultures of lymph node fragments. When the amount of T2 phage was increased 10^2-10^4 fold (6) Macro-T2-RNA was obtained (10) which gave rise to two waves of antibody formation, an early 19S phase which was followed on or after day 8 by the formation of antibody which was predominantly 7S. Treatment of such Macro-T2-RNA with RNAase in the proportion 100:1 yielded a product which elicited only a delayed 7S antibody response; higher concentrations of RNAase caused complete loss of immunogenicity.

The treatment of those Macro-T2-RNA preparations which were capable of eliciting 19S and 7S antibody with high-titered anti-T2 sera resulted in precipitation. Extraction of RNA from the supernatant and from the precipitate yielded immunogenic materials which differed from each other in that the RNA from the supernatant evoked only the 19S antibody whereas the RNA from the precipitate proved to be highly immunogenic and elicited a response which was predominantly 7S antibody. It seems reasonable to assume that the latter RNA is specifically precipitated by antibody because it is complexed to T2 antigen. Since Macro-T2-RNA of Macro-RNA forms varying amounts of precipitate not only with rabbit anti-T2 sera but also with other rabbit sera, the specificity of the precipitation is open to question.

In support of the concept of specificity are the following observations:

1. Precipitates from the reaction of Macro-T2-RNA with rabbit antisera against bovine serum albumin or with rabbit anti-T2 sera that had been exhaustively absorbed with T2 phage yielded no immunogenic material and the RNA extracted from the supernates of reaction mixtures still stimulated both 19S and 7S antibody formation.

2. Highly purified anti-T2 antibody preparations which caused only minimal precipitation with Macro-RNA effectively frac-

34

tionated Macro-T2-RNA into the two species of immunogenic material. Preliminary data suggest that the putative "superantigen" precipitated by antibody against T2 phage contains at most 2% of the total Macro-T2-RNA, yet this material proved to be active in 10 μg amounts, whereas 100 μg amounts of Macro-T2-RNA or supernate RNA were required to demonstrate biological activity.

A second line of investigation sought to determine whether Macro-T2-RNA contains preformed or newly synthesized RNA. That an RNA of unique base composition is formed by macrophages that have ingested antigen has indeed been reported recently (9). When actinomycin D, in concentrations of 1-5 μg/ml of medium, was present during the 30-minute incubation of macrophages and T2, a Macro-T2-RNA was obtained which engendered delayed 7S antibody formation but no longer evoked the early 19S response (6). In extension of these experiments it has been found that exposure of macrophages to actinomycin D for 2 hours in the dark prior to the addition of T2 phage caused a complete loss of their ability to form active Macro-T2-RNA. If actinomycin D acted under these conditions as a specific inhibitor or RNA synthesis it would then appear that the early 19S antibody response is mediated by RNA that is synthesized after ingestion and solubilization of T2 phage by macrophages, whereas 7S antibody is formed in response to a fraction of macrophage RNA, present before the ingestion of T2 phage, which has a relatively short half-life. This is presumably the RNA which complexes with antigenic fragments of the phage.

Experiments (5) in which the phage was opsonized with trace amounts of antibody led to the interesting observation that the greatly increased phagocytosis failed to result in more active Macro-T2-RNA preparations. Among several possible explanations one could assume that the opsonized phage is catabolized in a manner which is neither productive of new RNA synthesis nor of complex formation with Macro-RNA. However, peritoneal exudate cells from animals whose RE system had been stimulated non-specifically also failed to yield more active Macro-T2-RNA in spite of enhanced phagocytosis. Alternatively, one could assume that the population of peritoneal exudate cells which possess the ability of channeling antigen or a specific antigen into productive metabolic pathways is limited, and that opsonization merely brings into play unproductive cells. It has been shown by others that macrophages do indeed differ from each other in their reactivity with antigens (2, 13).

A third major line of investigation consists of attempts to fractionate Macro-T2-RNA by physical means. Density gradient centrifugation, employing sucrose, has failed to yield acceptable resolution of Macro-T2-RNA. Most often the bulk of the RNA was found in a zone containing 5-7S material and this RNA was active in evoking the early 19S antibody response (4). Observations from experiments with diffusion chambers suggested that the Macro-T2-RNA responsible for the later 7S antibody response diffused more slowly than that which caused the appearance of the early antibody (6). More recently methylated albumin columns (11) have been employed. Three fractions, representing 5-7S, 16S, and 28S RNA, can be routinely obtained from Macro-T2-RNA. All three fractions elicit antibody formation but the lightest fractions appear to favor the production of 19S antibody whereas the heaviest fraction led to the eventual formation of 7S antibody. Whether this fraction contains T2 antigen remains to be established.

Finally, the possible adjuvant role of Macro-RNA has been investigated (12). All the evidence obtained points against such a role in the system under study in our laboratory. This evidence includes (a) the requirement of an incubation of not less than a 10-minute period in the T2-macrophage interaction (3), (b) inhibition of the activity of Macro-T2-RNA by the addition of Macro-RNA (5), (c) the demonstration that addition of Macro-RNA to sonicated T2 phage neither increased the immunogenicity of amounts of disrupted phage which gave rise to antibody when given alone, nor did such RNA convert a subliminal dose of disrupted phage into an antigenic dose. These last experiments were done by the diffusion chamber technic in rats since T2 alone or mixed with RNA did not give rise to antibody when added to cultures of lymph node fragments from normal rats.

Table 1 summarizes the information herein and in earlier publications from our laboratory.

TABLE 1

Property of System	Early Product (Peak Day 5)	Late Product (Peak Day 12)
Sedimentation rate of Antibody	19S	7S
Macrophage:T2 Ratio		
100:1	present	absent
1:1 - 1:100	present	present
RNAase Inactivation of Macro-T2-RNA		
enzyme:substrate 1:100	absent	present
1:15	absent	absent
Macrophages Treated with Actinomycin D		
1-5µg/ml 30′	absent	present
120′	absent	absent
Macro-T2-RNA Treated with anti-T2		
supernate RNA	present	absent
precipitate RNA	absent	present
Methylated Albumin Fractions		
5-7S	present	absent
16S	present	absent
28S	absent	present

Acknowledgment: This work was supported by Grant 1 ROI-AI-06899-01 from the National Institute of Allergy and Infectious Diseases.

REFERENCES

1. Askonas, B. A., and Rhodes, J. M. (1965): Immunogenicity of antigen-containing ribonucleic acid preparations from macrophages. Nature *205*, 470.
2. Cohn, Z. A. (1964): The fate of bacteria within phagocytic cells. III. Destruction of an *E. coli* agglutinogen within polymorphonuclear leucocytes and macrophages. J. Exp. Med. *120*, 869.
3. Fishman, M. (1961): Antibody formation *in vitro*. J. Exp. Med. *114*, 837.
4. Fishman, M., and Adler, F. L. (1963): Antibody formation initiated *in vitro*. II. Antibody synthesis in x-irradiated recipients of diffusion chambers containing nucleic acid derived from macrophage incubated with antigen. J. Exp. Med. *117*, 595.
5. Fishman, M., Adler, F. L., van Rood, J. J., and Binet, J. L. (1964): Macrophage involvement in antibody formation *in vitro*. Proceedings of the IVth International Symposium of RES. Otsu and Kyoto, Japan. p. 229.
6. Fishman, M., van Rood, J. J., and Adler, F. L. (1964): The initiation of antibody formation by ribonucleic acid from specifically stimulated macrophages: Molecular and cellular basis of antibody formation. Proceedings of a Symposium. Prague, Czechoslovakia. p. 491.
7. Friedman, H. P., Stavitsky, A. B., and Solomon, J. M. (1965): Induction *in vitro* of antibodies to phage T2:antigens in the RNA extract employed. Science *149*, 1106.
8. Garvey, J. S., and Campbell, D. H. (1957): The retention of S^{35}-labelled bovine serum albumin in normal and immunized rabbit liver tissue. J. Exp. Med. *105*, 361.
9. Halec, E., Rife, U., and Rinaldini, L. M. (1964): Changes in composition of ribonucleic acid induced by antigenic stimulation. Nature *202*, 558.
10. Homma, M., and Graham, A. F. (1963): Synthesis of RNA in L cells infected with mengo virus. J. Cell. Comp. Physiol. *62*, 179.

11. Mandell, J. D., and Hershey, A. D. (1960): A fractionating column for analysis of nucleic acid. Anal. Biochem. *1*, 66.

12. Merritt, K., and Johnson, A. G. (1965): Studies on the adjuvant action of bacterial endotoxins on antibody formation. VI. Enhancement of antibody formation by nucleic acids. J. Immun. *94*, 416.

13. Nossal, G. J. V. (1965): Self-Recognition. Autoimmunity—Experimental and clinical aspects. Ann. N. Y. Acad. Sci. *124*, 37.

DISCUSSION

CEBRA: You have suggested that the "superantigen" may be formed by combination of partially degraded antigen with RNA which was already present in the macrophage prior to ingestion. Have you tried *in vitro* to duplicate what may occur in the cell by mixing antigen with RNA either isolated from macrophage or even with yeast or liver cell RNA? A kind of "superantigen" might be isolated from the mixture by precipitation of antigen with specific antiserum and then by extraction of any RNA that might be bound to antigen in the precipitate.

FISHMAN: At present we are trying to duplicate *in vitro* the preparation of RNA-antigen complexes.

JOHNSON: I am not surprised that your addition of normal RNA to suboptimal amounts of RNA-antigen complex did not enhance activity of the latter. Although the nucleic acids perform well as adjuvants *in vivo*, addition of undegraded nucleic acids to our own splenic organ culture system making antibody results in cessation of synthesis. It may be that nucleic acids are inhibitory, but are degraded *in vivo* to active oligo-nucleotides. The latter are also excellent adjuvants, but have not yet been tested on organ cultures.

With respect to your "superantigen," didn't Dr. Justine Garvey show enhanced activity of antigen when it was complexed with liver RNA and added *in vitro* as a challenge in the Schultz-Dale test?

FISHMAN: Dr. Garvey did indeed take RNA-antigen complex from the liver and got a secondary response when it was injected into primed animals.

SMITH: Garvey and I also showed in similar experiments that RNA-associated antigen obtained from the rabbit did not differ whether it was prepared in the tolerant or immune animal.

HILDEMANN: I understand Dr. Askonas argues that the macrophage RNA merely complexes with antigen to produce a "superantigen." Does your current evidence still leave open the possibility that some specific RNA codon or messenger is produced by appropriately stimulated macrophages?

FISHMAN: The antigen complexed to RNA is a "superantigen" by virtue of the very small amount of material that can give rise to an antibody response. There seems to be something unique about the RNA but not in the sense that it is "messenger RNA." It cannot be increased by opsonization and by creating more macrophage involvement; thus it does not appear to be present in every macrophage.

SMITH: Has the capability of RNA-associated antigens—such as can be obtained in large quantities from rabbit liver—to induce tolerance ever been assessed?

FISHMAN: I don't believe so.

GOOD: Is it not possible that at least with respect to your smaller RNA there is a messenger function and the possibility of information transfer?

FISHMAN: It is possible that there is an RNA which is not associated with demonstrable antigen and which can induce a response. The small size of this RNA, if it is messenger, would mean that it is only coding for a small piece of the total antibody protein.

EBERT: Dr. Fishman, you suggested that there may be little or no cell division upon stimulation of γM antibody production. What is the basis for this?

FISHMAN: Since plasma cells are not implicated in the γM response, it is possible that there is no need for differentiation to occur.

EBERT: Do you think that the differentiation may be already "incorporated" into the RNA? Is there really good evidence that no cell division occurs?

FISHMAN: There is a report by Sterzl that mitotic poisons prevent any kind of proliferation but still allow an early antibody response.

MIESCHER: Did you get cell division in the late response which you observed *in vitro*?

FISHMAN: We have not looked at cell division in our system.

CEBRA: When you prepare your superantigen by precipitation of the antigen-RNA with antibody and subsequent isolation of RNA, do you include in it any of the antibody used to isolate that particular complex? If some antigen could survive the phenol treatment, some antibody might also. Thus you may have antibody-antigen complexes which could potentiate the immune response. Have you used labelled antibody to rule out this possibility?

FISHMAN: We haven't used labelled antibody. We are relying on the 3 or 4 phenol extractions to minimize this effect.

EBERT: What do you know about the size of the RNA that is in the antigen-RNA complex?

FISHMAN: On the assumption that the complex is responsible for the late response, fractionation of the RNA with such activity suggests it sediments at a rate of 16 to 28S.

EBERT: Perhaps one could approach the identification of functional RNA in a cruder way. That is, to obtain a polyribosomal pellet and check its size in the electron microscope. Then, perhaps using chlorpromazine, by the methods described here by Braun, attempt to have the material incorporated by lymphocytes. If it would stimulate antibody production then more sophisticated attempts to isolate and characterize messenger RNA might be warranted.

MITCHISON: Let me make an experimental prediction and suggest a way of testing it. In an immune response, it would appear unlikely that an antigen is recognized twice. It is difficult not to have it recognized once. Thus, if there is something specific about the active RNA, that is, it has some messenger function, this implies recognition of antigen has taken place in the macrophage. Thus, there is probably no recognition in the lymphocyte for that antigen. There may be lymphocyte recognition of RNA but that is a different matter. Thus we could predict that one could not competitively inhibit the macrophage-lymphocyte interaction by any agent where competition depends on antigenic structure. We have been studying the inhibition of immunization with hapten-protein conjugates by haptens. The enhancing effect of macrophage in the macrophage-lymphocyte interaction is clearly susceptible to hapten competition. This seems to count very strongly against the probability that there is anything specific about the RNA coming out of the macrophage. Thus the recognition seems to be occurring on the lymphocyte rather than by the macrophage.

7

MICHAEL FELDMAN and RUTH GALLILY

The function of macrophages in the induction of antibody production in x-irradiated animals

THE CONDITIONS which determine whether the introduction of an antigen into an organism will stimulate antibody production or confer specific immunological tolerance have been extensively studied in recent years. These studies have led to continuous modifications of our concepts regarding the determining factors in tolerance induction. The original notion that the introduction of an antigen at the adult stage will result in antibody production whereas its application at the fetal or embryonic stage will confer tolerance has long been revised following the demonstration that adult animals can acquire tolerance. The stage of differentiation of the lymphoid cell seems to be no longer the only factor nor even a determining factor in tolerance induction. Analysis of the quantitative parameters for tolerance induction in the adult organism has introduced the notion of the antigen dose as a controlling factor. It was initially proposed that the probability of tolerance increases as a function of the amount of antigen per lymphoid cell. This concept has, again, been subjected recently to re-evaluation following Mitchison's demonstration of the two quantitative zones of tolerogenic activity of an antigen (18, and this volume, Part III, page 135).

In studies of tolerance induction in adult rabbits carried out in this laboratory, an experimental system was developed wherein immunological tolerance to serum proteins (i.e., human serum albumin) was induced by applying relatively low doses of antigen after total body irradiation at sublethal doses (19, 20). It appeared initially that the stage of differentiation of the lymphoid cell population, following exposure to x-rays, determined the acquisition of tolerance. However, further analysis demonstrated that tolerance was conferred on adult rabbits even when antigen was injected as late as 4 weeks following sublethal doses of irradiation. At this stage, the lymphoid elements *per se* appeared to have regenerated almost completely, yet the animals did not respond to the antigenic stimulation by antibody formation, but rather by acquiring specific immunological tolerance (21). Thus, a segregation was manifested between the histological recovery of the lymphoid system and its functional recovery as measured by the immunological reactivity. This could be explained on the basis of two alternative assumptions. Either the cytological regeneration of the lymphoid system does not reflect the functional recovery of the lymphoid cells, or the lymphoid cells *per se* have completely recovered both morphologically and functionally but a cell type other than the lymphoid cell may not have regained its functional properties, and this is the one which determines whether the antigen will induce antibody formation or tolerance.

Our attention was therefore turned to the function of the macrophages in the susceptibility of animals to the tolerogenic versus immunogenic effects of antigens. Macrophages have long been suspected to play a decisive role in inducing the immune response (10), yet their "immunogenic" capacity following irradiation has not been studied. From histological evidence, it appears that RES macrophages are radiation-resistant (5, 6). Most studies seem to indicate that the clearance of colloidal particles by the RES is unaffected by total body irradiation (2, 3, 4, 11, 17, 22). Similar observations have been made with regard to bacteria; here, however, it appears that although the initial clearance of bacteria is unaffected by x-rays, macrophages of irradiated animals are unable to kill or retain bacteria (15). Peritoneal macrophages of irradiated rabbits showed a reduced capacity to digest chicken red blood cells, as compared to those of non-irradiated donors (8). Since macrophage-antigen interaction may be an essential step in the induction of antibody production, the impaired capacity of macrophages of x-irradiated animals to degrade antigenic material could at least partly account for the impaired immunological reactivity of animals exposed to sublethal doses of x-rays.

In the present study, a comparison has been made of the capacity of macrophages from normal and x-irradiated mice to elicit antibody production in irradiated mice, when injected after an *in vitro* interaction with Shigella antigen (13).

Materials and Methods

Animals.—Female mice of C57BL/6 strain, 10-weeks-old, were used both as donors and recipients in all the experiments. The sera of these mice were tested for agglutinating "natural" antibody to Shigella. No measurable traces of antibody could be found.

X-irradiation.—Mice were exposed in lucite containers to total body x-irradiation of 550 r (unless otherwise stated), using a General Electric Maximar III X-Ray machine (250 KV, 15 mA). They were irradiated at a target distance of 50 cm (dose rate 65 r/min) with 0.5 mm Cu and 1 mm Al filters.

Peritoneal macrophages. — Macrophages were obtained from the peritoneal exudate by a modification of Bang's method (12). Each mouse was injected intraperitoneally with 3 ml thioglycolate medium (Difco Laboratories, Detroit, Mich.). Four days later the peritoneal cells were collected by washing out the peri-

toneum with 5 ml phosphate-buffered saline containing penicillin, streptomycin, and heparin (100 units, 50 μg, and 5 U.S.P. units/ml, respectively). The cells were counted with a hemocytometer and after centrifugation (1000 rpm for 8 min) were suspended in Hank's salt solution. Incubation of these cells with Shigella was then carried out in Erlenmeyer flasks containing 7.5 x 10^6 cells/ml of 0.005% Shigella in Hank's solution, on a shaking tray for one hour at 37°C. After incubation, the cells were centrifuged and washed in approximately 40 volumes of Hank's salt solution. They were then resuspended in Hank's solution at a concentration of 30 x 10^6 cells/ml and injected intraperitoneally at doses of 15 x 10^6 cells per recipient two days following exposure of the mice to x-rays.

Macrophages in tissue culture.—The macrophages were taken from the peritoneum as described previously. After sedimentation, the packed cells were resuspended in a tissue culture medium (horse or fetal calf serum 35%, chick embryo extract 5%, and Hank's salt solution). The cells were then transferred into 50 mm diameter petri dishes (6 x 10^6 cells/dish) which had been overlayed with reconstituted rat tail collagen substrate, prepared according to the method of Ehrman and Gey. After 48 hours in culture about 98% of the cells which adhered to the bottom of the dishes were macrophages. These macrophages were then washed twice with Hank's solution and Shigella was added (final concentration 0.005%) to the cell-containing medium which consisted of fetal calf serum (10%) and Hank's solution. The petri dishes were incubated for one hour at 37°C. The cultures were then washed with Hank's solution, and collagenase (0.025%-0.050%) was applied to remove the cells. Incubation with the enzyme was carried out for 15 minutes in a shaking tray at 37°C. The released cells were washed, resuspended, and after counting were injected intraperitoneally into the x-irradiated mice.

Lymphocytes.—The cervical, submaxillary axillary, brachial, inguinal, and mesenteric nodes were excised from normal mice. The nodes were cut in Tyrode's solution, filtered through a stainless steel filter (pore size of 0.6 x 0.6 mm), and washed twice. After centrifugation, the cells were suspended with the antigen in Hank's solution at a concentration of 7.5 x 10^6 cells/ml of 0.005% Shigella, and incubated for one hour at 37°C on a shaking tray. The cells were then washed, resuspended in Hank's solution, and injected intraperitoneally into x-irradiated mice.

Antigenic material.—The antigen used was Shigella *paradysenteriae*. The stock of bacteria was obtained by courtesy of Dr. T. N. Harris, and was prepared according to his description (16). A 10% suspension (v/v) of the alcohol-killed bacteria was kept at 4°C as a standard stock.

Anti-Shigella agglutinins. — Agglutinins were measured after serial two-fold dilutions of 0.1 ml volumes of mouse sera and a subsequent addition of 0.5 ml of 0.02% suspension of alcohol-treated Shigella per tube. After shaking and one hour of incubation at 37°C, the tubes were stored at 4°C for 48 hours, then read for agglutination by the pattern of sediment on the bottom of the tubes and also by shaking them under the agglutinoscope.

Cytologic examination.—Smears of cell suspension before incubation were prepared and stained by Giemsa or May-Grünwald-Giemsa. Differential counts were made of 400-600 cells in each test.

Experimental and Discussion

The first set of experiments was designed to test whether macrophages from normal donors could induce after *in vitro* interaction with Shigella antigen, an immune response in x-irradiated mice which did not respond to injection of the antigen alone. Macrophages from the peritoneal exudates of normal mice were incubated with Shigella, then injected at doses of 15 x 10^6 cells per animal into mice which had been exposed two days previously to a dose of 550 r total body irradiation. A second group of irradiated animals was inoculated with macrophages alone (without pre-incubation with antigen), and a third with Shigella alone. The animals were tested for agglutinins to Shigella, 5 and 8 days following treatment. The results of a number of such experiments are pooled and presented in Table 1. They indicate that macrophages from normal animals after interaction with the antigen elicited the formation of antibody in the x-irradiated mice, showing a $\log_2$ titer of 4.0 after 5 days which had risen to 7.5 when measured after 8 days. The agglutinating titer of the control groups did not rise above 1.6 (Table 1).

In a subsequent experiment, mice exposed to 550 r were inoculated two days later with different doses of macrophages which had been incubated with Shigella antigen. The results are recorded in Fig. 1. In view of the clear and sufficiently high immune response obtained in animals treated with 15 x 10^6 cells, this dose of macrophages was chosen as the standard one in all the following experiments.

The macrophage cell population of the peritoneal exudate was found to be contaminated with about 10% lymphocytes. The production of antibody in the irradiated recipients ob-

TABLE 1.—Antibody Production by Irradiated C57BL Mice Following Inoculation of Macrophages Incubated *in vitro* with Shigella Antigen

Treatment of irradiated recipients		Agglutinin titer					
	No. of experiments	5 DAYS			8 DAYS		
(per mouse)		No. of tested mice	$\log_2$ of titer (mean)	S.E.*	No. of tested mice	$\log_2$ of titer (mean)	S.E.*
15 x 10^6 macrophages incubated with Shigella	6	36	4.0†	0.10	54	7.5†	0.37
15 x 10^6 macrophages	4	19	0.1	0.07	30	0.8	0.29
Shigella (0.1 ml of 0.1% suspension)	6	27	0.7	0.30	40	1.6	0.30

*Standard error of the mean.

†The difference between this value and that of each of the two control experiments was checked according to the rank sum test and found significant at a level exceeding 99%.

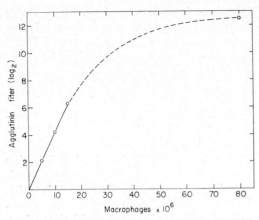

FIG. 1. Antibody production by irradiated C57BL mice as a function of macrophage dose.

tained in the previous experiments could therefore be attributed to the lymphoid components of the peritoneal exudates. To eliminate the question of participation of the lymphoid contaminants of the macrophage population in the immune reaction attempts were made to culture the macrophages *in vitro* and thereby to obtain lymphoid-free cell populations. Peritoneal macrophages were cultured on collagen, then removed by collagenase. Differential counts of the cells after 48 hours showed that 98% were macrophages (Table 2) while only 1% of cells seemed to be of lymphoid type. The macrophages were incubated in culture with Shigella antigen, then injected into x-irradiated mice (550 r) which were subsequently tested for antibody 5 and 8 days following cell inoculation. The results (Table 3) show that macrophages cultured *in vitro*, then interacted with Shigella, do elicit the production of agglutinin to the antigen in the irradiated recipients.

To determine whether lymphocytes are at all capable of producing antibody when similarly treated, the capacity of lymph node cells to elicit antibody production in irradiated mice was studied. Lymphocytes obtained from the lymph nodes of normal mice and incubated with Shigella under conditions similar to those of the macrophage-Shigella incubation were injected at various cell doses into C57BL mice that had been exposed 2 days previously to 550 r. The results (Table 4) show clearly that lymphocyte doses even greater by a factor of 7 than those corresponding to the lymphoid components of the peritoneal exudates elicited only a very low titer of antibody; less by a factor of 10 than the titer obtained following the inoculation of macrophages. It appears therefore that the macrophages of peritoneal exudates rather than the lymphocytes trigger the formation of antibodies in irradiated mice.

It could, however, be postulated that the donor macrophages "process" the antigen, and are then transformed to lymphocytes within the irradiated recipients, so that the donor rather than the recipient cells produce the antibody. If this were so, similar results to those reported above would be obtained if macrophages which had interacted with antigen were injected into animals exposed to irradiation doses higher than 550 r. On the other hand, if the macrophages "signal" the lymphocytes of the recipient animals which survived irradiation to produce antibodies, the higher the dose of irradiation, the lower should be the immune response of the host, since depletion of lymphocytes would leave less target cells for the macrophage "signal." To test this, mice exposed to 550 r, 750 r, and

TABLE 2.—DIFFERENTIAL COUNT OF PERITONEAL CELLS BEFORE AND AFTER CULTURING *in vitro*

Origin of cells	No. of cells counted	Macro- phages (%)	Granulo- cytes (%)	Lympho- cytes (%)	Unidentified cells (%)
Peritoneal exudate after withdrawal	4400	83	7	10	-
Peritoneal exudate in culture*	2100	98	-	1	1

*48 hours after seeding.

900 r were inoculated with macrophages following incubation with the antigen. The results (Fig. 2) show that animals exposed to 550 r responded with a titer of 7.5, as compared to 3.5 for mice exposed to 750 r and 1.0 for mice exposed to 900 r. It is therefore concluded that normal macrophages, following interaction with Shigella, "instruct" lymphoid elements of sublethally irradiated mice to produce antibodies.

TABLE 3.—ANTIBODY PRODUCTION FOLLOWING
INOCULATION OF MACROPHAGES CULTURED *in vitro*

Treatment of recipients (per mouse)	Agglutinin titer					
	5 DAYS			8 DAYS		
	No. of animals tested	$\log_2$ of titer (mean)	S.E.*	No. of animals tested	$\log_2$ of titer (mean)	S.E.*
8 x 10⁶ macrophages on collagen incubated with Shigella	4	0	-	6	3.0	1.31
13 x 10⁶ macrophages on collagen incubated with Shigella	7	0.6	0.23	11	4.3[a]†	0.72
15 x 10⁶ macrophages on collagen incubated with Shigella	4	0	-	7	6.1[b]	1.55
Shigella (0.1 ml of 0.1% susp.)	17	0.3	0.15	18	0.8[c]	0.28

*Standard error of the mean.
†The difference between the values of (a) and (c) as well as that between (b) and (c) was checked according to the rank sum test and found significant at a level between 95% and 99%.

TABLE 4.—ANTIBODY PRODUCTION BY IRRADIATED MICE
FOLLOWING INOCULATION OF MACROPHAGES OR
LYMPHOCYTES INCUBATED *in vitro* WITH SHIGELLA
ANTIGEN

Treatment of irradiated recipients (per mouse)	No. of experiments	Agglutinin titer					
		5 DAYS			8 DAYS		
		No. of tested mice	$\log_2$ of titer (mean)	S.E.*	No. of tested mice	$\log_2$ of titer (mean)	S.E.*
15 x 10⁶ macrophages incubated with Shigella	6	36	4[a]†	0.10	54	7.5[c]†	0.37
1.5 x 10⁶ lymphocytes incubated with Shigella	2	7	0	-	11	1.8	0.54
5 x 10⁶ lymphocytes incubated with Shigella	3	15	0.1	0.05	23	1.0	0.36
10 x 10⁶ lymphocytes incubated with Shigella	2	7	0[b]	-	10	1.6[d]	0.60
10 x 10⁶ lymphocytes	2	8	0	-	11	1.5	0.51
Shigella (0.1 ml of 0.1% suspension)	3	11	1.4	0.57	11	1.6	0.57

*Standard error of the mean.
†The difference between the values of (a) and (b) as well as that between (c) and (d) was checked according to the rank sum test and found significant at a level exceeding 99%.

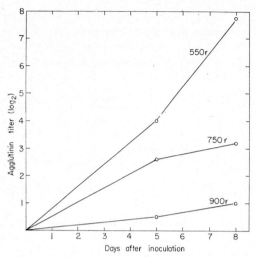

FIG. 2. The production of antibody by animals exposed to various doses of x-rays and inoculated with macrophages that had interacted *in vitro* with Shigella antigen.

It would then appear that macrophages of irradiated animals cannot "instruct" or trigger such reactions. Accordingly, it could be predicted that macrophages of x-irradiated mice after interaction with the antigen would be incapable of such immune-reactivation when injected into mice. To test this prediction, mice were exposed to 550 r, and after two days the peritoneal macrophages were withdrawn and incubated with Shigella. Controls consisted of macrophages from normal non-

irradiated donors otherwise treated similarly. X-irradiated animals were then injected with either type of macrophages, and a third control group was inoculated with Shigella. The results (Table 5) indicate that macrophages from normal animals elicited antibody production in the x-irradiated recipients, whereas those from x-irradiated donors did not. We conclude therefore that x-irradiation, at sublethal doses, impairs the immunological reactivity of the animal not only by depleting the lymphoid cell population, but to an even greater extent by damaging the capacity of the macrophages to process the antigen to an "immunogenic" state.

According to our unpublished observations, it appears that this defective capacity is not due to the inability of macrophages of irradiated animals to take up the Shigella. Previous studies have demonstrated that the initial clearance of bacteria was as great in irradiated animals as in non-irradiated ones (15). However, bacteria removed from the blood stream of x-irradiated mice were not destroyed, but released into the circulating blood. Thus, phagocytic cells of x-irradiated animals appear to be incapable of killing and carrying out intracellular digestion of microorganisms. The ability to degrade killed bacteria or chicken red blood cells is also impaired in macrophages of x-irradiated animals (9). The immunogenic properties of macrophages

TABLE 5.—THE EFFECT OF MACROPHAGES FROM NORMAL AND IRRADIATED DONORS ON THE PRODUCTION OF ANTIBODIES BY IRRADIATED MICE

Treatment of irradiated recipients (per mouse)	No. of experiments	Agglutinin titer					
		5 DAYS			8 DAYS		
		No. of tested mice	$\log_2$ of titer (mean)	S.E.*	No. of tested mice	$\log_2$ of titer (mean)	S.E.*
15 x 10⁶ macrophages from irradiated donors incubated with Shigella	2	22	0.4[a]†	0.17	54	0.9[c]†	0.26
15 x 10⁶ macrophages from normal donors incubated with Shigella	2	11	3.4[b]	0.24	13	8.2[d]	0.53
Shigella (0.1 ml of 0.1% suspension)	2	11	0.3	0.18	13	0.5	0.25

*Standard error of the mean.

†The difference between the values of (a) and (b) as well as that between (c) and (d) was checked according to the rank sum test and found significant at a level exceeding 99%.

that have interacted with bacterial antigen may depend on a specific degradation of the antigen, which may be followed by formation of a complex between the antigenic determinant and certain constituents of the macrophages (1, 10). The differences between the immunogenic properties of macrophages that have phagocytized *E. coli* and those of granulocytes which phagocytize the bacteria may be a function of the differences in the pattern of digestion of the antigen by the two cell types (7).

The demonstration that the injection of antigen alone did not elicit the production of antibody to Shigella by x-irradiated animals, while macrophage-antigen complexes did elicit this response, seems to indicate that mere interaction between antigen and a lymphoid cell, without the functional macrophage intermediate, may not result in antibody production. It has been suggested that such interactions will induce immunological tolerance rather than antibody production (14). The impaired capacity of macrophages of x-irradiated animals to "process" antigen may then be a determining factor in the induction of tolerance following total body x-irradiation.

SUMMARY

Experiments have demonstrated that peritoneal macrophages from normal mice that had interacted *in vitro* with Shigella triggered the production of agglutinating antibody to the bacterial antigen when injected into mice which had been exposed to 550 r total body x-irradiation. Such mice did not respond when injected with the antigen alone. The antibody formed was not produced by "contaminating" lymphocytes of peritoneal exudates, since pure populations of macrophages, obtained after *in vitro* culturing of the cells, were similarly effective in inducing antibody. Neither could the producton of antibody be attributed to the inoculated "macrophages" themselves having undergone "lymphoid transformation." This is deduced from the inverse relationship between the dose of irradiation to the recipient and the level of antibody obtained following macrophage inoculation. It was thus demonstrated that cells of the irradiated recipients produced antibody due to the triggering effect of macrophages from normal animals. Macrophages from irradiated donors, incubated with Shigella, were incapable of inducing antibody production in x-irradiated mice. It is, therefore, concluded that the immunological suppression obtained following sublethal doses of total body irradiation is at least partly due to the impaired capacity of macrophages to process the antigen. It is argued that this may explain the susceptibility of such animals to the induction of immunological tolerance.

Acknowledgments: This work was supported by a grant (C-6165) from the National Institutes of Health, United States Public Health Service, Bethesda, Maryland, and through National Institutes of Health Agreement No. 335105.

REFERENCES

1. Askonas, B. A., and Rhodes, J. M. (1965): Immunogenicity of antigen-containing ribonucleic acid preparations from macrophages. Nature *205*, 471.
2. Barrow, J., Tullis, J. L., and Chambers, F. (1951): Effect of x-radiation and antihistamine drugs on the reticulo-endothelial system measured with colloidal radiogold. Amer. J. Physiol. *164*, 822.
3. Benacerraf, B., Biozzi, G., Halpern, B. N., and Stiffel, C. (1957): The Physiopathology of the RES. Oxford, Blackwell Scientific Publications, Ltd.
4. Benacerraf, B., Kivy-Rosenberg, E., Sebestyen, M. M., and Zweifach, B. W. (1959): The effect of high doses of x-irradiation on the phagocytic, proliferative, and metabolic properties of the reticulo-endothelial system. J. Exp. Med. *110*, 49.
5. Bloom, W. (1948): Histopathology of Irradiation from External and Internal Sources. New York, McGraw-Hill Book Co., Inc.
6. Brecher, G. K., Endicott, H. G., and Broner, H. P. (1948): Effects of x-ray on lymphoid and hemopoietic tissues of albino mice. Blood *3*, 1259.
7. Cohn, Z. A. (1962): Influence of rabbit polymorphonuclear leucocytes and macrophages on

the immunogenicity of *Escherichia coli*. Nature *196*, 1066.

8. Donaldson, D. M., Marcus, S., Gyi, K. K., and Perkins, E. M. (1956): The influence of immunization and total body x-radiation on the intracellular digestion by peritoneal phagocytes. J. Immun. *76*, 192.

9. Donaldson, D. M., and Miller, M. L. (1959): Depression of normal serum bactericidal activity by nitrogen mustard. J. Immun. *82*, 69.

10. Fishman, M. (1961): Antibody formation *in vitro*. J. Exp. Med. *114*, 837.

11. Gabrieli, E. R., and Auskaps, A. A. (1953): The effect of whole body x-irradiation on the reticulo-endothelial system as demonstrated by the use of radioactive chromium phosphate. Yale J. Biol. Med. *26*, 159.

12. Gallily, R., Warwick, A., and Bang, F. B. (1964): Effect of cortisone on genetic resistance to mouse hepatitis virus *in vivo* and *in vitro*. Proc. Nat. Acad. Sci. *51*, 1159.

13. Gallily, R., and Feldman, M. (1966): The induction of antibody production in x-irradiated animals by macrophages that interacted with antigen. Israel J. Med. Sci., *2*, 358.

14. Glynn, L. E., and Holborow, E. J. (1965): Autoimmunity and Disease. Oxford, Blackwell Scientific Publications, Ltd. p. 18.

15. Gordon, L. E., Cooper, D. B., and Miller, C. P.

(1955): Clearance of bacteria from the blood of irradiated rabbits. Proc. Soc. Exp. Biol. Med. *89*, 577.

16. Harris, S., Harris, T. N., and Farber, M. B. (1954): Studies on the transfer of lymph node cells. I. Appearance of antibody in recipients of cells from donor rabbits injected with antigen. J. Immun. *72*, 148.

17. di Luzio, N. R. (1955): Effects of x-irradiation and choline on the reticulo-endothelial system of the rat. Amer. J. Physiol., *181*, 595.

18. Mitchison, N. A. (1964): Induction of immunological paralysis in two zones of dosage. Proc. Roy. Soc. (Biol.), *161*, 275.

19. Nachtigal, D., and Feldman, M. (1963): Immunological unresponsiveness to protein antigens in rabbits exposed to x-irradiation or 6-mercaptopurine treatment. Immunology *6*, 356.

20. Nachtigal, D., and Feldman, M. (1964): The immune response to azo-protein conjugates in rabbits unresponsive to the protein carriers. Immunology *7*, 616.

21. Nachtigal, D., Greenberg, E., and Feldman, M.: To be published in 1966.

22. Wish, L., Furth, J., Sheppard, C., and Storey, R. H. (1952): Disappearance rate of tagged substances from the circulation of roentgen-irradiated animals. Amer. J. Roentgen. Radium Therapy Nuclear Med. *67*, 628.

DISCUSSION

CEBRA: Have you irradiated macrophages *in vitro* before and after incubation with and ingestion of Shigella? Can you thus set up a system for studying damage or impairment of the "processing" of antigenic material?

FELDMAN: We are just beginning to do irradiation *in vitro*. We did not start these experiments until we had defined a proper tissue culture system for keeping macrophages for a long time.

BRAUN: Dr. Feldman's data appear to be complemented by observations cited recently by Cinader: Antigens injected into newborn animals that cannot react to such antigens will elicit antibodies if these antigens are supplied within the macrophages of adult animals.

MIESCHER: It is interesting to note that Metchnikoff made the statement that a substance which is not phagocytized by macrophages is a "bad" antigen. The method of Dresser to induce immunological tolerance may be related to the role of macrophages in immunity. Dresser showed that animals do not form antibodies to heterologous γ-globulins if the γ-globulin was first submitted to ultracentrifugation in order to eliminate larger or ag-

gregated material. Animals injected with such γ-globulin became tolerant. Benacerraf modified the Dresser method by injecting BSA into intact animals. The BSA was then recovered again one hour after injection, when the "aggregated" molecules had been cleared by the RES in the intact animals. BSA, "cleared" *in vivo* instead of by ultracentrifugation, also produced tolerance rather than immunization in recipient animals.

SILVERSTEIN: Did I understand you to say that the irradiated macrophages ingested antigen, but presumably did not digest it suitably?

FELDMAN: Yes.

SILVERSTEIN: If I may refer again to Metchnikoff; one of his students—Cantacuzène—demonstrated that macrophages could be intoxicated by opium to such an extent that they became sluggish and unable to phagocytize organisms. It would be interesting to repeat your experiment with such a system, in which presumably the digestive processes are normal, but the antigen does not enter the phagocyte.

FELDMAN: Certainly many approaches should be utilized to determine whether the simplified concept we have been discussing is correct: that whenever an animal is administered an immunogenic dose, under certain conditions part of its lymphoid cells will interact directly with the antigen and others will be bombarded with macrophage-processed antigen. Thus tolerant cells and antibody forming cells may be induced at the same time.

VAN FURTH: It would also be of interest to know whether change is observed in the hydrolytic enzymes of the macrophages obtained from x-irradiated animals.

FELDMAN: We have not made such studies.

HILDEMANN: Granted that macrophages may be necessary for preliminary digestion of particulate antigens like Shigella, your basic hypothesis requires that truly soluble antigens must also be processed by macrophages before antibody production ensues.

EBERT: It is not established, in my opinion, that the macrophages of embryos and newborn animals are, in fact, non-functional. One would want to specify precisely the species, the age of the embryo, and the antigens employed. Certainly the cells of early chick embryos have some phagocytic ability. We might lead ourselves astray if we looked at the problem as a failure to catabolize antigens. Possibly, as Humphrey and MacFarland suggested a number of years ago, embryonic macrophages break down antigens too far or too rapidly.

BRAUN: A difference between the ability to clear and the ability to process antigens is not distinguished by these experiments.

EBERT: I would agree if by processing you mean preparation of some "superantigen" or partial degradation to a still antigenic substance. But embryonic macrophage probably catabolizes ingested material to amino acids.

SMITH: Robbins has shown that there is no difference in the assayable content of various cathepsins in the spleens of adults or newborn rabbits. However, since the relative numbers of macrophages in the cell population of the two groups is unknown, these data regarding macrophages remain inconclusive.

GOOD: On this point, Peter Reade in Derrick Rowley's laboratory has carried out pertinent experiments. He found that, using opsonized bacteria in a chick embryo, he could identify a period in ontogeny when macrophage action was vigorous with respect to clearance but feeble with respect to digestion of the organism.

Reade has preliminary phylogenetic evidence that a similar situation exists. Certain gastropods and crayfish have been shown to be vigorous in their clearance of particulate material and even opsonized bacteria, but these animals do not have a capacity to digest these organisms. Thus, even though enzymes may develop ontogenetically early, there may be either a limited specificity of these enzymes or a requirement for maturation of their production or delivery.

Finstad and I have looked at the phylogenetic development of clearance and Condie has also carried out numerous studies relevant to the question. Primitive forms, including crabs and shrimp, can clear particulate material but clearance of so-called soluble antigens, including hemocyanin, correlates well phylogenetically with antibody-forming ability.

Enough data are available to indicate that antibody is induced in several animals by particulate antigen whereas antigen lacking a particulate nature induces tolerance. Dresser used two different antigens in two different hosts with the same results: bovine γ-globulin in the mouse, and hare albumin in the rabbit. Negative results may be difficult to interpret. If one injects bovine serum albumin into the Chimaera (the ratfish), this antigen circulates for some hours and then is eliminated by the liver macrophages without any antibody being formed. It appears that the host transforms, non-specifically, the albumin to an aggregated form and then elimination occurs. Failure to show the Dresser effect in this model may be due to the fact that, in the recipient host, aggregation of the centrifuged antigen may occur and induce antibody formation rather than tolerance.

COOPER: It would be of interest to give irradiated and thymectomized mice normal macrophages incubated with antigen. This would allow one to determine whether the thymus system lymphocytes are also necessary to initiate antibody synthesis versus tolerance. It would also be of interest to use thymectomized mice as donors for unirradiated macrophages. This would allow one to find if the peritoneal macrophages have been influenced in their development by the thymus.

STRAUSS: Along the same lines of Dr. Cooper's suggestion it would be of interest to study non-syngeneic macrophages and macro-phages in the chimeric circumstance.

MITCHISON: In a somewhat different system we found that 600 r does not impair macrophage function (actually it slightly enhances function) and also that allogeneic transfers do not work. In this system bovine serum albumin (BSA) taken up by macrophages was compared with free BSA for activity in primary immunization. The radiation is given *in vitro*, and this may possibly account for the result being different from Feldman's.

8

KURT HIRSCHHORN

Derepression and differentiation of human peripheral lymphocytes in vitro

THE DEMONSTRATION by Nowell in 1960 (32) that phytohemagglutinin (PHA), an extract of the kidney bean, is able to act as a mitotic stimulant for human peripheral blood leucocytes, and the later demonstration (17) that the cell being so stimulated is the small lymphocyte, have led to a great number of studies on these cells during the past few years. Also in recent years, primarily through the work of Gowans (16), the small lymphocyte has been shown to be a precursor of at least one form of immunologically competent cell. Others, primarily Yoffey (42), have postulated that it is the stem cell for all immunologically competent cells and have even implied the possibility that it is a potential precursor for all cells of the blood-forming organs. It has been demonstrated that PHA and antigens can convert the small peripheral blood lymphocyte *in vitro* to a large basophilic pyroninophilic cell (19, 28). Recent work with a mitogen prepared from the pokeweed (14) has extended the basis for the hypothesis that immunologically competent cells are produced in this system, since this substance causes a variable proportion of small lymphocytes to differentiate *in vitro* to cells containing significant amounts of rough endoplasmic reticulum (10). We have attempted to study the mechanisms of derepression and differentiation of lymphocytes by means of tissue culture techniques.

It has been shown by several groups (6, 31, 33) that the human peripheral blood lymphocyte is a long-lived cell, ranging in its life span

from a period of months to years without undergoing mitosis. This finding, of course, makes this cell a prime candidate for the immunologic memory cell. It is clear that the various types of stimulants used in tissue culture cause a derepression of these cells, causing them to begin rapid production of new RNA (29) and protein (2, 39). In a previous preliminary communication (2), it was indicated that some of this new protein consists of immunoglobulin. Other workers (25, 30, 38, 40) have also shown that circulating lymphocytes from man or other mammals are capable of producing γ-globulin, and several groups (7, 10, 11, 13, 15) have shown an increased production of immunoglobulins following stimulation by phytohemagglutinin or specific antigens. Another study (43) demonstrated the inactivation of T2 phage by cultured peripheral lymphocytes of T2 sensitized rabbits after 1 to 3 days of culture in the presence of T2 phage. One laboratory (37), on the other hand, has been unable to demonstrate γ-globulin production by stimulated or unstimulated lymphocytes. In a recently completed series of experiments (36) it was shown that a marked increase in immunoglobulin production and content occurs when the lymphocyte is stimulated with PHA or antigens to which the donor is sensitized. A proportion of this immunoglobulin consists of specific antibodies.

Two different methods were used. The first, that of immunofluorescence, was used to demonstrate the development and presence of immunoglobulins in these cells. The second, that of specific coprecipitation, was used to demonstrate that the immunoglobulins present in these cells are the result of new synthesis. The methodology in the immunofluorescent experiments has been previously described (18). The findings have in part been verified by other groups on both fixed (10) and unfixed (11) material. The results are summarized in Table 1. The anti-γ-globulins used include fluorescein-conjugated, monospecific, absorbed antisera against γG, γA and γM obtained from Behringwerke (Marburg a. Lahn), as well as anti-γG and anti-γM from Dr. Edward Franklin at New York University. The only antiserum showing any cross-reaction with other

antisera was the anti-γA material but this was not sufficient to stain cells from individuals who had no γA in their serum. Anti-κ chain and anti-fragment C of γG specificity, both obtained through the courtesy of Dr. Franklin, were also used. Antisera obtained from the two sources gave similar results. The materials used in the blocking experiments were identical, except that they were not conjugated with fluorescein. Immunofluorescence with anti-γ M began to appear at 24 hours and reached a peak at 48 hours after which it diminished. Immunofluorescence with anti-γG and anti-γA began to appear between 36 and 48 hours and reached a peak at 72 hours. The results in the table indicate that the great majority of

TABLE 1.—FLUORESCENCE EXPERIMENTS

		fl-anti-γG	fl-anti-γA	fl-anti-γM	fl-anti-goat γ or fl-anti-rabbit γG
I.	Normal lymphocytes (3 complete, 11 partial) Treated with:				
	Nothing; 0 days	0.1-0.5%	0.1%	0.1-0.5%	
	PHA*(1); 2-3 days	75-95	75-95	75-95	
	PHA + anti-γG*(2); 2-3 days	0-5	75-90	75-90	
	PHA + anti-γA; 2-3 days	75-95	0-5	75-90	
	PHA + anti-γM; 2-3 days	75-95	75-90	0-5	
	PHA; 2-3 days	-	-	-	0
	Nothing; 3 days	<5	<5	<5	
	Antigens (PCN*(1), PPD*(1)); 2-3 days	5-35	5-35	5-35	
II.	Congenital agammaglobulinemia with PHA (8 patients); 3 days	<1	<1	<1	
	Mothers of sex linked agammaglobulinemia with PHA (5); 3 days	50-65	50-65	50-65	
III.	Dysgammaglobulinemia with normal or elevated γG and γM and absent γA with PHA (2 patients); 3 days	85-95	<1	85-95	
IV.	Atypical agammaglobulinemia with PHA; 3 days	31	<1	40	
	(% of normal level in serum	γG: 20-30	γA: <3	γM: 40-50)	

*(1) PHA = phytohemagglutinin - M; 0.1 ml per 4 ml culture.
      PCN = penicillin; 100 units per 4 ml culture.
      PPD = purified protein derivative of tuberculin 2.5 x 10^{-3} mg per 4 ml culture.

*(2) Added at the end of culture period for blocking.

cells contain material binding these various anti-immunoglobulins after stimulation with PHA. Stimulation with antigens to which the donor was sensitized produced positive results in a proportion of cells similar to that which enlarged under these stimuli, generally in the range of approximately 15%. A number of different controls were used to demonstrate the specificity of fluorescence, as well as the lack of non-specific adherence of the fluorescein-conjugated materials to the cells. Blocking experiments showed that each conjugated antibody could be specifically blocked by the unconjugated material of the same type, but not by unconjugated material of different specificity. The use of fluorescein-conjugated anti-rabbit γ-globulin did not produce fluorescence of any of these cells. The cells of agammaglobulinemic individuals, although enlarging in culture with PHA to cells morphologically identical with those of normals, did not demonstrate fluorescence under these conditions.

Cells from mothers of boys with sex-linked congenital agammaglobulinemia showed fluorescence in only 50 to 65% of the cells, demonstrating the Lyon effect (27) of inactivation of one x-chromosome in female cells, and again indicating the lack of non-specific adherence of the fluorescent material. This group also eliminates the possibility of fluorescence caused by non-specific absorption of circulating γ-globulin. Also, no fluorescence is demonstrated in the earlier phases of the culture despite the cellular enlargement, and these cells are thoroughly washed and cultured with "agammaglobulinemic" serum. Cells from patients with specific agammaglobulinemias, obtained from Dr. Hugh Fudenberg, further confirmed the lack of non-specific absorption of the fluorescence material. This also confirmed the specificity of immunofluorescence in these experiments. For example, patients with normal or elevated γG and γM and absent γA demonstrated immunofluorescence with anti-γG and anti-γM, but not with anti-γA.

In a study of 20 patients with a history of penicillin allergy demonstrating a positive immediate reaction to a skin test with penicillin or benzyl-penicilloyl-polylysine (BPO), the lymphocytes of each of these patients showed stimulation when cultured in the presence of penicillin (35). The cells of several of these patients were studied for the production of specific anti-penicillin antibodies. The results are summarized in Table 2. The presence of penicillin-binding material in the cultured cells was determined through the use of fluorescein-conjugated anti-BPO obtained through the courtesy of Drs. Bernard Levine and Michael Fellner. In those experiments in which the cells were cultured in the presence of penicillin, only the conjugated anti-BPO was used at the end of the culture period, since penicillin could be presumed to be already attached to the pertinent cells.

In those experiments in which the cells were stimulated with PHA, the cells were incubated with penicillin at the end of the culture period, washed, and then exposed to the anti-BPO. Blocking experiments with non-conjugated anti-BPO demonstrated the specificity of this fluorescence, while the lack of fluorescence in non-allergic patients, as well as in PHA-stimulated cells from allergic patients without exposure of the cells to penicillin at the end of culture, demonstrated the lack of non-specific adherence of this material. In cells from two patients who had had their penicillin reactions one and seven years prior to the experiment, the proportion of cells binding penicillin after stimulation with penicillin was 3 to 7%, and after stimulation with PHA was 11 to 20%. Cells obtained from two patients toward the end of their serum sickness reaction to penicillin showed binding of penicillin in 18 to 20% of the cells stimulated with penicillin and in 54 to 70% of those stimulated by PHA. This unexpectedly large proportion of fluorescence-positive cells could be the result of their recent extrusion into the circulation from the central lymphatic tissues during the severe immunological reaction.

The fact that PHA-stimulated cells demonstrate visible fluorescence in a greater number of cells than does the specific antigen is compatible with the results of Forbes (15), who showed that PHA caused the production of three times as much material capable of binding thyroglobulin than did thyroglobulin itself, when used as a stimulant of cells from a patient with Hashimoto's disease.

This first group of studies has demonstrated that after culture and stimulation cells contain immunoglobulins and that some of this immunoglobin is in the form of specific antibody. These experiments suggest, but do not prove, that this material is newly synthesized. In order to prove new synthesis of γG, the cells were cultured in the presence of C-14 labelled l-leucine (final radioactivity: 1μC/ml). Replicate cultures were harvested at various time intervals. Cell extracts were prepared by freezing and thawing. To these extracts, human γG was added as a carrier and sufficient absorbed anti-human γG to result in slight antibody excess. The precipitates were washed, dissolved, and their radioactivity determined in a scintillation counter. In order to check for non-specific precipitation of radioactive material, the same experiments were performed at the same time intervals on replicate cultures, utilizing ovalbumin and anti-ovalbumin. These experiments were performed in the presence and absence of PHA in the cultures. The results, shown in Figure 1, are expressed as counts per minute after precipitating with anti-γG minus the counts per minute precipitated with ovalbumin—anti-ovalbumin and minus the background counts. In the presence of PHA, incorporation of a

TABLE 2.—PENICILLIN EXPERIMENTS

I. Penicillin allergic patients' lymphocytes (2 patients 1 and 7 years after serum sickness)

Treated with:	fl-anti-γG	fl-anti-γA	fl-anti-γM	fl-aBPO*[3]	PCN+ fl-aBPO
Nothing; 0 days	0.3	0.1	0.2	0	0
PHA*[1]; 3 days	88	86	82	0	11-20
PHA + PCN* [2] +aBPO*[4]; 3 days	-	-	-	0	-
PCN; 3 days	15-20	15-20	15-20	3-7	-
PCN+aBPO; 3 days	-	-	-	0	-
Nothing; 3 days	<5	<5	<5	-	-

II. Penicillin allergic patients' lymphocytes (2 patients 7 and 10 days after onset of serum sickness)

	fl-anti-γG	fl-anti-γA	fl-anti-γM	fl-aBPO	PCN+ fl-aBPO
Nothing; 0 days	0.3	3.9	5.0	0	0
PHA; 3 days	90	85	90	0	54-70
PHA + PCN + aBPO; 3 days	-	-	-	0	-
PCN; 3 days	25	35	55	18-20	-
PCN + aBPO; 3 days	-	-	-	0	-
Nothing; 3 days	<5	<5	<5	0	<5-10

III. Normal lymphocytes (non-allergic controls) (4 individuals)

	fl-anti-γG	fl-anti-γA	fl-anti-γM	fl-aBPO	PCN+ fl-aBPO
Nothing; 0 days	0.1-0.3	0.1	0.1-0.3	0	0
PHA; 3 days	90	80	85	0	0
PCN; 3 days	0	0	0	0	-

*(1) PHA = phytohemagglutinin - M; 0.1 ml per 4 ml culture.
   PCN = penicillin; 100 units per 4 ml culture.

*(2) Incubation with penicillin at the end of culture period.

*(3) fl-aBPO = fluorescein-conjugated anti-benzyl-penicilloyl-BAA.

*(4) Anti-benzyl-penicilloyl-BAA added at end of culture period directly or after incubation with penicillin.

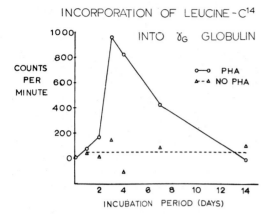

FIG. 1. Counts per minute of material from extracts of cells cultured with and without PHA, after precipitation with anti-human γG and after subtraction of counts per minute precipitated with ovalbumin—anti-ovalbumin and of background counts. C-14 l-leucine added to 1 μC per ml.

high number of counts into the material specifically precipitated by anti-human γG was found. This new material, presumably γG, shows a significant rise by the third day. This correlates with the time of maximum fluorescence with conjugated anti-γG described above. High quantities of this newly synthesized material are still found on the fourth day and then the counts diminish until there is no more new material by 14 days of culture, at which time the majority of cells are dead. In the absence of PHA, no significant amounts of such material could be found. Immunoelectrophoresis of the cell extract of 4 days of culture in the presence of C^{14}-l-leucine demonstrated a single precipitation line against rabbit anti-human γG. Autoradiography of the slide showed radioactivity over this line.

This experiment lends strong support to the evidence obtained from the fluorescence studies that the immunoglobulin found in these cells by the third day is newly synthesized under the influence of PHA. The small human peripheral blood lymphocyte, therefore, is apparently capable of being derepressed, not only to make structural proteins necessary for enlargement of the cell, but also to form immunoglobulin and specific antibodies.

The mechanisms active in the derepression of these cells and in their differentiation to dividing cells may represent a general biologic mechanism. The materials capable of non-specific stimulation of lymphocytes include streptolysin S (20) and staphylococcal exotoxins (26), agents which are capable of causing leakage of enzymes from lysosomes (5). It has been shown that chloroquine (23) and prednisolone (12), compounds which protect lysosomes from disruptive agents such as streptolysin S (41), inhibit stimulation of cultured lymphocytes by either non-specific or specific stimulants. Cooper and Rubin (8) have shown that within the first 30 minutes of exposure of lymphocytes to PHA there is not only rapid incorporation of uridine into new RNA but also rapid destruction of existing RNA. It appears that one of the events mediating derepression of a resting cell to one which produces new proteins rapidly may be the disruption of lysosomes and the release of their enzymes, such as RNAase. The purpose of this could be to provide the cell with the required large pool of precursors for new RNA and new protein production. The protein precursors would be produced by the action of lysosomal cathepsins. This mechanism could be brought about by direct action of agents such as streptolysin S or as a response to pinocytosis of antigen-antibody complexes or of PHA, with or without its binding site. Becker and Lane (3) have postulated a similar mechanism for the early events associated with the regeneration of rat liver.

It has been shown histochemically (1, 21) and verified electron microscopically (10, 34) that, beginning at about 12 hours after the exposure to PHA, new acid phosphatase-positive lysosome-like structures appear in the lymphocytes. These become very abundant at the time of mitosis and seem to collect near the nuclear membrane and the spindle fibers. Similar findings have been published for regenerating rat liver (4, 24). R. Hirschhorn and Weissmann (22) have extended these observations and have demonstrated net synthesis of two lysosomal enzymes, acid phosphatase and aryl sulfatase, in these cells. They have also shown that these enzymes are in structures which fit the biochemical definition of lysosomes. After obtaining a granular fraction by differential centrifugation of PHA-stimulated lymphocyte homogenates in a sucrose gradient, they showed that this granular fraction had the highest acid phosphatase content. The enzyme could be released from this fraction into the supernate upon exposure to lysolecithin, thus demonstrating latency, one of the properties of lysosomal enzymes. The appearance of new acid phosphatase demonstrating latency has also been demonstrated *in vivo* (9) in the cells of regional lymph nodes draining the site of an antigenic stimulus. Since a cell cannot properly divide without destruction of the nuclear membrane and the spindle fibers, it appears likely that cell division is aided by release of the appropriate destructive enzymes from the newly formed lysosomes.

The human peripheral blood lymphocytes thus may offer a model system for the study of derepression and differentiation. The nature of the antibody-like material representing immunological memory and capable of attaching the antigenic stimulus to the cell is, however, unknown. The mechanism of derepression of the part of the genome responsible for the production of new antibodies is not understood. The factors deciding which cells will divide during their process of differentiation are a mystery. This technically simple method of lymphocyte culture may aid in elucidating some of these problems.

Conclusion

Human peripheral blood lymphocytes are capable of synthesizing new immunoglobulin, some of which behaves as specific antibody after both specific and non-specific stimulation. Lysosomal enzymes may play a role in mediating derepression and differentiation of these cells. It is proposed that the small human peripheral blood lymphocyte represents a model system for the study of derepression, differentiation, and mitosis, with general biologic application, and for the specific study of cellular events occurring during the immune response.

Acknowledgments: The work described in this paper was done in collaboration with Dr. Carolyn S. Ripps and Dr. Rochelle Hirschhorn. It was supported by grants from U.S. Public Health Service (HD-00542); New York City Health Research Council (U-1030); American Heart Association; Career Scientist of the New York City Health Research Council (I-416).

REFERENCES

1. Allison, A. C., and Mallucci, L. (1964): Lysosomes in dividing cells, with special reference to lymphocytes. Lancet *ii,* 1371.
2. Bach, F., and Hirschhorn, K. (1963): Gamma globulin production by human lymphocytes. Exp. Cell Res. *32,* 592.
3. Becker, F. F., and Lane, B. P. (1965): Regeneration of the mammalian liver. I. Auto-phagocytosis during dedifferentiation of the liver cell in preparation for cell division. Amer. J. Path. *47,* 783.
4. Becker, F. F., and Lane, B. P. (1966): Regeneration of the mammalian liver. IV. Further evidence of the role of cell injury. Amer. J. Path. [In press]
5. Bernheimer, A. W., and Schwartz, L. L. (1964): Lysosomal disruption by bacterial toxins. J. Bact. *87,* 1100.
6. Buckton, K. E., Jacobs, P. A., Court Brown, W. M., and Doll, R. (1962): A study of the chromosome damage persisting after x-ray therapy for ankylosing spondylitis. Lancet *ii,* 676.
7. Ceppellini, R. (1965): Discussion. Histocompatibility Testing; Pub. 1229, National Academy of Science, Washington, D.C., p. 138.
8. Cooper, H. L., and Rubin, A. D. (1965): RNA metabolism in lymphocytes stimulated by phytohemagglutinin: initial responses to phytohemagglutinin. Blood *25,* 1014.
9. Diengdoh, J. V., and Turk, J. L. (1965): Immunological significance of lysosomes within lymphocytes *in vivo.* Nature *207,* 1405.
10. Douglas, S. D., Hoffman, P. F., Borjeson, J., and Chessin, L. N. (1966): Histochemical and fine structural studies of lymphocyte transformation with phytohemagglutinin and pokeweed mitogen. Anat. Rec. *154,* 340.
11. Eljsvoogel, V. P., and The, H.: Personal communications.
12. Elves, M. W., Gough, J., and Israels, M. C. C. (1964): The place of the lymphocyte in the reticulo-endothelial system: A study of the *in vitro* effect of prednisolone on lymphocytes. Acta Haemat. *32,* 100.
13. Elves, M. W., Roath, S., Taylor, G., and Israels, M. E. G. (1963): The *in vitro* production of antibody lymphocytes. Lancet *i,* 1292.
14. Farnes, P., Barker, B. E., Brownhill, L. E., and Fanger, H. (1964): Mitogenic activity in *Phytolacca americana* (pokeweed). Lancet *ii,* 1100.
15. Forbes, I. J. (1965): Specific and non-specific stimulation of antibody synthesis by human leucocytes *in vitro.* Lancet, *i,* 198.
16. Gowans, J. L., and McGregor, D. D. (1965): The immunological activities of lymphocytes. Progress in Allergy (Karger, Basel/N.Y.), *9,* 1.
17. Hastings, J., Freedman, S., Rendon, O.,

Cooper, H. L., and Hirschhorn, K. (1961): Culture of human white cells using differential leukocyte separation. Nature *192*, 1214.

18. Hirschhorn, K. (1965): Method for studying lymphocyte interaction and other immunologic and cytogenetic studies of human lymphocytes. Histocompatibility Testing, Pub. 1229, National Academy of Sciences, National Research Council, Washington, D.C., p. 177.

19. Hirschhorn, K., Bach, F., Kolodny, R. L., Firschein, I.L., and Hashem, N. (1963): Immune response and mitosis of human peripheral blood lymphocytes *in vitro*. Science *143*, 1185.

20. Hirschhorn, K., Schreibman, R. R., Verbo, S., and Gruskin, R. (1964): The action of streptolysin S on peripheral lymphocytes of normal subjects and patients with acute rheumatic fever. Proc. Nat. Acad. Sci. *52*, 1151.

21. Hirschhorn, R., Kaplan, J. M., Goldberg, A. F., Hirschhorn, K., and Weissmann, G. (1965): Acid phosphatase-rich granules in human lymphocytes induced by phytohemagglutinin. Science, *147*, 55.

22. Hirschhorn, R., and Weissmann, G.: The development of new lysosomes and lysosomal enzymes in cultured human peripheral blood lymphocytes. [In preparation]

23. Hurvitz, D., and Hirschhorn, K. (1965): Suppression of *in vitro* lymphocyte responses by chloroquine. New Eng. J. Med. *273*, 23.

24. Kent, G., Minick, O. T., Orfei. E., Volini, F. I., and Malera-Orsini, F. (1965): The movement of iron-laden lysosomes in rat liver during mitosis. Amer. J. Path. *47*, 783.

25. Landy, M., Sanderson, R. P., Bernstein, M. T., and Jackson, A. L. (1964): Antibody production by leucocytes in peripheral blood. Nature *204*, 1320.

26. Ling, N. R., and Husband, E. M. (1964): Specific and non-specific stimulation of peripheral lymphocytes. Lancet *i*, 363.

27. Lyon, M. F. (1962): Sex chromatin and gene action in the mammalian x-chromosome. Amer. J. Hum. Genet. *14*, 135.

28. Marshall, W. H., and Roberts, K. B. (1963): The growth and mitosis of human small lymphocytes after incubation with phytohemagglutinin. Quart. J. Exp. Physiol. *48*, 146.

29. McIntyre, O. R., and Ebaugh, F. G. J. (1962): The effect of phytohemagglutinin on leukocyte cultures as measured by P³² incorporation into the DNA, RNA and acid soluble fractions. Blood *19*, 443.

30. Möller, G. (1965): 19S antibody production against soluble lipopolysaccharide by individual lymphoid cells *in vitro*. Nature *207*, 1166.

31. Norman, A., Sasaki, M. S., Ottoman, R. E., and Fingerhut, A. G. (1965): Lymphocyte lifetime in women. Science *147*, 745.

32. Nowell, P. C. (1960): Phytohemagglutinin: an initiator of mitosis in cultures of normal human leukocytes. Cancer Res. *20*, 462.

33. Nowell, P. C. (1965): Unstable chromosome in tuberculin-stimulated leukocyte cultures from irradiated patients. Evidence for immunologically committed, long-lived lymphocytes in human blood. Blood *26*, 798.

34. Parker, J. W., Wakasa, H., and Lukes, R. J. (1965): The morphologic and cytochemical demonstration of lysosomes in lymphocytes incubated with phytohemagglutinin by electron microscopy. Lab. Invest. *14*, 1736.

35. Ripps, C., and Fellner, M.: The correlation of the *in vitro* lymphocyte response to penicillin and penicillin allergy. [In preparation]

36. Ripps, C., and Hirschhorn, K.: The production of immunoglobulins by cultured human peripheral blood lymphocytes. [In preparation]

37. Sell, S., Rowe, D. S., and Gell, P. G. H. (1965): Studies on rabbit lymphocytes *in vitro*. III. Protein, RNA, and DNA synthesis by lymphocyte cultures after stimulation with phytohemagglutinin, with staphylococcal filtrate, with antiallotype serum, and with heterologous antiserum to rabbit whole serum. J. Exp. Med. *122*, 823.

38. Thorbecke, G. J. (1964): Development of immune globulin formation in fetal, newborn and immature guinea pigs. Fed. Proc. *23*, 346.

39. Torelli, U., Grossi, G., Artusi, T., and Emilia, G. (1963): RNA and protein synthesis in normal peripheral mononuclear leukocytes. A radioautographic study. Acta Haemat. *30*, 129.

40. Van Furth, R. (1964): The formation of immunoglobulins by human tissues *in vitro*. Thesis, University of Leiden, p. 62.

41. Weissmann, G. (1964): Labilization and stabilization of lysosomes. Fed. Proc. *23*, 1038.

42. Yoffey, J. M. (1958): Cellular equilibria in blood and blood-forming tissues. Brookhaven Sympos. Biol. No. 10, 1.

43. Young, R., and Ruddle, F. H. (1965): Inactivation of T-2 bacteriophage by sensitized leucocytes *in vitro*. Nature *208*, 1105.

DISCUSSION

VAN FURTH: Do you have any explanation for the different results obtained with the immunofluorescence method when applied to either fixed or unfixed cells? Using unfixed cells we were almost unable to demonstrate immunoglobulin containing cells in peripheral blood, thoracic duct samples, and bone marrow cell suspensions which were not cultured. Considerable numbers of positive cells were observed in the *fixed* slides. (See Table.)

COMPARISON OF IMMUNOFLUORESCENCE ON FIXED AND UNFIXED CELLS

Source of cells	State of cells	Number of positive cells stained with		
		γG	γA	γM
Peripheral blood	fixed	3	25	3
	unfixed	0	0	1?
Bone marrow	fixed	79	78	13
	unfixed	0	0	0
Thoracic duct lymph	fixed	29	49	50
	unfixed	0	2	0

Does phytohemagglutinin alter the membrane of the lymphocyte in such a way that the conjugates or immunoglobulins present in the culture fluid penetrate the transformed cells? Even in the cultures restored without serum, small amounts of immunoglobulin will be produced. This protein might penetrate the cells and be detected by immunofluorescent staining.

HIRSCHHORN: We, as well as Drs. Chessin and Borjeson in Dr. Landy's laboratory, have obtained similar results with unfixed cells and those fixed by short exposure to cold methanol. Actually, we found quite the opposite of the effect which you described; namely, that we could not demonstrate fluorescence after culture of cells if they were prepared for staining by methods other than those employing methanol.

Regarding the question of altering the cell membranes and allowing penetration of fluorescent material, our controls eliminate this possibility. Firstly, the membranes of cells from agammaglobulinemics should become just as "leaky" as those derived from normals and yet the former, although they respond morphologically like normal cells, do not stain. Secondly, half the cells from putative heterozygotes of agammaglobulinemic families do not become fluorescent; yet they should become as "leaky" as the half that do stain. Also, cells from individuals who do not make γA-globulin fluoresce with all the immunoglobulin reagents except anti-γA-globulin. Finally, the fact that the anti-BPO does not adhere to any cells except those from penicillin-sensitive individuals in the presence of penicillin seems to eliminate non-specific

ingestion or adsorption of the fluorescein-conjugated material.

Concerning the possibility that human immunoglobulins released into the culture medium may get into most of the lymphocytes present, we have difficulty trying to demonstrate the presence of such globulin in the supernate since it is present in such small amounts. Also the experiments have been controlled by mixing normal cells with those from agammaglobulinemics and the latter still did not stain with the fluorescent antibody.

CEBRA: Since very large percentages of your PHA-stimulated cells stained positively for each of three classes of immunoglobulins, it would seem that the majority of the stimulated cells contained all classes of globulins. Using double fluorescent staining we have found a remarkable degree of differentiation of cells in spleen and lymph nodes in that almost all positive cells contain only one class of heavy chain and one type of light chain of the immunoglobulin molecule. Would you comment on the apparent polydispersity of the globulin contained in your PHA-stimulated cells?

HIRSCHHORN: Firstly, the time at which the different immunoglobulins are detectable in our cultured cells does appear to be somewhat different. Further, if PHA mediates nonspecific derepression of the cells, then they might synthesize all the globulins that they are capable of making. In your studies you are dealing with spleen cells from animals stimulated with specific antigens and thus you are selecting against total derepression of the cells. The peripheral lymphocytes which we are stimulating non-specifically with PHA presumably are expressing the whole range of their synthetic potential.

We do observe, however, using fluorescent anti-κ chain, that only about 30 to 40 per cent of the stimulated cells stain. This would indicate prior commitment for specific light chain synthesis but not for specific heavy chain production.

KIMMEL: I presume you meant that two different kinds of events, with respect to the lysosomes, occur in the cells after stimulation with PHA: (a) activation of lysosomes—and this would have to occur early—and (b) stimulation of the production of lysosomes.

What is the evidence that (a) actually happens? Has the direct experiment been done, i.e., the measurable increase in free activity of the enzymes in these cells, and (b) the demonstration of PHA release of enzymes from the particles isolated *in vitro?*

HIRSCHHORN: The data for the "activation" of lysosomes are inferential. Firstly, substances which can break lysosomes, such as streptolysin S, produce immediate stimulation similar to that induced by PHA. Secondly, substances which are known to protect lysosome membranes from these agents, such as prednisolone and chloroquin, inhibit their effects. But if the prednisolone or chloroquin is added only 10 to 30 minutes after the PHA it no longer has an inhibitory effect.

Apparently PHA does not affect *isolated* lysosomes. Thus, I would suggest that the mechanism for PHA action may resemble antigen-antibody stimulation. Thus, it would cause a response of lysosomal membrane and a release of hydrolytic enzymes in the cell which is akin to that observed during pinocytosis.

KIMMEL: Would such an "activation" of lysosomes not be deleterious to the cell? Presumably these pinocytotic vesicles are isolated from the nucleic acid of the cell.

HIRSCHHORN: The release of lysosomal enzymes does not necessarily kill a cell. I think these have many normal functions and one of these is to play a role in mitosis.

EBERT: You have limited your discussion to a few lysosomal enzymes, focusing attention on these which might break down the nuclear membrane and RNA. Yet you have made no mention of other enzymes, especially DNAase. Thus, you have implied a selective release of some lysosomal enzymes. Please comment on differential activity or localization of lysosomal enzymes in small lymphocytes.

HIRSCHHORN: There appear to be lysosomes with different contents of enzymes. For example, Dr. R. Hirschhorn found a marked increase in acid phosphatase and aryl sulfatase, but no increase in β-glucuronidase in cultured lymphocytes. As for release of DNAase, since the small lymphocyte has relatively

few lysosomes it may be that there is insufficient enzyme released to cross the nuclear membrane and do damage.

CEBRA: I am concerned about the "perfection" of the immunoglobulins synthesized by the PHA-stimulated lymphocytes. The mechanism for assembly of a complete molecule may be relatively simple and depend on initial non-covalent association of polypeptide chains if a cell only makes one type of light chain and one class of heavy chain. However, if cells are making at least three classes of heavy chains and possibly different light chains the problems of correct assembly would increase and "imperfect" molecules, which might be hybrids of several different chains, might be formed. Have you investigated this possibility, perhaps by carrying out some of your coprecipitation experiments sequentially, first with anti-γG-globulin and then with anti-γM-globulin and then vice versa? If hybrid molecules were formed, they might be precipitated by either specific antiserum.

HIRSCHHORN: We have not done sequential coprecipitations using antisera specific for the various classes of globulins. However, we are quite convinced that the radio-label we are coprecipitating is at least in human γG-globulin.

AUERBACH: Can you comment on why one might expect more than 50% positive cells in mothers of sex-linked agammaglobulinemics?

HIRSCHHORN: Perhaps this may partly be explained by selection *in vivo.* Those cells that can be stimulated by antigens may selectively replicate at a more rapid rate.

BLOCK: You have described a wide variety of antibodies developing in small lymphocytes cultured in phytohemagglutinin. Did any of these small lymphocytes develop into plasma cells?

HIRSCHHORN: If one looks at many PHA-stimulated cells with the electron microscope one can find a very few cells that have much organized endoplasmic reticulum. And if one looks at the general morphology perhaps 5% of the cells may look like "plasma cells."

R. VAN FURTH, H. R. E. SCHUIT, and W. HIJMANS

Differentiation of immunoglobulin-containing cells in human peripheral blood

IN A previous publication the formation of immunoglobulins by lymphoid cells from human peripheral blood has been reported (12, 15). In these studies lymphoid cells were incubated in a medium which contained ^{14}C amino acids. The synthesized immunoglobulins in the culture fluid were indicated by autoradiography of the immunoelectrophoretic pattern. The results of these studies revealed that lymphoid cells of normal peripheral blood synthesize a distinct amount of γG and smaller amounts of γA and γM (Table 1). Lymphocyte cultures from patients with infectious mononucleosis and also from patients with rubella (Fig. 1) show a greater synthesis during the first ten days of illness. Thereafter the synthesis of γM decreased significantly. In chronic lymphatic leukemia a characteristic pattern was found: labelling of γG, mainly restricted to the medium- and high-speed part of the line, labelling of the γM line and the consistent absence of the γA line (Table 1).

The antibody activity of the immunoglobulins synthesized *in vitro* was not determined in these studies. However, from other recent studies it is known that lymphoid cells of the peripheral blood can synthesize antibodies (9, 18, 19, 20, 21).

The cells which may be engaged in immunoglobulin synthesis have been studied by the immunofluorescent technique. In that study samples of normal peripheral blood and samples from patients with different diseases, as mentioned above, have been investigated, prior to incubation. The results have shown that a proportion of the medium-sized and

TABLE 1.—IMMUNOGLOBULIN FORMATION BY LYMPHOID CELLS OF HUMAN PERIPHERAL BLOOD

	Autoradiography*		
	γG	γA	γM
Normal peripheral blood	+	+	(+)
Infectious mononucleosis			
4th-10th day	++	+	++
11th-14th day	+	—	—
> 14th day	+	+	(+)
Chronic lymphatic leukemia	+	—	+

*The intensity of the autoradiographic image is graded from — = negative; (+) = just visible; + = clearly visible; to ++++ = very dark.

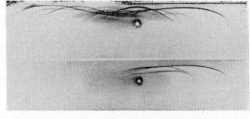

FIG. 1. Culture of lymphoid cells from patient with rubella. *Above*: Immunoelectrophoretic pattern of carrier serum and culture fluid developed with horse anti-human serum; *below*: Autoradiograph with intense labelling of γG, γA, and γM lines.

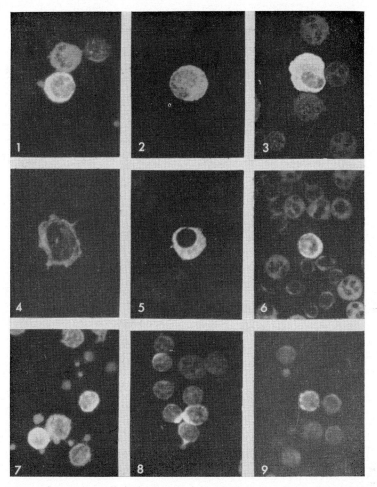

FIG. 2. Immunofluorescent cells in human peripheral blood. *Normal peripheral blood*: 1. γG positive medium-sized lymphocyte. 2. γM positive large lymphocyte. 3. γG positive plasma cell. *Rubella*: 4. γM positive atypical lymphoid cell. 5. γM positive plasma cell. *Chronic lymphatic leukemia*: 6. γG positive medium-sized cell. *γM positive small lymphocytes*: 7. Normal peripheral blood. 8. Infectious mononucleosis. 9. Fetal blood.

large lymphocytes and occasionally a plasma cell is positive for γG, γA, or γM, whereas small lymphocytes were only found positive for γM (12, 15) (Fig. 2).

To obtain more information about the number of positive cells, obtained from different conditions, a more quantitative approach of the immunofluorescent staining was attempted. Some preliminary results will be presented here.

MATERIALS AND METHODS

Blood samples were taken from healthy donors, from patients with infectious mono-nucleosis, and from patients with a definite rheumatoid arthritis.

A detailed description of the preparation of the blood samples for immunofluorescent staining, the preparation of the conjugates, and the staining procedure have been published previously (14). Fig. 3 shows an outline of the technique.

The sedimentation apparatus (Fig. 4) provides a very suitable method to prepare slides with well-exposed cells. A drop of the cell suspension is put into the hole of the plastic block. When a pressure of about 3 kg is applied, the fluid diffuses into the filter paper,

Blood collected in 5% EDTA solution

↓

Centrifugation 3 min, 175 g at 4° (twice)

↓

Combined supernatants centrifuged 10 min, 175 g at 4°

↓

Sediment suspended in 30 ml 5% bovine albumin + 1% EDTA in buffered saline

↓

Centrifugation 10 min, 175 g at 4°

↓

Sediment resuspended in 0.5 ml bovine albumin solution

↓

Slides prepared in sedimentation apparatus

↓

Fixation with 5% acetic acid in 96% ethanol, 15 min at —20°

↓

Slides washed in buffered saline for 60 min at 4°

Fig. 3. Preparation of peripheral blood lymphocytes for immunofluorescence.

leaving the cells spread on the microscopic slide.

For morphological examination slides, made with the sedimentation apparatus, were stained with Giemsa stain. The lymphocytic

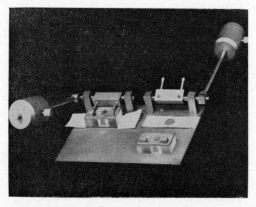

Fig. 4. Sedimentation apparatus.

cells were classified (25) into small lymphocytes (diameter < 7 μ), medium-sized lymphocytes (diameter 8-9 μ), and large lymphocytes (diameter > 10 μ).

The globulin fractions of the antisera, at a protein content of at least 20 mg/ml, were conjugated either with an equal volume of a solution of fluorescein-isothiocyanate (FITC), or tetramethyl-rhodamine-isothiocyanate (TRITC, Baltimore Biological Laboratories) in 2% $NaHCO_3$ at pH 9.0, and adsorbed with calf-liver powder. The protein concentration of the different conjugates, in the dilution as used in the staining procedure, and the optical density ratio (4) are given in Table 2; the protein concentration of the globulin fraction is estimated by the biuret method.

TABLE 2.—CHARACTERISTICS OF CONJUGATED ANTISERA IN THE DILUTION USED FOR STAINING

Conjugate	Protein concentration mg/ml	Optical Density ratio	
		280/495 mμ	280/550 mμ
FITC anti-γG	3.3	2.30	
FITC anti-γA	3.9	4.45	
FITC anti-γM	2.0	2.25	
FITC anti-κ	3.9	3.00	
TRITC anti-λ	4.4		1.75

To obtain a better contrast and to facilitate the counting, the FITC labeled conjugates were mixed with a TRITC labelled bovine albumin solution. The ratio of κ and λ positive cells was estimated with a mixture of the FITC labelled anti-κ conjugate and the TRITC labelled anti-λ conjugate. All mixtures were centrifuged for 30 minutes at 3,000 rpm immediately before use. The fixed slides (Fig. 3) were stained for 30 minutes at room temperature, washed again, and mounted in buffered glycerol.

RESULTS

The differentiation of the lymphoid cells in peripheral blood samples is given in Table 3. The percentage distribution of the total number of fluorescent cells, positive for γG, γA, and γM, are shown in Table 4. There was no significant difference in the percentage distri-

TABLE 3.—PERCENTAGE DISTRIBUTION OF LYMPHOID CELLS IN PERIPHERAL BLOOD*

	Number of individuals	Lymphocytes			Plasma cells
		small	medium	large	
Normal	13	13.2	78.6	7.5	0.7
Infectious mononucleosis†	7	8.8	84.7	5.9	0.6
Rheumatoid arthritis	9	14	71.5	13.5	1

*From Giemsa-stained preparations.
†Duration of disease 2 weeks or more.

TABLE 4.—PERCENTAGE DISTRIBUTION OF TOTAL NUMBER OF FLUORESCENT CELLS IN PERIPHERAL BLOOD

Origin	Number of individuals	Lymphocytes		Plasma cells
		medium	large	
Normal	13	76.1	15.7	8.2
Infectious mononucleosis*	7	81.4	7.6	11.0
Rheumatoid arthritis	9	81.2	8.9	9.9

The small lymphocytes are not incorporated in these tables because they were only positive for γM.
*Duration of disease 2 weeks or more.

TABLE 5.—PERCENTAGE DISTRIBUTION γ, α, μ, κ, AND λ POLYPEPTIDE CHAINS IN LYMPHOID CELLS OF PERIPHERAL BLOOD

	Number of individuals	Chains			Ratio κ/λ	Ratio H/L
		γ	α	μ		
Normal	13	36.1	35.8	28.1	2.9:1	1.1:1
Infectious mononucleosis*	7	8.0	42.2	49.8	2.6:1	2.7:1
Rheumatoid arthritis	9	33.9	46.4	19.7	8.1:1	4.9:1

*Duration of disease 2 weeks or more.

the κ/λ ratio and the H/L ratio. The latter ratio is also increased in infectious mononucleosis.

DISCUSSION

Previous studies have shown that peripheral blood samples which contain 0.5×10^8 lymphoid cells synthesize in vitro γG, γA, and γM (12, 15). The main amount of immunoglobulins is synthesized during the first 6-12 hours of incubation (13). It is therefore justified to assume that cells which synthesize immunoglobulins in vitro do not transform into another morphological type during this period of incubation. The immunofluorescent staining performed on samples prior to incubation may thus indicate the cells which synthesize immunoglobulins in vitro.

The results of the quantitative immunofluorescent studies have clearly shown that mainly the medium-sized lymphocytes are immunoglobulin-containing cells. These cells conceivably provide a major contribution of immunoglobulin synthesis in vitro by normal peripheral blood samples. The contribution of the plasma cells in normal peripheral blood may be of minor importance.

These conclusions are based on the following calculations, using the data of Tables 3 and 4. A sample of 0.5×10^8 lymphoid cells contains about 40×10^6 medium-sized lymphocytes, 4×10^6 large lymphocytes, and 0.4×10^6 plasma cells. The number of immunoglobulin-containing cells in these sample amounts were 30×10^6 medium-sized lymphocytes, 0.6×10^6 large lymphocytes, and 3×10^4 plasma cells. If 5×10^8 lymphoid cells weigh 1 g wet weight (25), the immunoglobulin-containing medium-sized cells weigh

bution of total number of fluorescent cells in peripheral blood of the three groups of individuals. In all three the major contribution was formed by the medium-sized lymphocytes regardless of whether the cells were investigated for the presence of H or L chains. The percentage of plasma cells in peripheral blood varies between 0 and 3 of the total of mononuclear cells. The activity of this type of cell is evident from the figures presented in Table 4, where it can be seen that the plasma cells constitute about 10% of the total number of fluorescent cells. The distribution of the different polypeptide H chains (γ, α, μ) and the ratio of κ/λ chains in the lymphoid cells are given in Table 5. The ratio of H/L chains was calculated from the total number of cells positive for γ, α, and μ chain and the number of cells, which were positive with the anti-L chain conjugates. The results show that in infectious mononucleosis the percentage of γM-containing cells is increased and the percentage of γG-containing cells is about one-fourth of that found in normal samples. In rheumatoid arthritis there is a marked increase in

60 mg, but the positive plasma cells only 0.06 mg. This amount corresponds with the experience that about 50-100 mg lymphoid tissues is optimal for the detection of immunoglobulin synthesis *in vitro* (12, 17).

The frequency distribution of the different H chains in normal peripheral blood samples corresponds roughly with the results found in human spleen and lymph nodes (2, 3). These authors already discussed that the distribution of the heavy chains among the positive cells does not correlate with the ratio of the different immunoglobulins in the serum (7). In infectious mononucleosis, an acute disease probably of viral origin, there is a preponderance of γM-containing cells. These samples contain a large number of lymphoid cells which are the result of active proliferation in the lymphoid organs (16, 22). It may be possible that these cells are antigen-stimulated and mainly synthesize γM as expression of primary response. A combined autoradiographic and immunofluorescent study may elucidate this question.

The ratio of κ/λ chains of about 3:1 in lymphoid cells of normal peripheral blood and infectious mononucleosis samples corresponds well with the ratio of these molecules in the serum (6, 8, 23). In rheumatoid arthritis a κ/λ ratio of 8.1:1 was found. Although it is reported that the rheumatoid factor consists of mainly type κ molecules (10, 11), this cannot explain the present findings, because the rheumatoid factor is only a minor constituent of the immunoglobulins in the serum. It is likely that in rheumatoid arthritis more immunoglobulins of type κ are synthesized. This may be the result of a reactive process or the expression of a genetic factor. Immunofluorescent studies of bone marrow samples and quantitative determinations of serum immunoglobulins from patients with rheumatoid arthritis are in progress to determine if also here the preponderance of type κ molecules can be established.

In normal peripheral blood the ratio H/L chains is 1.1:1. A ratio of 1 is expected if both chains are synchronously synthesized in the lymphoid cells. From the data of Fahey and McKelvey (7), the H/L ratio of serum immunoglobulins in normal individuals can be calculated to be 1.1 or 1.3:1. In infectious mononucleosis and rheumatoid arthritis much higher ratios, e.g., 2.1:1 and 4.9:1, were found in our immunofluorescent studies. As the same antisera were used throughout, it is very unlikely that the results depend on the difference in the amount of antibodies in anti-H and anti-L sera. An increased H/L ratio can be expected if individual cells contain more than one class of immunoglobulins, but even in the extreme situation where all cells would contain all three major immunoglobulins one would never reach the value found in rheumatoid arthritis in this study. It is known, however, that in general one cell contains only one type and one class of immunoglobulin (1, 2, 3, 5, 24, 26).

Another possibility is that in infectious mononucleosis and in rheumatoid arthritis an excess of H chains is synthesized as a result of antigenic stimulation. At the present time no information is available on the presence of free H chains in the serum or urine of these patients.

Finally consideration should be given to the possibility that in the diseases studied here the antigenic determinants of the L chains are not as easily accessible to the relevant antisera as in the normal controls.

Acknowledgment.—The technical assistance of Dr. F. Klein, Mrs. M. Diesselhoff-den Dulk, and Miss Thedel van Zwet is acknowledged with sincere gratitude.

REFERENCES

1. Bernier, G. M., and Cebra, J. J. (1964): Polypeptide chains of human gamma-globulin: cellular localization by fluorescent antibody. Science, *144,* 1590.
2. Bernier, G. M., and Cebra, J. J. (1965): Frequency distribution of α, γ, κ, and λ polypeptide chains in human lymphoid tissues. J. Immun. *95,* 246.
3. Cebra, J. J. (1966): This volume.
4. Cebra, J. J., and Goldstein, G. (1965): Chromatographic purification of tetramethylrhodamine-immune globulin conjugates and their use in the cellular localization of rabbit γ-globulin polypeptide chains. J. Immun. *95,* 230.
5. Chiappino, G., and Pernis, B. (1964): Demonstration with immunofluorescence of 19S macroglobulins and 7S γ-globulins in different cells in the human spleen. Path. Microbiol. *27,* 8.

6. Fahey, J. L. (1963): Two types of 6.6S γ-globulins, β₂A-globulins and 18S γ-macroglobulins in normal serum and γ-microglobulins in normal urine. J. Immun. *91,* 438.

7. Fahey, J. L., and McKelvey, E. M. (1964): Quantitative determination of serum immunoglobulins in antibody agar plates. J. Immun. *94,* 84.

8. Fahey, J. L., and Lawrence, M. E. (1963): Quantitative determination of 6.6S γ-globulins, β₂A-globulins and γ₁-macroglobulins in human serum. J. Immun. *91,* 597.

9. Forbes, I. J. (1965): Specific and non-specific stimulation of antibody synthesis by human leucocytes *in vitro.* Lancet *i,* 198.

10. Franklin, E. C., and Fudenberg, H. H. (1964): Antigenic heterogeneity of rheumatoid factors and Rh antibodies. Arch. Biochem. *104,* 433.

11. Franklin, E. C., and Fudenberg, H. H. (1965): The heterogeneity of rheumatoid factors and the genetic control of polypeptide chains of γ-globulins. Ann. N.Y. Acad. Sci. *124,* 873.

12. Van Furth, R. (1964): The formation of immunoglobulins by human tissues *in vitro.* Thesis, University of Leiden, pp. 62.

13. Van Furth, R. (1966): The formation of immunoglobulins by human tissues *in vitro.* II. Quantitative studies. Immunology *11,* 13.

14. Van Furth, R., Schuit, H. R. E., and Hijmans, W. (1966a): The formation of immunoglobulins by human tissues *in vitro.* I. The methods and their specificity. Immunology *11,* 1.

15. Van Furth, R., Schuit, H. R. E., and Hijmans, W. (1966b): The formation of immunoglobulins by human tissues *in vitro.* IV. Circulating lymphocytes in normal and pathological conditions. Immunology *11,* 29.

16. Hale, A. J., and Cooper, E. H. (1963): DNA synthesis in infectious mononucleosis and acute leukaemia. Acta Haemat. *29,* 257.

17. Hochwald, G. M., Thorbecke, G. J., and Asofsky, R. (1961): A new technique for the demonstration of the synthesis of individual serum proteins by tissues *in vitro.* J. Exp. Med. *114,* 459.

18. Hulliger, L., and Sorkin, E. (1963): Synthesis of antibodies by blood leucocytes of the rabbit. Nature *198,* 299.

19. Hulliger, L., and Sorkin, E. (1965): Formation of specific antibody by circulating cells. Immunology *9,* 391.

20. Landy, M., Sanderson, R. P., Bernstein, M. T., and Jackson, A. L. (1964): Antibody production by leucocytes in peripheral blood. Nature *204,* 1320.

21. Landy, M., Sanderson, R. P., and Jackson, A. L. (1965): Humoral and cellular aspects of the immune response to somatic antigen of *Salmonella* enteriditis. J. Exp. Med. *122,* 483.

22. MacKinney, A. A. (1965): Tissue culture of cells already in DNA synthesis from patients with infectious mononucleosis. Blood *26,* 36.

23. Mannik, M., and Kunkel, H. G. (1963): Two major types of normal 7S γ-globulin. J. Exp. Med. *117,* 213.

24. Mellors, R. C., and Korngold, L. J. (1963): The cellular origin of human immunoglobulins (γ₂, γ₁M, γ₁A). J. Exp. Med. *118,* 387.

25. Nossal, G. J. V., and Mäkelä, O. (1962): Elaboration of antibodies by single cells. Ann. Rev. Microbiol. *16,* 53.

26. Pernis, B., and Chiappino, G. (1964): Identification in human lymphoid tissues of cells that produce group 1 or group 2 γ-globulins. Immunology *7,* 500.

DISCUSSION

JOHNSON: There is a γG antibody appearing at the same time as the γM antibody in the primary antibody response. It has been detected by the Farr test by several investigators and we also have evidence for it. Consequently the γM to γG temporal sequence may not be valid.

VAN FURTH: We were never able to detect small lymphocytes staining positively for γG-globulins. Only γM-globulin could be detected in these cells.

SMITH: What is your evidence that the small lymphocytes are synthesizing the γM-globulin? Staining with fluorescent antisera for γM-globulin doesn't necessarily indicate synthesis of that protein by the cell.

VAN FURTH: Incubation of cells from agammaglobulinemic individuals with serum containing high concentrations of γM-globulin does not cause them to stain positively for γM.

MITCHISON: Do you have any comment on the discrepancy in number between the lymphocytes that you see γM-globulin in, and those that have been transformed by Sell and Gell?

Do you think that any lymphocyte is really "virgin"—i.e., not descended from a cell that participated in an immune response?

VAN FURTH: Sell and Gell found that as many as half of the small lymphocytes in peripheral blood could be "transformed" with a given anti-allotype serum. However, they could not detect appreciable synthesis of immunoglobulins by these transformed cells, perhaps because they incubated much smaller numbers of cells in the radio-labelled medium. The minimum number of cells adequate for detection of incorporation of label into globulin was 10^7 in our experience.

MITCHISON: Sell and Gell found that a given anti-allotype serum caused transformation of only some of the small rabbit lymphocytes of a heterozygous animal. A second anti-allotype serum of the other appropriate specificity added along with the first caused an increase in number of transformed cells. Thus, considering the high frequency of transformation, a high proportion of small lymphocytes appeared to contain a little bit of antibody of a given allotype. Yet you found only a few small lymphocytes to contain detectable immunoglobulin by immunofluorescence. Is "transformation" a more sensitive way of detecting immunoglobulin on or in cells than fluorescent antibody methods?

HIRSCHHORN: In answer to Dr. Mitchison's question:

1. The cells defined as "small" lymphocytes by Dr. van Furth represent only 13% of those in his peripheral human blood samples. These may not be the ones from rabbit blood stimulated by the anti-allotype sera of Sell and Gell. They very probably stimulate what Dr. van Furth calls "medium" lymphocytes which he has indicated do contain γG-globulin.

2. We have experiments using peripheral blood lymphocytes from a human donor who was sensitized to several antigens. We added the antigens to the culture singly, doubly, in threes, and in fours. There was a non-additive significant increase in enlarged cells at 5 days of culture with three and even more with four antigens, as compared with one or two antigens. The results indicate (a) multipotentiality of lymphocytes for recognition of antigens and (b) that most of the circulative lymphocytes are precommitted cells.

GOOD: I would like to caution against thinking of all small round cells in the peripheral blood as being all of one population. Increasing evidence suggests that small lymphocytes in the peripheral blood may include several distinct populations of cells. Among these cells may be elements which have no immunological potential but only potential for

producing hematological elements such as red blood cells, platelets, and granulocytes. Other small round cells have perhaps differentiated in a direction which will permit only the expression we relate to the cellular forms of immunity. Finally there may be a population of small round cells which have differentiated in a direction that will permit synthesis of one or another of the several immunoglobulins. Largely because of the postulates of Warner and Szenberg and the experiments of Cooper et al., we view the lymphoid cell populations as being distributed into the cells originating in the central lymphoid tissues or peripheral lymphoid tissue, and also divisible depending upon the direction of their differentiation. The point is that all of the cells that look like small lymphocytes may not be functionally identical.

HILDEMANN: From where do you postulate the antigenic stimuli may come that cause up to 20% of fetal spleen cells to form γM-globulin?

VAN FURTH: We do not know which particular antigens may pass the placenta. However, maternal γ-globulin can be found circulating in the fetus and might act as an antigenic stimulus.

SMITH: The evidence recently described by Epstein and colleague identifies at least one prenatal antigenic stimulus which stimulates γM synthesis. They found that a high proportion of cord sera contain anti-λ chains and that these antibodies are γM globulins. Anti-κ chains were uncommon.

BLOCK: Would you not expect that the small lymphocytes in the spleen of sheep or cattle embryos (ungulates) with a relatively impermeable placenta would have a lesser percentage of small lymphocytes containing γM antibody than you found among small lymphocytes in the spleen of the embryonic human?

SILVERSTEIN: (Answering Dr. Block)

As far as I know, no adult λ or other chains cross the ovine placenta to the fetus, and yet the fetal lamb forms γM and γG in utero, the former predominating.

JOHN CEBRA and GEORGE M. BERNIER

Quantitative relationships among lymphoid cells differentiated with respect to class of heavy chain, type of light chain, and allotypic markers

IMMUNOGLOBULIN MOLECULES occur in most vertebrates in a variety of different molecular forms (1). Earlier, these forms were differentiated on the basis of differences in some of their antigenic determinants. Now they can also be classified on the basis of chemical and structural differences. However, the immunoglobulins all seem to be assembled according to the same general pattern and are comprised of pairs of polypeptide chains, one member of which is a "light" and the other a "heavy" chain (2). The "classes" of immunoglobulins, γG, γA, and γM, are differentiated on the basis of their heavy polypeptide chains, called γ, α, and μ chain, respectively (3). These heavy chains have different molecular weights of 50,000, 65,000, and 70,000, for γ, α, and μ chain, respectively, and presumably they have different primary sequences as judged from their differing tryptic peptide "fingerprints" (4, 5, 6).

The same variety of light chains is found in all classes of immunoglobulins (2). These chains, derived from human globulins, can occur in at least two different molecular forms, called κ and λ chain, and these differ markedly in primary sequence (7, 8). Thus the immunoglobulins can be represented as aggregates of subunits, such as $(\gamma L)_2$ for γG-immunoglobulin; $(\mu L)_{10}$ for γM-immunoglobulin, $(\alpha L)_4$ for γA-immunoglobulin from colostrum, etc., where L is either all κ chain or all λ chain in a given human immunoglobulin molecule.

Upon immunization, an animal may re-spond by synthesizing some specific antibody of all classes and types (9). Thus, though the molecular forms of the immunoglobulins differ, they all may possess the same antibody specificity. To explore the synthesis of the various forms of immunoglobulin at a cellular level, the technique of double fluorescent staining was employed (10). This approach seemed suited to the revelation of each of the two polypeptide chains of a given immunoglobulin in the cytoplasmic milieu and to the discrimination between heavy chains of different classes or light chains of different types occurring in individual elements of a population of lymphoid cells.

Reagent antibody was prepared in an alternate species to each of several of the polypeptide chains from which the different classes and types of human and rabbit immunoglobulins are assembled. Reagent antisera were obtained in rabbits to the κ, λ, α, and γ polypeptide chains of human globulins by immunization with purified Bence-Jones proteins of type I and II, with the heavy chain of a γA-myeloma protein (Langston), and with a purified abnormal protein (Crawford) from a patient with "heavy chain disease," respectively (11,12). Goats were used to provide reagent antisera for the light, α, μ, any γ polypeptide chains of the rabbit by immunization with light chains, γA-immunoglobulin from colostrum, purified γM-antibody, and the Fc-fragment of γ chain (10,13). Rabbit antisera for either the Aa1 or Aa2 allotypic markers were prepared in Aa^3/Aa^3 homozygous animals (13). The reagent antibodies for subclasses of human γ chain were prepared by absorption of rabbit serum to the abnormal protein Zucker (Zu), from a patient with "heavy chain disease," with Crawford protein (Cr), and vice versa (14).

The reagent globulins were then conjugated with one or the other of the contrasting fluorochromes, fluorescein and tetramethylrhodamine (10, 15). Recent technical improvements in fluorescent antibody preparation and application were utilized, which facilitated simultaneous staining with mixtures of antibodies conjugated with contrasting fluorochromes and the enumeration of lymphoid cells containing each of any two immunoglobulin polypeptide chains (10). The fluorescent reagents, when applied to tissue imprints or sections at concentrations of 0.2-2.0 mg globulin per milliliter (30-300 μg antibody/ml) gave bright specific staining accompanied by negligible non-specific fluorescence. Differentiation of cells stained with the fluorescein (green) labelled reagent, the rhodamine (red) labelled reagent, or both reagents (yellow) was made by sequential observation with the yellow K2 filter, followed by the Kodak Wratten filters 57A (green window filter) and 23A (red barrier filter) (10). To determine the relative number of cells stained with either or both fluorescent reagents of a given pair, from 100 to 500 fluorescing cells were evaluated. Differential cell counts made on different imprints or sections of the same tissue or by different individuals on the same specimen were in close agreement.

Human lymphoid tissue was obtained at surgery or autopsy. None of the patients providing material suffered from a paraproteinemia. Imprints were made from either splenic tissue or lymph nodes and these were stained for either the two types (κ and λ) of light chain, two classes of heavy chains (γ and α), or for one particular type of light chain and one particular class of heavy chain. In some instances, imprints were also stained with a mixture of the two reagents for κ and λ light chains, both conjugated with the same fluorochrome (rhodamine), and the reagent for γ chain, conjugated with the contrasting fluorochrome (fluorescein).

In general, single cells were found to contain detectable amounts of only one type of light chain (11). Similarly, cells were differentiated with respect to their content of α and γ chain, and separate cellular localization of these heavy chains was observed (12). Not more than 3% of the fluorescing cells appeared to stain for both types of light chain and not more than 1% appeared to stain for both classes of heavy chain (11,12). Figure 1 presents schematically the result of staining splenic tissue of a particular patient with the various pairs of fluorescent reagents. The relative number of cells stained for κ chain $vs.$ λ chain was 62:38. When the lymphoid tissue was stained for both types of light chains (κ and λ) and the γ heavy chain, slightly less than half of the fluorescing cells appeared yellow and were doubly stained. These doubly stained cells thus contained both component parts of some type of γG-immunoglobulin, i.e., a light chain and the γ chain. The balance of the cells, which stained for light chains alone, presumably could have contained another class of heavy chain. The results of staining for the γ chain $vs.$ the α chain indicated that most of these cells in question probably contained the components of γA-immunoglobulin. By direct staining, the relative numbers of fluorescing cells containing α $vs.$ γ chain were 43:57. Double staining experiments, in which a particular type of light chain and a particular class of heavy chain were revealed, permitted the inferential determination of the distribution of κ and λ chains among that group of cells containing a particular class of heavy chain. These experiments also permitted the estimation of the proportion of cells which contained a given class of immunoglobulin among those cells containing a particular type of light chain. Thus, the fraction of κ or λ chain-containing cells which were synthesizing γG-immunoglobulin could be determined and compared with the corresponding fraction found for the whole population of cells which stained for light chain. The lower row of Fig. 1 illustrates the inferential estimations just described and attests to the internal consistency of the data obtained by counting cells.

In Table 1, quantitative data for the proportions of the various differentiated lymphoid cells from four of the nine human sources previously described (11,12) are presented. The same kind of differentiation just described

DISTRIBUTION OF IMMUNOGLOBULIN POLYPEPTIDE
CHAINS AMONG HUMAN LYMPHOID CELLS

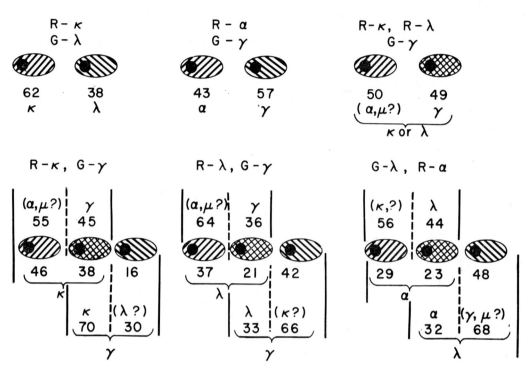

FIG. 1. Schematic representation of the various cell counts obtained for spleen tissue from a single human individual. For simplicity, the few per cent of doubly stained cells observed after staining with the reagent pairs rhodamine labelled anti-κ (R-κ) plus fluorescein labelled anti-γ (G-λ) or with rhodamine labelled anti-α (R-α) plus fluorescein labelled anti-γ (G-γ) were omitted. Likewise, the few cells fluorescing green after staining with R-κ, R-λ, and G-γ were omitted. (Cross-hatch = yellow or doubly stained; slanted lines up to right = red; slanted lines up to left = green)

was observed for all subjects, whether the lymphoid tissue was derived from lymph nodes or spleen. In general, cells seemed confined to the production of both component chains of only one class and type of immunoglobulin. In instances where cells were stained for κ, λ, and γ chains, a few cells (0-8%) appeared to stain only for the γ heavy chain. Such cells could represent cases of asynchronous chain production or they could contain a minor type of light chain, different from either κ or λ chain.

From the data of Table 1 the relative number of cells containing each class of immunoglobulin could be calculated. The relative number of μ chain-containing cells was estimated by difference, since these cells were not directly identified. In general, γG-immunoglobulin cells predominated, followed by γA-

and γM-immunoglobulin cells in decreasing order of abundance. The serum concentrations of three classes of immunoglobulins stand in about the same order as the relative abundance of the cells containing them. However, the contribution of γA-immunoglobulin to the total serum immunoglobulin concentration is only 17% (16), while the relative proportion of spleen cells which contained this immunoglobulin rather than γG-immunoglobulin ranges from 28 to 51% (12). Presumably, rates of passage to extravascular spaces and rates of catabolism, as well as number of synthesizing cells, would also be reflected in the serum steady state levels.

Table 1 also shows that cells containing κ chain predominated over those containing λ chain by about 3:2 in almost all specimens

TABLE 1.—FREQUENCY DISTRIBUTION OF α, γ, κ, AND λ CHAINS AMONG HUMAN LYMPHOID CELLS

Stains	R-κ + G-λ		R-κ + G-γ			R-λ + G-γ			G-λ + R-α			R-κ + R-λ + G-γ		R-α + G-γ		Inferential		
Chain	κ	λ	κ	κ+γ	γ	γ	γ+λ	λ	α	α+λ	λ	κ or λ	κ+γ or λ+γ	α	γ	α	γ	Other (μ?)
Patient No. 8	62	38	46 * 55	38 70 45λ	16 30λ?	42 67κ?	21 33 33γ	37 * 64	29 56κ?	23 44 32α	48 * 68	50	49γ	43	57	37	49	14
Patient No. 6	55	44	51 * 64	29 59 36γ	20 41λ?	28 44κ?	35 56 43γ	37 * 57	39 51κ?	30 49 57α	31 * 43	58	43γ	48	51	40	43	17
Patient No. 5	68	32	39 * 50	39 64 50γ	22 36λ?				59 74κ?	21 26 51α	20 * 49			51	48			
Lymph Node	68	31	24 * 31	53 69 69γ	23 31λ?	43 60κ?	29 40 51γ	28 * 49				35	59γ					
Patient No. 3	66	32	28 * 37	47 65 63γ	25 35γ?	39 48κ?	41 52 67γ	20 * 33										
Spleen												27	73γ					

Adapted from Bernier and Cebra (1964 and 1965).
*Relative number of cells containing κ vs. λ-chain inferred from data for that group of cells containing a particular class of heavy chain (γ or α).

examined (11,12). In fact, the over-all ratio of cells containing each of the two types of light chain was 63:37 for $\kappa:\lambda$. Table 2 presents

TABLE 2.—RELATIVE FREQUENCY OF κ (TYPE I) AND λ (TYPE II) CHAINS

Light	Serum (%)				Myeloma	2,500
Chain	γG*	γG†	γA†	γM†	Globulins‡	Cells
Type I (κ)	60	69	62	68	69%	63%
Type II (λ)	30	31	38	32	31%	37%

*Mannik and Kunkel (43).
†Fahey (44).
‡Korngold (45).

some correlations of this ratio with the relative serum concentrations of each of the types of a particular class of immunoglobulin. The incidence of the various types of myeloma may reflect the proportions of already differentiated cells at risk at the time of oncogenesis. Likewise, the proportions of the different types of differentiated cells seem to be reflected in the serum concentrations of their products.

Human γG-immunoglobulin can itself be resolved into at least four subclasses, differentiable on the basis of antigenic differences on its heavy chain (17,18). Normal human serum contains a mixture of these molecules, designated γ_{2a}-, γ_{2b}-, γ_{2c}-, and γ_{2d}-globulins (18). In certain cases of "heavy chain disease," described by Franklin, a protein is produced in abundance which resembles the γ chain of only one or another subclass of γG-immunoglobulin (19). Two samples of such proteins, from patients Crawford (Cr) and Zucker (Zu), were used to prepare reagent antisera. Specific anti-Zu essentially constituted a reagent for the γ_{2c}-subclass of γG-immunoglobu-

lins (20), while the anti-Cr, after absorption with Zu protein, reacted with the other subclasses of γG-immunoglobulins. Table 3 shows that the subclasses of the γ-chain are separately localized in lymphoid cells. Again there seems to be a good correspondence between the relative number of cells containing the γ_{2c}-subclass of γG-immunoglobulin and (a) the incidence of multiple myeloma of this subclass, and (b) the relative serum concentration of γ_{2c}-globulin.

A similar study of the extent of differentiation of lymphoid cells with respect to their content of the classes of heavy chains was made in the rabbit. Indeed, the rabbit was used as the donor of lymphoid tissue during the development of the methods for double fluorescent staining and in the assessment of their reliability for determining the quantitative distribution of particular polypeptide chains (10) (Fig. 2). Table 4 shows that 63-78% of all fluorescing cells present in rabbit spleen contained both component chains of γG-immunoglobulin. The balance of these cells, stained with anti-light chain alone, presumably contained heavy chains of another class. The proportion of cells containing γG-immunoglobulin was similar in non-immunized rabbits and in those immunized with either lysozyme or sheep erythrocytes.

When fluorescent antibody reagents became available for rabbit α, μ, and γ chains, the distribution of each class of immunoglobulin among the lymphoid cells of an experimental animal could be directly determined (13). Table 5 indicates how, by staining alternate spleen sections or imprints with contrasting fluorescent reagents for any two heavy chains, the distribution of all three chains could be

TABLE 3.—PER CENT OF PROTEINS OR CELLS WITH SPECIFIC ANTIGENIC DETERMINANTS

γG-Immuno-globulin (Subclass)	Pooled γG-globulin	Normal individual γG-globulin	γG-myeloma globulins*	Cells containing markers in normal individuals		
				#1	#2	#3
"Cr"	72	75	82	94	86	91
"Zu"	8	6	7	6	14	9

Adapted from Bernier et al. (1967).
*Per cent of individual myeloma proteins bearing "Zu" or "Cr" determinants (108 specimens examined, 10% were "Cr variant," and 1 was not classified).

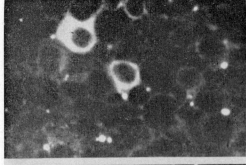

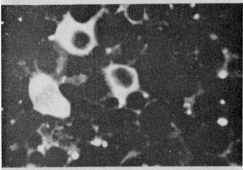

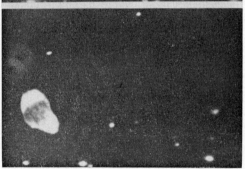

Fig. 2. Photomicrographs of cells present in a spleen imprint of a hyperimmune rabbit. The three pictures are of the same field viewed through the red barrier filter No. 23A (top), the neutral filter No. K2 (middle), and the green window filter No. 57A (bottom). The cells were stained with a mixture of rhodamine labelled anti-γ chain and fluorescein labelled anti-μ chain. The middle picture shows four fluorescent cells. Three of these cells are stained only with the anti-γ chain and can also be seen through the red filter (top). The cell in the lower left is stained only with the anti-μ chain and it can also be seen through the green filter (bottom). From Cebra *et al.* (1966). Magnification X650.

calculated. The lymphoid cell donors were hyperimmunized to either dinitrophenylated ferritin, Salmonella, or a mixture of proteins. In general, each class of heavy chain was separately localized in cells. A similar kind of cellular differentiation was found in the popliteal and mesenteric lymph nodes, where often great clusters of fluorescing cells were observed in the medullary cords. Frequently cells staining for only one particular heavy chain predominated in these clusters; however, cells staining only for the other heavy chain were always scattered throughout these areas in apparent random fashion. The frequency distribution of cells containing each heavy chain in popliteal and mesenteric nodes was usually similar to that found in spleen (13,21). Table 5 shows that cells containing γ chain usually predominated over those containing α chain by about 10:1. Similarly, the γ chain-containing cells ordinarily outnumbered those con-

TABLE 4.—RELATIVE NUMBER OF RABBIT SPLEEN CELLS CONTAINING DETECTABLE AMOUNTS OF EITHER γ CHAIN, LIGHT CHAIN, OR BOTH CHAINS

Spleen Imprint	Immuno-globulin Chain	Anti-Lysozyme			Normal		Anti-Sheep RBC	
		A	B	C	A	B	A	B
#1	γ	3	0	1	3	3	0	0
	Light	31	27	21	34	24	33	30
	γ+Light	66	73	78	63	73	67	70
#2	γ	1	1	4	4	3	0	0
	Light	26	26	24	31	27	22	31
	γ+Light	73	73	72	65	70	78	69

Adapted from Cebra and Goldstein (1965).

TABLE 5.—DISTRIBUTION OF α, γ, AND μ HEAVY CHAINS AND OF ALLOTYPIC MARKERS Aa1 AND Aa2 AMONG RABBIT SPLEEN CELLS

Pairs of Stains / Rabbits	Relative Number of Cells Stained by Each or Both of the following Reagents				Calculated Distribution %	Average Distribution %	Relative Serum Conc. %
	G-α + R-γ	G-μ + R-γ	R-α + G-μ	G-A1 + R-A2			
	α γ α+γ	μ γ μ+γ	α μ α+μ	Aa1 Aa2 Mix	α γ μ	Aa1 Aa2	Aa1 Aa2
Anti-DNP #1	7 93 — / 10 90 —	25 75 — / 32 68 —	22 78 — / 23 77 —	72 28 1 / 72 27 1 / 65 34 1 / 71 28 1	7 67 26	70 29	—
Anti-DNP #2	15 85 —	23 77 — / 22 77 1	22 78 — / 17 83 —	Homozygote	9 70 21	—	—
Anti-DNP #3	12 88 —	29 70 1		81 19 — / 86 14 —	9 64 27	84 16	80 20
Anti-Salmonella #1	5 95 — / 6 94 —	13 87 — / 16 83 1	29 71 — / 30 70 —	81 19 — / 79 21 — / 79 21 — / 86 14 —	6 80 14	81 19	—
Anti-Proteins #1*		15 85 — / 12 88 —		90 10 — / 86 14 —		88 12	91 9
Anti-Proteins #2*		16 84 — / 13 87 —	16 84 —	82 18 — / 84 16 —	3 82 15	83 17	87 13

Adapted in part from Cebra et al. (1966).

*Rabbits received 2mg each of hen ovalbumin, horse ferritin, and bovine γ-globulin in complete Freund's adjuvant intramuscularly 2 weeks before sacrifice.

taining μ chain by about 3:1. Consistently, cells in which the μ chain could be identified were more numerous than those staining for α chain by about 3:1. The over-all relative number of cells containing each heavy chain was calculated (13) and, as shown in Table 5, was found to be 3-9% for α chain, 14-27% for μ chain, and 64-82% for γ chain. Thus it would appear that the 22-37% of fluorescing cells which contain light chains in the absence of γ chain, found in the spleens of the seven rabbits listed in Table 4, indeed were synthesizing either γA- or γM-immunoglobulin.

The relative proportions of cells containing α, μ, or γ chain stand in the same order as the relative serum concentrations of the corresponding classes of immunoglobulins. However, there is not a direct proportionality between cell numbers and serum concentrations of their product. For instance, the concentration of γA-immunoglobulin in rabbit serum is only about 180 μg/ml, or about 1.5% of the total serum immunoglobulins (22), while this protein is found in 3-9% of the fluorescing cells. Similarly, 14-27% of positive cells contain μ chain while the rabbit serum macroglobulin concentration is probably relatively much lower. In one case, the anti-DNP antibody from rabbit #2 was purified and the γM-component was found to be only 6% of the total (13). Thus, the serum concentrations of the immunoglobulins may reflect their rates of degradation and escape from the vascular system and the quantity of cells containing and presumably synthesizing each immunoglobulin may reflect the number necessary to maintain a given steady state level of their product.

Table 5 also indicates that lymphoid cell differentiation even appears to extend to content of particular heavy chains which are products of allelic cistrons. In rabbits, the a locus controls a set of antigenic sites, called allotypic markers, which have been located on the γ chain (23,24). It is not yet clear whether this set of antigenic sites can be present on all classes of heavy chains (22), as had been suggested by some reports (25,26,27). At any rate, five of the rabbits analyzed in Table 5 were a locus heterozygotes (Aa^1/Aa^2). The allotypic markers, Aa1 and Aa2, were found mainly in separate splenic cells and also in separate cells of popliteal and mesenteric lymph nodes (13). In general, cells containing the Aa1 marker outnumbered those with the Aa2 marker by about 4:1. The serum obtained from some of these rabbits at the time of sacrifice was analyzed for relative concentrations of Aa1 and Aa2 molecules by Dr. Rose Mage, who used a quantitative gel diffusion method (28). Table 5 indicates that there is a good correspondence between relative serum concentrations of Aa1 and Aa2 molecule and their relative occurrence in lymphoid cells.

Another locus (b) in rabbits controls a set of allotypic markers present on light chains (23,24). Pernis et $al.$ have shown that the two allotypic variants of light chain present in animals heterozygous at the b locus can be

TABLE 6.—DISTRIBUTION OF Ab4 AND Ab5 ALLOTYPIC MARKERS AMONG
SPLEEN CELLS OF Ab^4/Ab^5 RABBITS

Rabbit	Relative Serum Concentration		Relative Number of Cells Containing Allotypic Markers Stained by:					
			R-γ, μ, α+ G-A4		G-A4 then R-A5		R-A5 then G-A4	
	Ab4	Ab5	Ab4	Ab5	Ab4	Ab5	Ab4	Ab5
Anti-proteins #2	69	31	60	40	53	47	—	—
Anti-proteins #3	66	34	60	40	36	64	68	32
Anti-proteins #4	87	13	90	10	88	12	73	27

Adapted from Lummus (1966).

localized to separate lymphoid cells (29). This differentiation of lymphoid cells of Ab^4/Ab^5 heterozygotes with respect to their content of the Ab4 and Ab5 markers was confirmed (30). The relative number of cells containing each marker in spleens of a group of heterozygotes is shown in Table 6. The cells staining for the Ab4 markers usually outnumbered those with Ab5 markers by about 2:1. Again, relative serum concentrations of molecules bearing one or the other of these markers, determined by Mage, accorded well with the relative number of cells containing each marker.

In Table 7, the distribution of the various heavy chains and of allotypic markers Aa1 and Aa2 among the cells in the popliteal node, spleen, mesenteric node, and intestines of a single hyperimmune rabbit is given. The rabbit was injected with *Salmonella* in the footpads and the data suggest a shift in the balance of differentiated cells in the draining popliteal node in favor of those containing μ chain. These nodes also show an increase in the relative number of cells containing the Aa2 marker, compared with the proportion of Aa2 containing cells in spleen or lymph nodes.

Those cells staining for α chain predominate in intestine (21), as indicated in Table 7. The large number of cells apparently synthesizing γA-immunoglobulin in rabbit intestine accords with similar observations made on human intestine (31). The remainder of the fluorescing lymphoid cells of intestines likewise seem differentiated, with approximately equal numbers of cells staining separately for the Aa1 and Aa2 markers (13) and those cells containing γ chain outnumbering those containing macroglobulin. Recently, an instance of a shift in the population of differentiated intestinal lymphoid cells after stimulation by antigen has been described (21). At 8-12 days following a primary trichina infection, a relative increase in cells with μ chain is observed throughout the intestines. Later, when the parasite has encysted in muscle tissue, such as diaphragm, differentiated plasma cells containing either μ or γ chain are observed in the region of inflammation surrounding the sites (21).

The sum of the data presented gives a comprehensive demonstration that lymphoid cells can be differentiated with respect to their content of class or subclass of heavy chain, type of light chain, and even with respect to their content of allotypic markers on chains presumably controlled by allelic cistrons. This kind of cellular differentiation is in accord with earlier observations by Mellors and Korngold, who found mainly separate cellular localization of the different classes of human immunoglobulins (32). Pernis and coworkers have also independently demonstrated the differentiation of rabbit and human cells, in spleen and in the medullary cords of lymph nodes, with respect

TABLE 7.—DISTRIBUTION OF γ, μ, AND α HEAVY CHAINS AND OF ALLOTYPIC MARKERS Aa1 AND Aa2 IN LYMPHOID CELLS OF DIFFERENT ORGANS FROM A SINGLE HYPERIMMUNE RABBIT*

Tissue	R-Anti-γ+ G-Anti-μ		R-Anti-γ+ G-Anti-α		R-Anti-α+ G-Anti-μ		R-Anti-Aa2+ G-Anti-Aa1		Relative No. of Cells Containing:			Relative No. of Cells Containing:	
	γ	μ	γ	α	α	μ	Aa1	Aa2	γ	μ	α	Aa1	Aa2
Popliteal	36	64	96	4	7	93	60	40					
Lymph node	35	65	97	3	3	97	53	47	35	62	3	56	44
							54	46					
Spleen	53	47			25	75	75	25					
	55	45	——		23	78	78	22	49	39	12	74	26
	60	40					69	31					
Mesenteric Lymph node	71	29	——		25	75	69	31	65	26	9	69	31
Intestine	91	9	20	80	98	2	51	49	22	2	76	50	50
			15	85	98	2	49	51					

*Adapted from Cebra *et al.* (1966) and from Crandall *et al.* (1966).

to their content of type of light chain (33) and of allotypic markers controlled by the *a* or *b* locus (29). Thus, with respect to the apparent monodispersity of their product, fluorescing cells of "normal" humans and rabbits bear a striking resemblance to those cells which synthesize myeloma proteins in patients with paraproteinemias (34).

If the "normal" differentiated cells revealed by fluorescent staining are representative of actively synthesizing cells, then the polydispersity of immunoglobulins must reflect the simultaneous production of many differentiable proteins, each by a separate set of cells. The good agreement between the relative numbers of cells found to contain a given immunoglobulin chain and the relative serum concentration of that polypeptide suggests that the fluorescing cells at least reflect the size of the particular synthetic "plants" and may be representative of a particular synthesizing population. The cells at issue probably no longer were synthesizing DNA (35). However, it is now obviously important to determine whether those cells revealed by their fluorescence were still synthesizing RNA and protein just prior to fixation. If they indeed were still capable of RNA synthesis, then they each may represent cells making a highly restricted kind of immunoglobulin, presumably following a very limited expression of particular cistrons.

Those cistrons controlling synthesis of certain classes and subclasses of heavy chain have been examined in the mouse. By crossing individuals from various inbred strains of mice, which differ in part by certain antigenic determinants on a particular heavy chain, the close linkage of the cistrons controlling the α and one subclass of γ chain (36) and also two subclasses of γ chain (37) has been shown. Thus, barring some sort of reduction division, a very selective activation must occur at a particular heavy chain cistron preceding protein synthesis. To account for the observed differentiation of cells with respect to the Aa1 and Aa2 markers in a consistent way, one must likewise postulate selective expression of one of two allelic cistrons.

The influence of antigen on the differentiation of lymphoid cells with respect to variety of polypeptide chain remains enigmatic. Evidence for the summation of lymphoblast transformations caused by two antisera to different allotypic markers acting on the small lymphocyte of heterozygous rabbits may indicate a cellular differentiation prior to specific antibody synthesis (38). Similarly, one interpretation of specific immunosuppression of the production of one allotypic marker by treated, heterozygous newborn rabbits would imply the destruction of a group of cells that had been committed to the synthesis of a particular globulin allotype even before antigen exposure (39). Thus, the antigen at most may cause the selective stimulation of cells which are "precommitted" with respect to class, subclass, type, allotype, etc. of polypeptide which they can produce. Alternately, the antigen may only stimulate cells "precommitted" in the above sense by chance, and if the number of cells stimulated is small, may elicit antibodies of restricted kind (29). At any rate, antigen does seem to affect the proportions of the various molecular forms of antibody produced. For instance, purified antibodies to a particular antigen or hapten may show an imbalance in their content of antigenic markers (40) or even the deletion of some of these markers (41) with respect to those found on the total population of serum molecules.

The data presented above (Table 7), showing the differences in cellular distributions of classes and allotypes of immunoglobulin chains in different organs of the same animal, may be interpreted as reflecting the influence of antigen. Thus, the popliteal lymph node draining the site of injection of Salmonella shows a marked shift in the ratio of μ *vs.* γ and Aa1 *vs.* Aa2 containing cells, compared with nodes of other animals (13) or with its own mesenteric node and spleen. One might thus envision fluctuations in the serum concentrations of the molecular forms of immunoglobulins and transient "dysgammaglobulinemias" caused by local shifts in the synthesizing cell populations, which in turn may be influenced by antigens.

Many problems concerning lymphoid cell differentiation with respect to variety of chain persist, aside from the question of antigen influence. Among these are (a) the actuality of simultaneous synthesis of more than one type or class of chain by single cells, especially those in lymphoid follicles (32,33); (b) the conversion of cells from μ chain to γ chain production (42); and (c) the broader consideration of the survival value of the multiplicity of molecular forms of the immunoglobulins. The latter issue is now partly understood as the wide disparity in biologic activities of the immunoglobulins becomes apparent.

Acknowledgments: The work reported here was supported by Public Health Service Research Grant AI-05042 from the National Institute of Allergy and Infectious Diseases. Dr. Cebra is recipient of a Public Health Service Research Career Development Award (K3-AI-11, 469) from the National Institute of Allergy and Infectious Diseases.

REFERENCES

1. Smith, R. T., Miescher, P. A., and Good, R. A., eds. (1966): Phylogeny of Immunity. Gainesville, Univ. of Florida Press.
2. Cohen, S., and Porter, R. R. (1964): Structure and biologic activity of immunoglobulins, in: Dixon, F. J., and Humphrey, J. A., eds.: Advances in Immunology. New York, Academic Press, 4, 287.
3. Nomenclature for human immunoglobulins (1964): Bull. W.H.O. 30, 447.
4. Small, P. A., Jr., and Lamm, M. E. (1966): Polypeptide chain structure of rabbit immunoglobulins. I. γG-immunoglobulin. Biochemistry 5, 259.
5. Lamm, M. E., and Small, P. A., Jr. (1966): Polypeptide chain structure of rabbit immunoglobulins. II. γM-immunoglobulin. Biochemistry 5, 267.
6. Cebra, J. J., and Small, P. A. In preparation.
7. Hilschmann, N., and Craig, L. C. (1965): Amino acid sequence studies with Bence-Jones proteins. Proc. Nat. Acad. Sci. 53, 1403.
8. Titani, K., Whitley E., Jr., Avogardo, L., and Putnam, F. W. (1965): Immunoglobulin structure. Partial amino acid sequence of a Bence-Jones protein. Science 149, 1090.
9. Fahey, J. L., and Goodman, H. (1964): Antibody activity in six classes of human immunoglobulins. Science 143, 588.
10. Cebra, J. J. and Goldstein, G. (1964): Chromatographic purification of tetramethylrhodamine-immune globulin conjugates and their use in cellular localization of rabbit γ-globulin polypeptide chains. J. Immun. 95, 230.
11. Bernier, G., and Cebra, J. J. (1964): Polypeptide chains of human gamma globulin: Cellular localization by fluorescent antibody. Science 144, 1590.
12. Bernier, G., and Cebra, J. J. (1965): Frequency distribution of α, γ, κ, and λ polypeptide chains in human lymphoid tissues. J. Immun. 95, 246.
13. Cebra, J. J., Colberg, J. E., and Dray, S. (1966): Rabbit lymphoid cells differentiated with respect to α-, γ-, and μ- heavy polypeptide chains and to allotypic markers Aa1 and Aa2. J. Exp. Med. 123, 547.
14. Bernier, G., Ballieux, R. E., Tominaga, K., Easley, C. W., and Putnam, F. W.: J. Exp. Med. [In press]
15. Wood, B. T., Thompson, S. H., and Goldstein, G. (1965): Fluorescent antibody staining. III. Preparation of fluorescein-isothiocyanate labeled antibodies. J. Immun. 95, 225.
16. Fahey, J. L., and Lawrence, M. E. (1963): Quantitative determination of 6.6S γ-globulins, B₂A-globulins and γ₁-macroglobulins in human serum. J. Immun. 91, 597.
17. Grey, H. M., and Kunkel, H. G. (1964): H-chain subgroups of myeloma proteins and normal 7S γ-globulin. J. Exp. Med. 120, 253.
18. Terry, W. D., and Fahey, J. L. (1964): Subclasses of human γ₂-globulin based on differences in the heavy polypeptide chains. Science 146, 400.
19. Franklin, E. C. (1964): Structural studies of human 7S γ-globulin (G-immunoglobulin). J. Exp. Med. 120, 691.
20. Terry, W. D. (1965): Skin sensitizing activity related to γ-polypeptide chain characteristics of human IgG. J. Immun. 95, 1041.
21. Crandall, R. E., Cebra, J. J., and Crandall, C. A.: The relative proportions of γG-, γM-, and γA-immunoglobulin containing cells in rabbit tissues during experimental trichinosis. Immunology. [In press]
22. Cebra, J. J., and Robbins, J. B.: γA-immunoglobulin from rabbit colostrum. J. Immun. 97, 12.
23. Kelus, A. S. (1963): γ-globulin allotypes in the rabbit. Biochem. J. 88, 4 p.
24. Stemke, G. W. (1964): Allotypic specificities of A- and B-chains of rabbit gamma globulin. Science 145, 403.
25. Todd, C. W. (1963): Allotypy in rabbit 19S protein. Biochem. Biophys. Res. Commun. 11, 170.
26. Feinstein, A. (1963): Character and allotypy of an immune globulin in rabbit colostrum. Nature 99, 1197.
27. Stemke, G. W., and Fisher, R. J. (1965): Rabbit 19S antibodies and allotypic specifications of the a-locus group. Science 150, 1298.
28. Fahey, J. L., and McKelvey, E. M. (1965): Quantitative determination of serum immunoglobulins in antibody-agar plates. J. Immun. 94, 84.
29. Pernis, B., Chiappino, G., Kelus, A. S., and Gell, P.G.H. (1965): Cellular localization of immuno-

globulins with different allotype specifications in rabbit lymphoid tissues. J. Exp. Med. *122*, 853.

30. Lummus, Z. (1966): Properties and synthesis of light chains from rabbit γ-globulin. Dissertation, University of Florida.
31. Crabbé, P. A., Carbonara, A. O., and Heremans, J. (1965): The normal human intestinal mucosa as a major source of plasma cells containing γA-immunoglobulin. Lab. Invest. *14*, 235.
32. Mellors, R. C., and Korngold, L. (1963): The cellular origin of human immunoglobulins. J. Exp. Med. *118*, 387.
33. Pernis, B., and Chiappino, G. (1964): Identification in human lymphoid tissues of cells that produce group 1 or group 2 gamma-globulins. Immunology *7*, 500.
34. Solomon, A., Fahey, J. L., and Malmgren, R. A. (1963): Immunohistologic localization of gamma-1-macroglobulins, beta-2A-myeloma proteins, 6.6S gamma-myeloma proteins and Bence-Jones proteins. Blood *22*, 403.
35. Cohen, E. P., and Talmage, D. W. (1965): Onset and duration of DNA-synthesis in antibody forming cells after antigen. J. Exp. Med. *121*, 125.
36. Herzenberg, L. A. (1964): A chromosome region for gamma-2A and beta-2A globulin H-chain isoantigens in the mouse. Cold Spring Harbor Symposia on Quantitative Biology *29*, 455.
37. Lieberman, R., Dray, S., and Potter, M. (1965): Linkage in control of allotypic specifi-

cities on two different γG-immunoglobulins. Science *148*, 460.
38. Gell, P. G. H., and Sell, S. (1965): Studies on rabbit lymphocytes in vitro. II. Induction of blast transformation with antisera to six IgG allotypes and summation with mixtures of antisera to different allotypes. J. Exp. Med. *122*, 813.
39. Mage, R., and Dray, S. (1965): Persistent altered phenotypic expression of allelic γG-immunoglobulin allotypes in heterozygous rabbits exposed to isoantibodies in fetal and neonatal life. J. Immun. *95*, 525.
40. Rieder, R. F., and Oudin, J. (1963): Studies on the relationship of allotypic specificities to antibody specificities in the rabbit. J. Exp. Med. *118*, 625.
41. Gell, P. G. H., and Kelus, A. (1962): Deletions of allotypic γ-globulins in antibodies. Nature *195*, 44.
42. Nossal, G. J. V., Szenberg, A., Ada, G. L., and Austin, C. M. (1964): Single cell studies on 19S antibody production. J. Exp. Med. *119*, 485.
43. Mannik, M., and Kunkel, H. G. (1963): Two major types of normal 7S γ-globulin. J. Exp. Med. *117*, 213.
44. Fahey, J. L. (1963): Two types of 6.6S γ-globulins, B₂A-globulins and 18S γ₁-macroglobulins in normal serum and γ-microglobulins in normal urine. J. Immun. *91*, 438.
45. Korngold, L. (1961): Abnormal plasma components and their significance in disease. Ann. N.Y. Acad. Sci. *94*, 110.

DISCUSSION

COOPER: (1) Did the morphology of cells staining with various heavy chain antisera vary?

(2) Did cells of the intestinal lymphoid aggregates, i.e., Peyer's patches, sacculus rofundus, and appendix exhibit γ-globulin synthesis?

CEBRA: We did not observe any consistent morphologic differences which could be correlated with the particular heavy chain (α, γ, or μ) which the cells contained. Positive cells ranging from those with a large amount of cytoplasm to those with a thin rim of cytoplasm around the nucleus were observed when either fluorescent anti-α, anti-γ, or anti-μ reagent was applied.

Dr. Crandall has found α chain-containing cells of the rabbit gut to be numerous in the lamina propria of the villi, where they often appear as compact strands or groups which extended into the core of the villus. In contrast, cells staining for γ or μ chains were usually found scattered in the lamina propria

and were more concentrated in the basal areas near the muscularis mucosa. Immunoglobulin containing cells in lesser numbers were also observed in the rabbit appendix. The Peyer's patches were not investigated.

VAN FURTH: In studies done on circulating lymphocytes from three groups of people—healthy donors, patients with infectious mononucleosis, and rheumatoid arthritis patients—we found the μ chain to occur in 28% of the fluorescent cells from normals and in 50% of the positive cells in infectious mononucleosis patients. The increase in cells with μ chain in infectious mononucleosis patients correlated with the increase in circulating γM-antibody in the serum. We found ratios of κ:λ chain of about 3:1 in cells from normal and infectious mononucleosis patients, but a ratio of κ:λ of 8:1 in the rheumatoid patients. Can you explain this departure from the κ:λ ratio of 3:2 which you have observed in lymph nodes and spleen of normal individuals?

CEBRA: Rheumatoid factor is a macroglobulin with a very restricted antibody specificity, that of anti-human γG-globulin. In rheumatoid patients, cells from a restricted number of clones may be stimulated to proliferate and these may produce γM-antibody of mainly one particular type and this may comprise enough of the total globulin population to affect the $\kappa:\lambda$ ratio. It would be interesting to note whether other rheumatoid patients occur which have an imbalance of globulin types in favor of the λ chain.

HIRSCHHORN: In our studies using fluorescein-conjugated anti-κ chain, obtained from Dr. Franklin, we found 30-40% of the cultured lymphocytes stained. Therefore, light chain individuality of cells appears to remain stable in the culture system, while heavy chain (α, γ, μ) individuality seems to be lost as PHA-stimulated cells express all classes of globulin.

GOOD: In the lymph nodes did you find any special distribution of the staining for μ or γ chains? I am concerned here with distribution in the germinal centers and medullary cords.

CEBRA: Cells containing γ chain had about the same distribution as those containing μ chain. Indeed, the two classes of cells were usually interspersed throughout the medullary cords. Clusters of cells were observed made up predominantly of cells containing only γ chain or only μ chain. However, cells containing the other chain were always intermingled. The rabbit donors were mainly hyperimmunized animals. Essentially no cells differentiated with respect to globulin chain content were observed in the follicles.

BLOCK: Were any stainable cells observed in the bone marrow?

CEBRA: We examined human marrow smears for the two types of light chain and found cells differentiated with respect to κ or λ chain in about the same ratio as found for spleen and lymph node cells.

MITCHISON: Are the odd double $\gamma + \mu$ producers real? You haven't discussed them much. Are you sure that they are not due to a piece of macrophage getting smeared onto a plasma cell or to cytophilic antibody?

CEBRA: Very few cells stained for two different heavy chains were observed. Of the 1-2% of such cells which we did count, some could have been explained by artifacts such as you mention, but some of them certainly looked like doubly stained plasma cells and lymphocytes. To determine whether such "double producers" are real certainly merits further investigation.

II

ROSE G. MAGE

The quantitative expression of allelic allotypes in normal and "allotype-suppressed" heterozygous rabbits

THE PRODUCTION OF IMMUNOGLOBULINS and, in particular, antibody immunoglobulins, is a model system with great potentiality for the study of the mechanisms of cellular differentiation. The rabbit has probably been the experimental animal most intensively studied by immunologists and its immunoglobulins are among the most well-characterized chemically and immunochemically. We are therefore fortunate to have available for our work, rabbits from controlled breedings in closed colonies which were developed by Dr. Sheldon Dray, while he was at the National Institutes of Health. These rabbits are defined at two genetic loci known to contribute to the control of immunoglobulin structure. The genes of the a locus, a^1, a^2, and a^{3*}, control structural features of the heavy chains of the immunoglobulins which we detect as antigenic determinants (allotypic specificities), using antisera prepared by isoimmunizing rabbits of a given allotypic genotype with purified γG-immunoglobulin from rabbits of another type (4). The genes of the b locus, b^4, b^5, and b^6, control structural features on the light polypeptide chains which we detect with isoantisera (4), but which can also in some instances be distinguished by heteroantisera, for example, from goats (1, 7). Chemical studies of light chains from homozygous b4 and homozygous

b5 rabbits have revealed reproducible differences in total amino acid compositions (13) and in peptide maps (14) which suggest that the genes of the b locus are directly involved in determining at least a part of the light chains' amino acid sequences.

In rabbits heterozygous at a given allotypic locus, allelic specificities, although both expressed in the animals' sera, are not found together on the same molecules (3). On the other hand, in double heterozygotes, specificities of both loci are found together on the same molecules, and in studies thus far, the assortment appears compatible with random association of the non-allelic specificities (5); however, more extensive studies will be necessary to establish this point.

This paper will review the information obtained in our laboratory on the control of the relative quantities of immunoglobulins bearing allelic allotypic markers found in the sera of heterozygous rabbits.

In the newborn rabbit, there is very little γG-immunoglobulin synthesis (15) so that at least by the usual precipitation methods used for typing animals, for the first three or four weeks the young have the allotypic phenotype of their mothers regardless of what their fathers' allotype might be. When the father and mother differ in allotype, the appearance of the father's type in the serum of the offspring can be taken as an indication of immunoglobulin production by the young animal. In 1962, Dray (2) reported this, and also

*Allotype specificities Aa1, Aa2, Aa3, Ab4, Ab5, and Ab6 as well as the genes Aa^1, Aa^2, Aa^3, Ab^4, Ab^5, and Ab^6 will be abbreviated by omitting the capital A.

showed that in appropriate matings, allotypic specificities on the immunoglobulins could serve as natural markers for the disappearance of passively transferred maternal immunoglobulins as well as for the appearance of newly synthesized immunoglobulin in the serum of the young rabbit. At the same time, he reported that if the does were immunized against an allotype of the bucks (in the original report, b5), the maternal isoantibodies to the b5 type affected the ability of the developing young to express that allotype in the serum. Compensatory increased levels of the alternative allelic type, b4, appeared in the sera of these animals. Our work with Dray confirmed these findings and provided additional quantitative information about this phenomenon, named "allotype-suppression" (8).

The effect of maternal antibody on the

phenotypic expression of the b5 allotype lasts for at least three years. The data presented in Table 1 were obtained using a microquantitative precipitin method for the determination of the quantities of b4- and b5-immunoglobulins in the offspring of a b4 mother making anti-b5 mated with a b5 father. The b4 and b5 contents of the sera are calculated as per cent of b4+b5 immunoglobulin rather than as per cent of γG-immunoglobulin in the serum, although we always estimated this independently using either a sheep anti-γG or goat anti-Fc-fragment antiserum. The tube diffusion method of Oudin (12) was also used for the analysis of similar offspring of immunized mothers, and most recently, a modified radial diffusion method in gel (6, 9, 10, 11) has been employed for determinations of total γG and allotype contents of sera. Normal b4b5 heterozygotes generally have 20-40% b5 and 60-80% b4, but the offspring of the immunized mother (Table 1) were making less than 6% of b5 even at two to three years of age. The total γG and the b4 + b5 levels in animals suppressed for the b5 allotype were indistinguishable from the levels found in normal animals so that in this situation increased b4 levels appear to have compensated for decreased b5 levels.

Exposure of heterozygous offspring to anti-b5 at birth was sufficient to produce an effect upon the expression of the b5 allotype. Fig. 1

TABLE 1.—EFFECT OF MATERNAL ANTI-b5 UPON EXPRESSION OF ALLELIC b4 AND b5 ALLOTYPES IN HETEROZYGOUS OFFSPRING

Animal	Age months	b5 / b4+b5	b4 / b4+b5	b4+b5*	γG†
		%	%	mg N/ml	mg N/ml
14FZ-4	5	0.6	99.4	1.01	1.1
-5		0.3	99.7	1.25	1.4
-4	12	1.3	98.7	1.22	1.3
-5		1.4	98.6	2.03	2.1
-4	23	5.8	94.2	1.91	2.2
-5		1.6	98.2	1.93	1.7
-4	26	4.6	95.4	2.41	1.9
-5		2.0	98.0	1.53	1.7
-5	35	5.1	94.9	4.32	5.5

*Sum of separate determinations of b4 and b5 using microquantitative precipitin method.
†Independent determination of γG using microquantitative precipitin method. Although there is often close agreement between total γG and b4+b5 values, there are several reasons why one should not expect them to be identical. In both heterozygotes and homozygotes, some γG molecules appear to lack determinants controlled by the b locus (b negative molecules); the per cent is variable but averages approximately 15% (1, 3, 7, and 8). In addition, immunoglobulins other than γG may precipitate with our antisera. Finally, there are inherent analytical errors in each of the independent determinations. These considerations have been discussed in detail (8).

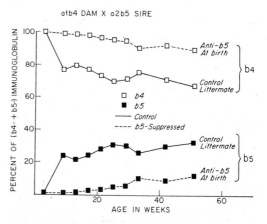

FIG. 1. The b4 and b5 levels in a non-injected littermate and in one of three animals which received 1 ml of antiserum containing 0.9 mg precipitable anti-b5 antibody protein at birth. Antigen concentrations were determined by a microquantitative precipitin method.

shows the development of the normal b5 levels by a control animal and the suppressed development of b5 in its littermate which received anti-b5. Although total γG-immunoglobulin levels varied greatly from time to time during the first year of life in these animals, the relative allotype contents were maintained with a striking constancy. In this mating, the father was of the a2 allotype and the mother a1. The injected antiserum happened to have been made in an $a^1a^2b^4b^4$ animal so that some paternal type a2 antigen was injected when we injected the anti-b5 antiserum. The a1 and a2 levels in two of the injected animals and in their non-injected littermate were measured using the radial diffusion method (Fig. 2). Whereas the control

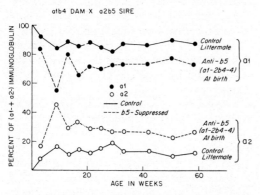

FIG. 2. The a1 and a2 levels in a non-injected littermate and in one of three animals which received 1 ml of anti-b5 antiserum. The antiserum contained paternal a2 antigen, approximately 2 mg/ml. Antigen concentrations were determined by a radial diffusion method in gel.

animal developed 10-20% a2, the two injected animals maintained levels of 20-30% a2. This suggests that possibly the composition of the passively received immunoglobulin present in the young animal during its first month of life has a lasting effect upon the relative levels at which the allelic allotypes are expressed; perhaps some feedback mechanism is initiated at the time of commencement of immunoglobulin production. Attempts are underway to test these possibilities experimentally.

The possible priming effect of the antigenic composition of the serum during the early weeks of life was also suggested when the b4b5 heterozygous offspring of

a b5 dam and b4 sire were studied. A tendency was noted for normal control offspring to maintain average b5 levels slightly higher than similar offspring of b4 mothers, but a sufficient number of such heterozygotes has not been studied to consider the difference significant. As shown in Fig. 3, for the first few weeks the normal offspring of such a b5 mother have large relative amounts of maternal b5. This decreases and the paternal b4 appears during the first 10 weeks. A littermate which received anti-b4 antiserum soon after birth (5 mg of precipitable anti-b4 antibody protein) maintained strikingly higher b5 levels and lower b4 levels (Fig. 3). Again in this situation, suppression of the b4 allotype did not appear to affect the total γG-immunoglobulin levels in the serum.

Using sensitive microprecipitin determinations of antigen concentrations, a quantitative rather than all-or-none nature of the "allotype-suppression" phenomenon was demonstrated by the time the affected animals were eight or nine weeks old. The normal control littermates in the mating of a b5 dam and b4 sire (Fig. 3) expressed the paternal b4 type as early as three weeks of age. At eight weeks the paternal type in the "allotype-suppressed" animals was detected but in concentrations (2-6 μgN/ml) representing about 0.4% of the total b4+b5 immunoglobulin, instead of the 53 and 61% b4 found in two controls.

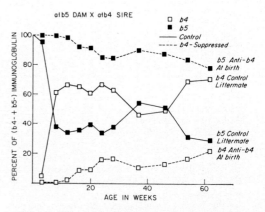

FIG. 3. The b4 and b5 levels in a non-injected littermate and in an animal injected with 5 ml of anti-b4 antiserum containing approximately 5 mg of precipitable anti-b4 antibody protein. Antigen concentrations were determined by a microquantitative precipitin method.

Information about the persistence of the injected antiserum was obtained by using an anti-b4 antiserum containing an a2 allotypic marker not present in either parent. When anti-b4 antiserum containing approximately 50 mg of immunoglobulin with a2 marker was injected at birth, precipitable a2 was still detectable six weeks later, but in a concentration ($<20\mu gN/ml$) probably representing less than 2% of the originally injected protein. By this time anti-b4 activity was apparently no longer present in the circulation since b4 antigen was already detectable.

It is clear then, that the products of allelic genes are found in the sera of heterozygous rabbits at controlled but not necessarily equal levels. The relative quantities of a1 and a2 are the most unequal found so far in non-injected animals. Three of the four animals listed in Table 2 are normal heterozygous offspring of an a1b4 mother. The fourth received anti-b5 antiserum at birth. In all of them, a1 is the major component with a2 representing 8-16% of the total. These values are similar to the 10-20% values found for a control littermate from a similar mating shown in Fig. 2. These animals were all offspring of homozygous a1 mothers. The question whether maternal a2 antigen or early exposure to passively administered a2 antigen will have an effect upon the subsequent expression of the a1 and a2 alleles is under investigation.

In recent experiments analogous to those described involving allotypes of the *b* locus (9), suppression of the expression of one of allelic genes at the *a* locus was found in heterozygous offspring of mothers, actively producing anti-a1, -a2, or -a3, mated with a buck of the appropriate type. In this system the alternative allele which is not suppressed accounts for most of the γG-immunoglobulin found in the sera, but it may turn out that the compensation is not entirely successful in maintaining normal γG-immunoglobulin levels. To be sure of this large numbers of "allotype-suppressed" and normal animals of similar background must be studied, in view of the large variability in serum γG-immunoglobulin

TABLE 2.—EXPRESSION OF ALLELIC GENES AT TWO LOCI IN NORMAL AND "ALLOTYPE-SUPPRESSED" DOUBLY HETEROZYGOUS OFFSPRING OF A NON-IMMUNIZED MOTHER. 45FZ-6 INJECTED WITH ANTI-b5 AT BIRTH

Animal	Age months	$\frac{b5}{b4+b5}$	$\frac{b4}{b4+b5}$	$\frac{a2}{a1+a2}$	$\frac{a1}{a1+a2}$	b4+b5*	a1+a2†
		%	%	%	%	mg N/ml	mg N/ml
45FZ-3	13	39	61	13	87	1.3	1.3
-5		35	65	14	86	1.2	1.2
-6		7	93	14	86	0.7	0.7
-7		39	61	14	86	1.6	1.4
-5	20	28	72	16	84	1.4	1.2
-6		6	94	12	88	0.7	0.7
-7		36	64	15	85	1.7	1.9
-5	35	28	72	9	91	3.2	4.1
-6		10	90	9	91	2.1	2.2
-3	38	27	73	8	92	2.2	2.6
-5		30	70	8	92	3.2	3.6
-6		10	90	10	90	1.7	2.0
-7		19	81	9	91	2.0	2.2
-3	42	31	69	13	87	3.0	4.3
-5		34	66	9	91	3.3	4.6
-6		13	87	9	91	1.9	2.4
-7		21	79	10	90	2.4	2.7

*Sum of separate determinations of b4 and b5 using the radial diffusion method in gel (see text).

†Independent sum of separate determinations of a1 and a2 using the radial diffusion method in gel.

levels among different rabbits and in the same rabbit at different times. The *a* locus determinants are associated with the *heavy* chains of the immunoglobulins, under the control of genes apparently unlinked to those of the *b* locus. Since the products of these two loci are assembled into a single molecule of immunoglobulin, it is possible that an effect upon the expression of alleles at one locus will influence the control of levels of allelic products of the other locus.

CONCLUSION

Studies to date demonstrate that there is in the rabbit a remarkable control of the relative quantities of total immunoglobulin which are

of a given allelic allotype. The level at which this control is exerted is not clear. As Cebra discussed in the preceding paper there is increasing evidence that the serum immunoglobulins that we are measuring are being produced by cells differentiated to produce only one of alternative types. If this is indeed so, then the number of cells differentiating in one of the alternative directions is reflected in the serum levels. The problem then becomes one of determining what chemical information directs a given cell toward one alternative rather than the other.

Acknowledgment.—The interest and collaboration of Dr. Sheldon Dray and Miss Glendowlyn O. Young are gratefully acknowledged.

REFERENCES

1. Bornstein, P., and Oudin, J. (1964): A study of rabbit γ-globulin allotypy by means of heteroimmunizations. J. Exp. Med. *120*, 655.
2. Dray, S. (1962): Effect of maternal isoantibodies on the quantitative expression of two allelic genes controlling the γ-globulin allotypic specificities. Nature (London) *195*, 677.
3. Dray, S., and Nisonoff, A. (1965): Relationship of genetic control of allotypic specificities to the structure and biosynthesis of rabbit γ-globulin, in: Molecular and Cellular Basis of Antibody Formation. Proceedings of a Symposium Held in Prague on June 1-5, 1964. New York, Academic Press, 1965, p. 175.
4. Dray, S., Young, G. O., and Gerald, L. (1963): Immunochemical identification and genetics of rabbit γ-globulin allotypes. J. Immun. *91*, 403.
5. Dray, S., Young, G. O., and Nisonoff, A. (1963): Distribution of allotypic specificities among rabbit γ-globulin molecules defined at two loci. Nature (London) *199*, 52.
6. Fahey, J. L., and McKelvey, E. M. (1965): Quantitative determination of serum immunoglobulins in antibody-agar plates. J. Immun. *94*, 84.
7. Leskowitz, S. (1963): Immunochemical study of rabbit γ-globulin allotypes. J. Immun. *90*, 98.
8. Mage, R., and Dray, S. (1965): Persistent altered phenotypic expression of allelic γG-immunoglobulin allotypes in heterozygous rabbits exposed to isoantibodies in fetal and neonatal life. J.

Immunol. *95*, 525.
9. Mage, R., Young, G. O., and Dray, S.: In preparation.
10. Mancini, G., Carbonara, A. O., and Heremans, J. F. (1965): Immunochemical quantitation of antigens by single radial immunodiffusion. Immunochem. *2*, 235.
11. Mancini, G., Vaerman, J. P., Carbonara, A. O., and Heremans, J. F. (1964): A single-radial-diffusion method for the immunological quantitation of proteins, in: Protides of the Biological Fluids, 1963. Proceedings of the Eleventh Colloquium, Bruges, 1963. Elsevier Pub. Co.
12. Oudin, J. (1952): Methods in Medical Research, Vol. 5. Corcoran, A. C., ed.: Specific Precipitation in Gels and its Application to Immunochemical Analysis. Chicago, Ill., The Yearbook Publishers, Inc., p. 335.
13. Reisfeld, R. A., Dray, S., and Nisonoff, A. (1965): Differences in amino acid composition of rabbit γG-immunoglobulin light polypeptide chains controlled by allelic genes. Immunochem. *2*, 155.
14. Small, P. A., Jr., Reisfeld, R. A., and Dray, S. (1965): Peptide differences of rabbit γG-immunoglobulin light chains controlled by allelic genes. J. Molec. Biol. *11*, 713.
15. Wainer, A., Robbins, J., Bellanti, J., Eitzman, D., and Smith, R. T. (1963): Synthesis of gamma-globulin in the newborn rabbit. Nature (London) *198*, 487.

DISCUSSION

HIRSCHHORN: The observations from your suppression experiments can be explained either by assuming that those cells which were potentially capable of producing a given allotypic marker have been lost from the animals or by assuming that these cells still survive, but are not producing their product. In the latter case, presumably other cells are making a compensatory amount of γ-globulin of the allotype not suppressed.

In the cases where only 5% of the suppressed allotype can be detected, I wonder whether an attempt to transform cells by the method of Sell and Gell, using antibody to that allotype, would show only 5% transformed cells. If a significantly greater per cent of cells were transformed this would indicate that the cells potentially capable of making the allotype were still present but were not functioning.

Which explanation of the observations do you consider most likely? Also, concerning the compensatory rise in γ-globulin of the allotype not suppressed, do you think that more cells are present making this allotype or that the normal number of cells are making protein at an increased rate or with a longer half-life?

MAGE: I think the most likely explanation will be, in the first instance, that the different levels of the two allotypes directly reflect the relative numbers of cells capable of making the respective proteins. It is probable that we are observing a feedback mechanism of some kind which determines the direction of cellular differentiation from undifferentiated cells which have the potential to develop into producers of either allotype.

CEBRA: Hirschhorn's suggestion to quantitate cellular transformation in suppressed animals with anti-allotype sera seems quite appropriate. There seems to be a relationship between your ability to immunologically suppress the expression of the paternal allotype very early in a rabbit's life and the ability of Sell and Gell to transform cells of a heterozygote early in life with antibody to the paternal allotype, even before molecules of this allotype are detectable in the circulation. It would seem that the cells may already be committed soon after birth to the production of a particular allotype and they may already be "marked" with its antigenic determinants.

MAGE: Sell and Gell's experiments were done when the expression of the father's allotype was already apparent in the serum, although its demonstration would require a more sensitive assay than Dray originally used for this purpose.

HIRSCHHORN: In the injection of anti-b5 serum you are also injecting b4 molecules which carry the antibody specificity. What happens if you inject an equivalent amount of b4 globulin without anti-b5 activity?

MAGE: When we inject one milliliter of anti-allotype serum we are adding to the newborn only about 20% more of the b4 molecules it has already obtained from the maternal circulation. However, we are now examining the effects of allotype levels in the newborn on its own expression of allotypes.

GOOD: It is not clear to me whether or not you can prolong the suppression of the suppressed allotype by administering additional antiserum against the suppressed allotype of γ-globulin. In the converse, can you speed up the recovery of the normal allotype balance by administration early in life of the allotype of γ-globulin which has been suppressed? There is a clinical situation that may be remotely related. I am referring here to a transient form of hypogammaglobulinemia of infancy. In this condition a delay occurs in γ-globulin synthesis which may be quite long lasting, in many instances more than a year. Hugh Fudenberg presented evidence to indicate that mothers of babies with this syndrome may have γ-globulins that differ in Gm allotype from those of the offspring. The mother is postulated to be immunized against her offspring's Gm allotype, analogous to erythroblastosis fetalis. In several such families Fudenberg found the mother and baby to be different in Gm γ-globulin allotypes and also found the mother to have anti-γ-globulin antibodies. Further studies of these relationships are surely indicated.

MAGE: The pertinent experiments have not yet been carried out using rabbits.

PETERSON: To your knowledge, has anyone tested the effect of antibody to an enzyme upon the ability of an inducer to call forth that enzyme?

MAGE: Presumably you have in mind the

tryptophan pyrrolase system as it is affected by the administration of tryptophan. I don't believe the effect of antibody to the enzyme has been assessed in this system.

HILDEMANN: Assuming interallelic suppression at autosomal loci, the effect of passive antibody in causing suppression of the corresponding allotype is reminiscent of serotype transformation in ciliate protozoans. Do you have any basis for knowing whether this suppression is reversible? Does the suppression persist in the absence of residual anti-allotype antibody?

MAGE: Presumably the suppressed level of an allotype is maintained not by residual antibody, but perhaps by the continual production of immunoglobulin being controlled by the existing relative antigen levels of b4 and b5 molecules in the serum. This mechanism would require a specific kind of feedback of marked molecules. The antiserum's effect would be to remove the paternal markers in a critical period of early life and the continued presence of the anti-allotype molecules would not be necessary to maintain the effect.

CEBRA: You described a compensatory rise in molecules of the allotype not suppressed. Is there a concomitant rise in molecules without detectable allotypic markers, the so-called "b-negative" molecules?

MAGE: It is difficult to quantitate b-negative molecules. However, we have no evidence of a rise in these molecules upon suppression, using the similarity of values for concentration of b4 molecules relative to either total γ-globulin or b4 plus b5 as a criterion.

MITCHISON: The question arises whether the choice of allotype made by a heterozygous cell is irreversible. If it is, then the kinetics of recovery from suppression should be precisely the same as the kinetics of recovery from tolerance. You would then expect (a) faster recovery in younger animals, (b) no effect of x-radiation, and (c) slower recovery after thymectomy. If it is reversible, you should see faster recovery after hyperimmunization.

MAGE: Thus far we have done experiments directed only to your last point. We have immunized both normal and suppressed b4/b5 heterozygotes with arsanilic acid conjugated to edestin. We then purified the anti-hapten antibodies by the immuno-absorbent method and recovered a large proportion of the antibody detectable in the serum by precipitation. Although the normal animal and the animal suppressed for b4 molecules had milligrams of antibody per ml of serum, the allotype markers were present in the antibody in about the same relative amounts as in the serum before immunization.

MIESCHER: H. Numbel tried some 5 years ago to produce agammaglobulinemic rabbits by injecting anti-gammaglobulin-serum to newborn rabbits. It may be worthwhile using your system and to try to suppress not only part of γG, but all of it, by administering both anti-b4 and anti-b5 serum. This may become a model of a- or hypogammaglobulinemia, as postulated by Numbel.

MAGE: This model is presently under investigation, using b4/b5 rabbit mothers in which b5 is depressed and b5/b5 male rabbits. The offspring b5/b5 which do not contain much of the maternal b5 will be treated with anti-b5.

PART III

EMBRYONIC DEVELOPMENT OF FORM AND FUNCTION OF THE LYMPHORETICULAR SYSTEM

12

EDWIN L. COOPER

Some aspects of the histogenesis of the amphibian lymphomyeloid system and its role in immunity

THE DEVELOPMENT AND MAINTENANCE of immune competence is dependent in part upon the thymus, formerly an organ of mysterious function. It is found in the more primitive fishes as a loosely disorganized aggregation of lymphoid cells, while in the higher vertebrates thus far examined it has a well-defined cortical and medullary region (21). In mammals, the thymus has recently been examined with respect to morphogenetic interactions occurring during its development (3) and its role in the maturation of the immune response capacity (33, 34). In birds, immunity to cellular antigens (e.g., skin grafts) is controlled by the thymus, while the bursa of Fabricius, another lymphoid organ located in the cloacal region, appears to be involved in immunity to soluble and particulate antigens (2, 23).

Thus, active work from several approaches is being directed towards an understanding of the role of the thymus and other lymphoid aggregations in homothermic vertebrates (15, 20). Yet the older literature reveals a considerable number of accurate investigations involving the thymus and other lymphomyeloid organs in poikilotherms. For example, some of the earlier descriptions of the thymus, its later influence on the peripheral centers, and its role as a possible source of all lymphoid cells were described from studies of the cartilaginous fish, *Raja batis,* by Beard (5) while others dealt with the nature of the interactions of precursor cells in the differentiation of the thymus in Amphibia (16, 17, 30). Neverthe-

less, these detailed studies were strictly morphological and they can profitably be re-examined in light of newer concepts relative to the development of lymphoid organs and immune competence.

Several structures in bullfrogs which, for lack of better terminology, will be referred to as lymphomyeloid organs have been studied recently. The microscopic anatomy of these organs suggests their involvement in the immune response like analogous structures in homotherms. From the studies of Kent *et al.* (27) it appears that structures in a similar anatomic position in *Bufo marinus* are involved in antibody synthesis. The term "lymphomyeloid" to describe specific organs like the thymus, spleen, bone marrow, or perhaps the liver and kidney will not be employed here even though these structures, at some time during the life of the bullfrog, function in hemopoiesis. This use of the term "lymphomyeloid" is supported by observations of von Braunmühl (7) and Yoffey (44).

The term lympho-epithelial will be used to denote the cells of these organs exclusive of the reticulo-endothelial cells, while the organs themselves will be referred to generally as lymphomyeloid with an occasional reference to specific names employed by earlier investigators.

Von Braunmühl's review of lymphomyeloid and lympho-epithelial organs mentions that "the corpus propericardiale and corpus procoracoidale were examined for the first time

87

by Gaupp" (19). He described the corpus pro-pericardiale, observed by Simon (38), as "a thymus lying on the pericardium next to other pericardial fat conglomerations, or a lymphoid structure of young frogs, which supposedly in its morphological formation resembles the so-called ventral gill remnant (jugular body). It retrogresses in earlier post-larval development under assumption of fat, its origin is unclear and it is a richly vascularized organ permeated with cells."

"Fleische (18) and Toldt (41) believed with Mayer (31) that the jugular body is a lymphocyte-forming organ and they categorized it with the lymph glands of mammals, structures which they assumed were not found in frogs. Similarly, Krause (28) thought that the jugular body was analogous to the lymphatic system of mammals. As in mammalian lymph glands he found a strand-like parenchyma which proved to be a reticulum with lymphocytic elements. Of these lymphocytes he only separated the large reticulum cells with chromatin-poorer nuclei from the small cells with a compact lymphocytic nucleus. Krause assumed the function of this body to be the formation of lymphocytes which then reach the blood by diapedesis. He did not present any newer information regarding the development of this organ, but only added, probably in support of Maurer (29), that they originated by the retrogression of the gills during metamorphosis."

Yoffey (44) defined the lymphomyeloid complex as the total mass of tissue concerned with the formation of blood cells, and also to a large extent with antibody formation. It is found throughout the vertebrate series. In the cyclostomes, for example, one can speak of a true lymphomyeloid complex where lymphoid and myeloid elements are closely intermingled. In the higher fishes the thymus and spleen are separate organs developmentally. The next big step in the evolution of the lymphomyeloid complex occurs in Amphibia where the bone marrow first appears as a clear-cut entity. Yoffey further cited the observations by other workers that only in birds and mammals does one find typical lymphoid tissues, in the form of lymph glands in mammals, and diffuse lymphoid deposits in birds.

The purpose of this presentation is to review some aspects of the embryogenesis of the thymus in the Anura and to consider the function of the thymus in American bullfrog (*Rana catesbeiana*) larvae, and leopard frog (*Rana pipiens*) adults. Finally, a historical survey of the lymphomyeloid organs in the Amphibia will be presented emphasizing observations of their structure during larval and adult stages of *R. catesbeiana*.

EXPERIMENTAL PROCEDURES

General.—*R. catesbeiana* and *R. pipiens* were obtained in all stages (newly hatched larvae to sexually mature adults) from Brescia's Animal Farm, Compton, California. Larvae were maintained according to the procedures outlined by Hildemann and Haas (26). A large wooden tank provided with constantly running water housed the adult bullfrogs which were fed small live rodents; the adult *R. pipiens* were kept in tubs and fed meal worms. An adult Caecilian, *Typhlonectes compressicauda* (Apoda), was obtained from South America by the Hermosa Reptile Farm, Hermosa Beach, California (identified by Philip J. Regal, Department of Zoology, UCLA) and kept in the same manner as the frog larvae (37).

Histology.—Tissues were removed and fixed in 10% neutral formalin, sectioned at 5-7 μ, and stained with hematoxylin and eosin. Larvae were anesthetized in MS 222 (tricane methanesulfonate 42 mg/L) prior to fixation, while ether was used to anesthetize the adults (Anura and Apoda). Blood smears were made in the usual manner and prepared with Wright's blood stain. Intraperitoneal injections of bullfrog larvae and adults with India ink in a 1:1 dilution (0.05-0.1 cc) were made to facilitate visualization of the lymphomyeloid organs.

Thymectomy.—The technique of removing the thymus from young bullfrog larvae has been described earlier (12). Thymectomy of adult *R. pipiens* and *R. catesbeiana* involved making a narrow incision with a sharp sterile scalpel on the posterior edge of the tympanic membrane and removing the thymus from the surrounding musculature. The open area was sprayed with tetracycline and the wound closed with two sutures.

Skin grafting.—The successful techniques for exchanging skin allografts between bullfrog larvae were developed by Hildemann and

Haas (26) and have been used throughout these investigations on both larval and adult anurans. The method for skin grafting Caecilians (10) was similar to that described for Anura except that the grafts were sutured in place.

Irradiation.—In order to understand the role of the adult anuran thymus and to look for a possible relationship between the thymus and bone marrow, an experiment using adult *R. pipiens* was performed. Frogs were exposed to doses of Cobalt-60 γ-irradiation ranging from 750 r to 5,000 r. Since syngeneic marrow for protection is not available in this species, the right hind limb was either shielded completely or partially so that each shielded leg received approximately 20 r. Skin allografts were exchanged five days after irradiation, a time when lymphocyte levels in irradiated frogs were lowest (39). Animals thymectomized prior to irradiation were replanted subcutaneously with autogeneic thymus glands (750 r-3,000 r), but the thymus was not removed in another group irradiated at 5,000 r. Certain histological parameters have not been determined yet, i.e., condition of replanted thymus glands, estimation of the number of bone marrow cells, and condition of other organs, nor were the frogs challenged with other antigens.

CHANGES IN THE STRUCTURE OF THE
THYMUS IN *Rana catesbeiana* DURING
DEVELOPMENT AND MATURATION

Larvae (2-10 days posthatching, stages 24-25).—At 2-4 days the thymus primordium (Figs. 1-4) is composed of a homogeneous mass of basophilic lympho-epithelial cells ventral to the developing ear and separated from the outer epidermis by a layer of pigment cells. It is surrounded by a loose collection of mesenchymal cells, and acidophilic yolk droplets are found interspersed between the epithelial components. At this time the primordium is still connected to the entodermal epithelium of the pharynx. Only a few cells in the thymus were dividing while numerous cells in the surrounding connective tissue were in active mitosis.

At 5-10 days the thymus epithelium and the

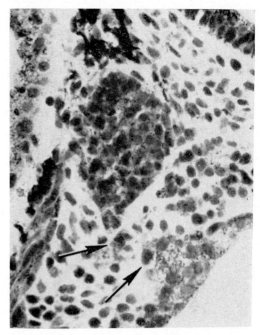

FIG. 1. Transverse section through the head of a bullfrog tadpole at stages 24-25, 2 days posthatching. The thymus primordium is composed of numerous lympho-epithelial cells and interspersed between them are pigment cells and yolk granules. Note the region indicated by the arrow which shows the connection between thymic cells and pharyngeal epithelium. The epithelium of the developing ear is seen at the left. x 640

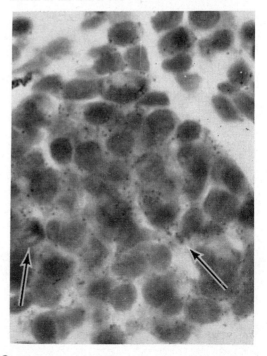

FIG. 2. The thymus here is taken from a tadpole during the same stage as Fig. 1. Note the mitotic figure and the pigment granules. x 1600

89

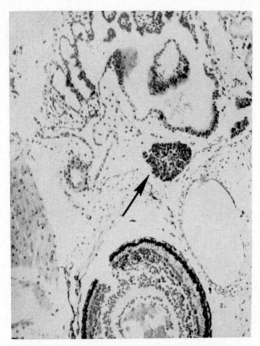

FIG. 3. This section represents a tadpole at 4 days posthatching stages 24-25. Note the location of the thymus and its relationship to the eye, ear, and pharyngeal epithelium. Developing head muscles can be seen in the lower portion of the section. x 160

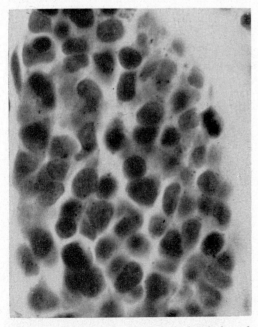

FIG. 4. Frontal section through the head of a tadpole 4 days posthatching. A comparison with Fig. 2 reveals an increased cellular basophilia during the older stages. x 1500

pharyngeal epithelium are less associated than at earlier stages (Figs. 5-11). Moreover, yolk and pigment stores decrease, while the number of dividing lympho-epithelial cells increases. Another feature at this period is the presence of three cellular types: large lymphocytes, lymphoblasts, and epithelial cells. Small thymocytes were not observed at this time. The thymus at 7 days has increased in mass as evidenced by an abundance of mitotic figures. There is further differentiation into the various cell types with cortical cells appearing toward the periphery and medullary material at the center. It is surrounded by mesenchymal cells and variable amounts of pigment cells. At 8 days the basophilia in the outer region of the thymus increased and the first indications of lobulation in the cortical region were observed. At 9 days the division into two regions, i.e., cortex and medulla, was plainly seen, and dividing thymocytes were still present around the periphery. Generally, however, the number of mitotic figures appeared to be less than on previous days. At 10 days the essential features were the same as those of the 9th day.

Larvae (36-51 days posthatching, stage 25). —At this stage there is a division into capsule, cortex, and medulla. With this distinction, a further separation into the definitive cell types of the organ occurs which is not as clearly defined as the condition in later larval stages (6-24 months). The thin mesenchyme surrounding the parenchyma has thickened and the framework of reticular cells and fibers can be distinguished.

Cortex.—In the cortex there is a large number of thymocytes in comparison with older larvae and adults. In the medulla, thymocytes of all sizes are present, as well as reticular cells and lymphoblasts. An occasional macrophage can be found but far fewer mitotic figures were present when compared with earlier stages (Fig. 12).

Bullfrog larvae 6-24 months posthatching, early metamorphic frogs, stages 25-33, and sexually mature adults.—The condition of the thymus (Figs. 21, 22) during these three stages is essentially the same except that with increasing age there is a corresponding decrease in lymphoid cells in the cortex, an increase in the collagenous connective tissue in the medulla, and the appearance of a greater number of blood vessels throughout both regions. For

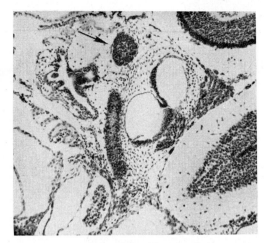

FIG. 5. At 5 days posthatching the thymus can be seen, in this section, in close proximity to the eye, ear, and gill epithelium. x 160

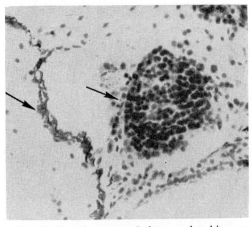

FIG. 7. The thymus at 6 days posthatching can be seen in relation to the outer epidermis and the pigment layer. Note the mesenchymal cells surrounding the thymus. x 384

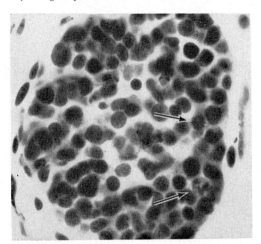

FIG. 6. At 5 days posthatching mitotic figures increase and there is differentiation into an outer darker staining area and an inner lighter region. x 1500

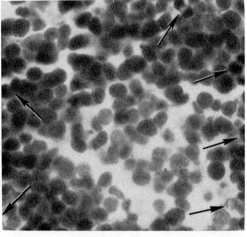

FIG. 8. A greater number of mitotic figures were observed at 6 days posthatching than earlier periods. The dividing cells are located primarily in the outermost region. x 1250

the sake of brevity, therefore, one general description will suffice for all three stages.

The whole organ is surrounded by a connective tissue capsule consisting of collagen fibers and fibroblasts, and at points surrounding it, the connective tissue penetrates deep into the parenchyma separating the cortex and medulla into smaller lobules (20-30/lobe). Usually accompanying these partitions are capillaries that take a tortuous course, especially in the medulla. The entire framework of the thymus is composed of reticular cells and fibers which may be recognized faintly with hema-

toxylin and eosin in the cortex between a greater number of thymocytes, but in the medulla where thymocytes are fewer the reticular elements appear predominantly.

Medulla.—Found in the medulla in addition to the usual reticular cells are a number of pale staining hyalinized corpuscles which are numerous and appear as structures analogous to Hassall's corpuscles in mammals. These bodies are acidophilic with a lamellar arrangement encircling a pale blue region, possibly the remaining nucleus of a reticular cell (Figs. 12-13).

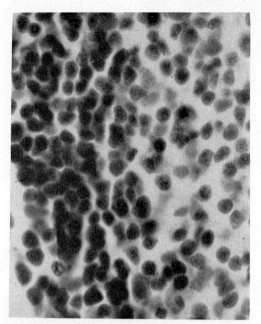

FIG. 9. At 8 days posthatching there is further distinction into cortex and medulla. x 1000

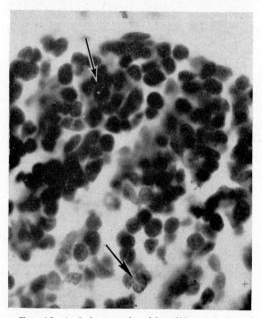

FIG. 10. At 9 days posthatching differentiation of cortical lymphocytes and reticular cells of the medulla is obvious. x 1000

ROLE OF THE THYMUS IN IMMUNITY IN *Rana catesbeiana* LARVAE

Investigations aimed at understanding the function of the thymus in Amphibia closely

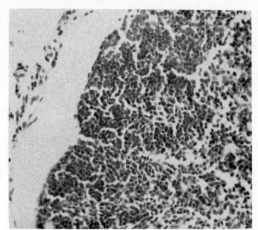

FIG. 11. At 32 days posthatching the thymus now contains typical cellular components and can be divided into cortex and medulla. Some of the capsule can be viewed extending down into the cortical lobules. x 384.

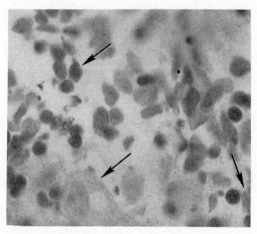

FIG. 12. The section represents part of the thymic medulla of a tadpole 6-24 months of age. Note the reticular elements and the sparse number of lymphoid cells in this region. In the lower portion of the figure note the hyalinized structure that resembles a Hassall's corpuscle. x 360

paralleled those in mammals and other vertebrates, i.e., the great interest during the latter part of the nineteenth century centered on morphology and description. Early work was not concerned with immunity, rather the role of the thymus in amphibians emphasized (a) its retrogression during later stages (36), (b) its essential role in the maintenance of life, especially during the adult stages (24), and (c) its possible function as an endocrine organ and its relation to other endocrines (1).

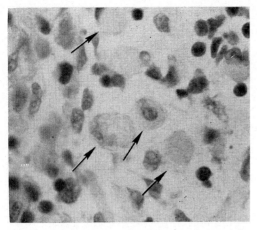

FIG. 13. Medullary region in the thymus of a sexually mature adult bullfrog. Note the numerous hyalinized bodies which appear to be different stages in the development of structures analogous to Hassall's corpuscles. x 1500

pared to sham-thymectomized controls. Thymectomy after 30 days appeared not to affect skin allograft survival but did weaken the immune response to diverse soluble antigens. Table 1 summarizes the effect of thymectomy on skin allograft survival in bullfrog larvae. The results again agree with earlier observations that the first month is the period in larval life when the thymus exerts its greatest influence.

REGENERATION OF THE THYMUS IN BULLFROG LARVAE

In bullfrog larvae, no attempts have been made yet to examine experimentally the possibility that the thymus will regenerate when completely or partially extirpated or whether the contralateral organ will undergo compensatory hypertrophy after removal of the opposite one. Yet after performing numerous thymectomies prior to skin grafting in young larvae and executing later biopsies, thymic tissue was found in varying amounts in animals in which thymectomy had been complete. Table 2 summarizes the condition of the thymus in a group of tadpoles which had been previously thymectomized. Thus, assuming that regeneration of the thymus can occur in bullfrog larvae, it might be expected that im-

A first attempt was made to define the role of the thymus in immunity in anuran amphibians by using bullfrog larvae (9, 12). These studies revealed that larvae thymectomized during the first month of life showed a prolonged survival of skin allografts when com-

TABLE 1.—PRESENCE OF THYMIC TISSUE IN PREVIOUSLY THYMECTOMIZED BULLFROG LARVAE

Number of Tadpoles	Age at Thymectomy in Days	Condition of the Thymus at Biopsy*				
		Unilateral		Bilateral		Absent
		Left	Right	Left	Right	
2	16-35			++	+	
1	16-35		+			
2	20-31			+	+	
1	20-31					0
1	20-31		+++			
2	20-31			+++	+++	
1	20-31			+	+	
1	20-31		++			
2	20-31		++			
1	20-31	++				
3	27-40			++	+	
5	27-40			++	++	
3	27-40			+	+	
1	27-40		+			
1	27-40			+++	+++	

*Age of bullfrog larvae at biopsy was 222-227 days posthatching.
+ = 1/3 present
++ = 2/3 present
+++ = present entirely
0 = absent

TABLE 2.—SUMMARY OF THE RELATIONSHIP BETWEEN THYMECTOMY,
THYMIC REGENERATION AND SKIN ALLOGRAFT SURVIVAL IN BULLFROG LARVAE

Animal Number	Larval Age at Thymectomy (Days)	Larval Age at Skin Grafting (Days)	Condition of Thymus at Biopsy		First Set Skin* Graft Survival (Days)			Second Set‡ Skin Graft Survival (Days)		
			Left	Right	<10	10-23	>23	<5	5-10	>10
1	20-31	125-130	+++	+++			>50			
2	20-31	145-155	0	+++			>35			
3	20-31	125-140	+	+			(28)		(5)	
4	27-40	130-150	0	0			>45#			
5	20-31	125-140	++	++			(26)		(9)	
6	27-40	130-150	0	0			(24)			
7	27-40	130-150	0	0			>45#			
8	27-40	145-155	0	0			>35#			
9	20-31	125-130	0	+++		(19)			(7)	
10	27-40	125-140	++	++		(19)			(5)	
11	27-40	130-150	0	0		(16)				
12	27-40	125-140	++	++		(14)			(7)	
13	27-40	130-150	+	+		(14)			(8)	
14	20-31	145-155	0	++		(12)			(7)	
15	27-40	130-150	0	++		(13)			(9)	
16	20-31	145-155	0	0		(11)				
17	27-40	130-150	0	+	(9)					
18	20-31	145-155	0	0	(8)					
19	20-31	145-155	0	0	(7)					(9)§
20	20-31	145-155	0	+	(7)			(3)		
21	27-40	145-155	0	+	(7)					
22	20-31	120-140	+	++	(7)				(2)	
23	20-31	120-140	+++	+++	(5)			(3)		

Note: The survival times greatly exceeded the 95% confidence limits (>2D). The MSTS with their 95% confidence limits reflect subacute rejection of numerous grafts with time mortality distributions skewed to the right. Thus, the upper confidence limits are higher and the standard deviations are generally greater than previously found in non-thymectomized larvae after 70 days of age (12, 26).

#Grafts still intact, no biopsy performed.

*First set range of survival times (days) 5 to >50 days. Median survival time (days) ± SE, 10.2 ± 3.0. SD = 7.

‡Second set range of survival time (days) 2 to 9. Median survival time (days) ± SE, 5.3 ± 0.2. SD = 6.7.

mune competence would be restored after regeneration. Of the eight tadpoles with prolonged graft survival times, four had no thymus present on later biopsy and three still had grafts intact; the risk of trauma from biopsy was not taken, instead the tadpoles were left undisturbed which had grafts with obvious prolonged survival times.

RELATIONSHIP OF BONE MARROW AND IMMUNITY IN ADULT Rana pipiens

Investigations involving certain mammals have shown that the thymus influences the differentiation of the lymphoid system during early stages in development. Similarly, thy-

mectomized adult mice were incapable of reacting to a variety of antigens after their immune system was damaged by lethal doses of irradiation (33). Thus, the reorganization of a damaged immune system during adult stages is apparently thymus dependent. In an attempt to ascertain whether the adult amphibian thymus influences the immune system after damage by total body irradiation, an experiment was designed using adult frogs.

Median survival time (MST) of skin allografts (700 r-3,000 r) was approximately 13 days in the control group (sham-operated, unirradiated) and 17 days in one experimental group (marrow protected, irradiated). Even though these experimental animals were severely debilitated as a result of irradiation (half died by 35 days) the remaining survivors were still capable of rejecting skin allografts, with a slight delay, in an apparently normal fashion. Frogs given total body irradiation without marrow protection showed prolonged allograft survival times; however, most of the animals died with grafts intact at approximately 15-25 days postirradiation. Further, there was no significant difference in the MST of skin allografts in thymectomized animals whose immunological mechanism was suppressed by irradiation and a comparable group in which the thymus was replanted subcutaneously immediately after irradiation. Differential counts of peripheral blood smears after irradiation showed a lymphopenia of approximately 50% of the normal values within 24 hours and successive fluctuations until the time of death. Approximately 28 days after irradiation, a striking increase in monocyte-like cells appeared in the peripheral blood smears, and at the same time the mortality rate began to increase.

At a still higher dosage (5,000 r) the unshielded marrow affected the immune response. (a) Grafts on control unirradiated animals showed an MST of 14 days. (b) In frogs subjected to total body irradiation, allografts were completely intact at the time of death, the final death occurring on the 15th day after grafting (20th day postirradiation). On the other hand, in the shielded group, graft rejection occurred at a similar rate to control animals, but there was a delay of approximately 2 days, a difference which was insignificant when compared to the controls. Of these animals 14% survived beyond 30 days. These experiments suggest that bone marrow from the shielded leg, in varying quantities, is capable of maintaining the life of the animals and that it may provide immunologically competent cells so that when the shielded animals were challenged with skin allografts these were rejected similarly to those of the unirradiated controls.

Lymphomyeloid Organs in Anura

Bullfrog larvae.—There are two major lymphomyeloid organs in bullfrog larvae, the lymph gland and the ventral cavity body. The lymph gland is a bilateral structure in the branchial chamber near the developing anterior limb (42). The exact role of this organ in immune competence has not been determined (13) but the structure, in some respects, is similar to a mammalian lymph node (Fig. 23). More precisely, it bears a striking resemblance to the hemal nodes of mammals (43). The lymph gland, histologically, shows no lines of demarcation between components such as the cortical and medullary regions of the thymus and mammalian lymph nodes. However, the lymph gland is composed of an outer connective tissue capsule, like the thymus, which surrounds a parenchyma that consists of numerous "lobules" of lympho-epithelial cells (Figs. 14, 15, 16). Surrounding

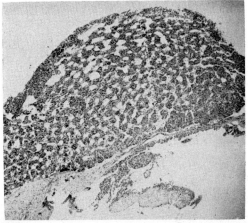

Fig. 14. This section shows the lymph gland of a tadpole 6-24 months of age. The connective tissue capsule is seen surrounding the parenchyma and the "lobules" of lympho-epithelial cells are easily distinguished. Between these cell groups are the sinusoids lined by reticulo-endothelial cells. x 150

the lymphoid elements and lining the sinusoids are reticuloendothelial cells which actively take up India ink. This observation suggests that it functions to filter foreign material from the circulation (11, 40). Occasionally, many small lymphocytes are detectable in the spaces between the "lobules." In addition to the predominant lymphoid cell and the phagocytic cell there are three other cell types: erythrocytes, hemocytoblasts, and plasma cells. The presence of plasma cells strongly suggests that the lymph gland plays a role in antibody synthesis. Presumably, this organ is strictly larval, for it is apparent that it disappears during metamorphosis.

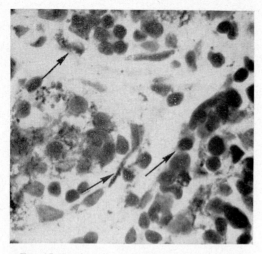

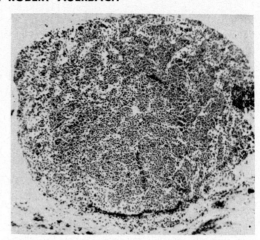

Fig. 15. Section through three groups of lympho-epithelial cells in the lymph gland of a tadpole 6-24 months posthatching. Note that the reticulo-endo-thelial cells which line the sinusoids contain India ink. x 1500

Fig. 17. This section represents an entire ventral cavity body from a tadpole. Note that the paren-chyma is generally homogeneous when compared to the lymph gland; yet a few sinusoids are present between groups of lympho-epithelial cells. x 150

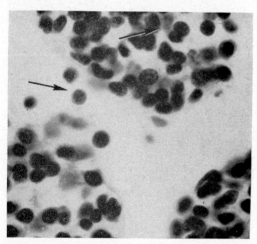

Fig. 16. Some specific cell types can be recognized among this group of lympho-epithelial cells. A few lymphocytes have escaped into the sinusoids and the reticular cells that form the framework of the parenchyma can be seen interspersed between the lymphoid cells. Note the processes of the fixed reticulo-endothelial cells which surround the lympho-epithelial components. x 1500

The ventral cavity body, another lympho-myeloid structure, is situated in the ventral portion of the branchial region and usually consists of three organs bilaterally located on the floor of the branchial cavity near the gills. These are smaller than the lymph glands and appear to be essentially a replica of a lobule of a lymph gland (Fig. 17).

Adult bullfrogs.—The adult bullfrog has four paired lymphomyeloid organs. These structures are found only in the adult; how-ever, some appear at different times following metamorphosis (Fig. 24). These are the pre-pericardial body located on either side of the larynx (a location similar to that of the mam-malian tonsil); the procoracoid body situated anterior to the truncus arteriosus and near the coracoid bone; the small epithelial body lo-cated in close proximity to the parathyroid glands and medial to the omohyoid muscle; the large pear-shaped jugular body ventrally located on either side of the sternohyoid muscle.

The jugular body, the prepericardial body, and the propericardial body are quite similar in that they are composed of "lobules." How-ever, the epithelial body, like the ventral cavity body, is smaller and less complex morphologi-cally. The first three, like the larval lymph gland, are composed of "lobules" of lympho-epithelial cells which are separated by spaces or sinusoids lined with reticulo-endothelial cells. In addition to some mature lymphoid cells, cells resembling lymphoblasts are found as well as plasma cells and erythrocytes. The parenchyma is supported by a framework of reticular cells and fibers (Figs. 18-20).

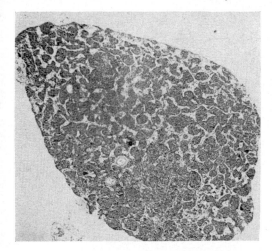

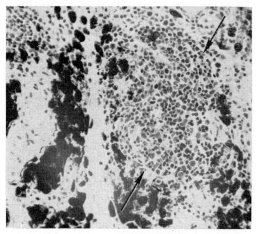

FIG. 18. This figure represents the jugular body of an adult frog which is located lateral to the sternohyoid muscle. This section is an example of the generalized microscopic structure of the procoracoid body and the prepericardial body. The gross shapes of these three adult structures differ; however, all three are similar to the lymph gland of tadpoles. Numerous lympho-epithelial cells are grouped together separated by sinusoids lined with reticulo-endothelial cells. x 64

FIG. 20. This section is an epithelial body of an adult bullfrog. Note the small size of this aggregation of lympho-epithelial cells when compared to the other larger organs described previously. x 300

THE THYMUS, LYMPHOMYELOID ORGANS, AND SKIN ALLOGRAFT IMMUNITY IN APODA AND URODELA

According to Noble (35), the thymus glands in most Amphibia originate from the dorsal portion of the pharyngeal pouches but eventually lose their connection. In the Apoda (e.g., Caecilians), thymus buds are located on either side of and develop from the first six visceral pouches. The first and last pair of buds degenerate and the four remaining pairs fuse to form a single-lobed structure. Baldwin (4) found that the thymus in the adult urodele originated from the first five buds but that the first two degenerate. Presumably the three-lobed structure in the adult resulted from the fusion of three pairs of buds on either side. Further reviews of the embryological development of the thymus in the Apoda and Urodela can be found by consulting Maurer (29), Bolau (6), and Maximov (30).

The lymphomyeloid organs in the Apoda and Urodela do not appear to be as well developed as those of the Anura. These are designated generally as gill remnants in the Urodela but more specifically as carotid glands and epithelial bodies. Maurer (29) believed that the carotid glands developed with the retrogression of the gill apparatus while the epithelial bodies remained as remnants of the third and fourth gill slits. Maurer further observed that other gill remnants which were

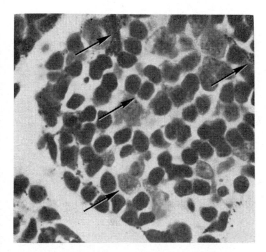

FIG. 19. This section of a jugular body represents one similar to that of the larval lymph gland in Fig. 17. It is taken through four groups of lympho-epithelial cells surrounding a central one. Note the dark staining lymphoid cells held together in a framework composed of reticular elements. The phagocytic cells can be seen surrounding the lymphoid cells especially after injections of India ink. x 1500

97

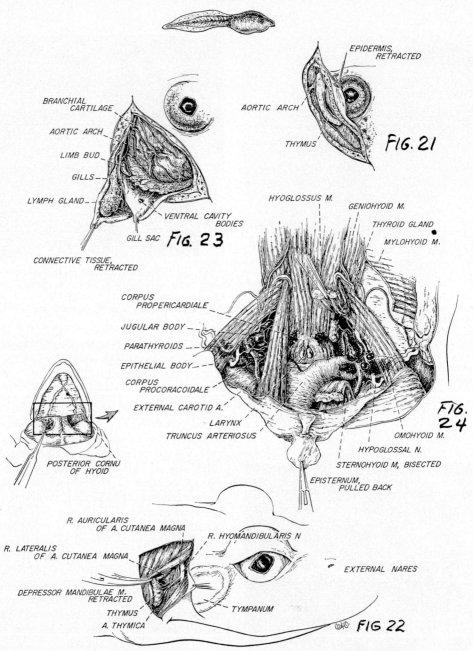

FIG. 21. This figure shows the location of the thymus in bullfrog larvae at stage 25. Note the relationship of the thymus to other branchial structures, ear and eye. x 10; FIG. 22. The thymus in the adult frog is located in close proximity to the muscles of the head and pectoral girdle and the tympanic membrane. x 5; FIG. 23. In this figure the branchial region reveals two types of lymphomyeloid organs found in bullfrog larvae at stage 25. Note the large pear-shaped lymph gland located close to the developing anterior limb. Also enclosed within the gill basket in the ventral region are several smaller nodules (ventral cavity bodies). In the same region can be seen the gills and aortic arches. x 10; FIG. 24. In this section the lymphomyeloid organs are located in the neck and lower jaw region of an adult bullfrog. One pair (prepericardial bodies) lies anterior and lateral to the larynx. A second pair (procoracoid bodies) is located just anterior to the truncus arteriosus. Lateral to the sternohyoid muscle near the insertion of the geniohyoid and posterior end of the hyoid apparatus are the large jugular bodies. The fourth pair (epithelial bodies) is lateral to the previous organ near the parathyroid glands. x 5

usually found in the Anura (presumably, jugular, prepericardial, and procoracoid bodies) were lacking in the Urodela. With regard to the Apoda, there seems to be no available information on the existence of lymphomyeloid structures.

The immune response to skin allografts in our Caecilians showed acute to chronic rejection as evidenced by first set survival times ranging from 7 to 75 days. Presently, second set grafts are being studied and only two animals, so far, have shown the typical second set phenomenon.

The rather short rejection time of 7 days may have resulted from technical difficulties encountered during the beginning stages of perfecting the technique of skin grafting. In the Urodela, according to Cohen (8), rejection of skin allografts in *Triturus (Diemictylus) viridescens* is chronic with a range of survival times from 20 to 40 days. Using this genus, he observed specificity of anamnesis, temperature sensitivity, and inhibition of rejection with x-irradiation. The relationship between the immune response, the thymus, and various lymphomyeloid organs in the Urodela and Apoda has yet to be determined.

Discussion and Conclusions

This presentation was aimed at drawing attention to the lymphoid and myeloid organs in three groups of Amphibia by citing our morphologic and experimental studies of immune competence. Emphasis was placed on the thymus, recently observed lymphomyeloid organs, and bone marrow without considering the spleen, liver, and kidney which, at some time during the life history of these animals, function in hemopoiesis.

On the basis of numerous regeneration experiments involving the Amphibia, particularly the adult urodeles (22), it seems predictable that certain tissues of larval anurans may regenerate under appropriate conditions. The limited data from this work suggest that the thymus can regenerate when removed and that the restoration of immune competence in the case of allografts was dependent upon a regenerated thymus. In mice, for example, the thymus in the AKR strain regenerates when small pieces are left after thymectomy of newborns (25).

Current observations suggest that the thymus in adult anurans may not be essential for restoration of immune competence to skin allografts. Thus, one or two factors should be considered when differences are pointed out between the present experiments involving adult frogs and those of Miller *et al.* (33). Firstly, the frogs may have been at an age, when compared with the adult mice, that was entirely different; i.e., the frog thymus had reached some point in development when it could no longer affect the immune system rendered non-functional by x-irradiation. To test this assumption, the thymus from recently metamorphosed frogs should be used in a similar experiment instead of frogs approximately two years old. Although the thymus morphologically at the early postmetamorphic period is essentially like that of the sexually mature forms, there are still fewer numbers of lymphocytes and a greater amount of connective tissue during later ages. Since some uncertainty still remains about the nature of the separation of lymphoid and myeloid elements in Amphibia, there may be still remaining in the marrow (unshielded leg) immunologically competent cells in greater quantity than in the marrow of mice. In addition, the population of cells in the marrow of amphibians may be equivalent to that of the thymus, which would suggest similar and perhaps independent functions. In rats, Craddock (14) believes, on the basis of DNA labelling experiments, that a population of lymphocytes is found in the marrow which show the same kinetics of labelling with triated thymidine as small lymphocytes in the thymus cortex. He suggested that if this population of "thymus-like" lymphocytes is self-sustaining, then removal of the thymus would be expected to have limited or variable effect on the lymphoid system.

Much is to be learned now from studies of the immune system of this group, especially in view of the finding of additional organs in the lymphomyeloid complex. This adds to the complexity of this system with the recognition that certain interrelationships may be existent. It may well turn out that the anuran lymphomyeloid organs can be classified as central lymphoid organs like the thymus, bursa of Fabricius, and appendix in mammals. The thymus and lymphomyeloid organs in Amphibia share some common morphological features; yet larval and adult differences do exist which may, no doubt, be responsible for undiscovered functional differences.

Acknowledgments.—This research was supported mainly by funds from U.S. Public Health Service Grant AM-09030 from the National Institute of Arthritis and Metabolic Diseases.

The author is grateful to Mrs. Eileen B. Gitin for technical assistance, Mrs. Crista Osterberg for executing the drawings, and Michael L. Mandell and D. William Schaefer for performing the irradiation experiments. Stimulating discussions with Drs. William H. Hildemann and Nicholas Cohen are also acknowledged.

REFERENCES

1. Adler, L. O. (1914): Metamorphosenstudien an Batrachierlarven. Arch. f. Entwicklungsmechanik (Leipz.) *40,* 1.
2. Aspinall, R. L., Meyer, R. K., Graetzer, M. A., and Wolfe, H. R. (1963): Effect of thymectomy and bursectomy on the survival of skin homografts in chickens. J. Immun. *90,* 872.
3. Auerbach, R. (1960): Morphogenetic interactions in the development of the mouse thymus gland. Develop. Biol. *2,* 271.
4. Baldwin, T. M. (1918): Pharyngeal derivatives of Amblystoma. J. Morph. *30,* 605.
5. Beard, J. (1903): The origin and histogenesis of the thymus in *Raja batis.* Zool. Jb. *17,* 403.
6. Bolau, H. (1899): Glandula Thyroidea und Glandula Thymus der Amphibien. Zool. Jahrb. Abth. f. Anat. Bd. 12.
7. Braunmühl, A. von (1926): Über einige myelolymphoide und lymphoepitheliale Organe der Anuren. Leitschr. Mikr. Anat. Forsch. *4,* 635.
8. Cohen, N. (1965): Skin homograft rejection in the adult newt *Triturus (Diemictylus) viridescens.* Amer. Zool. *5,* 227.
9. Cooper, E. L., Pinkerton, W., and Hildemann, W. H. (1964): Serum antibody synthesis in larvae of the bullfrog *Rana catesbeiana.* Biol. Bull. *127,* 231.
10. Cooper, E. L. (1965): Unpublished.
11. Cooper, E. L. (1965): Some aspects of the reticuloendothelial system in *Rana catesbeiana.* Anat. Rec. *151,* 448.
12. Cooper, E. L., and Hildemann, W. H. (1965a): Allograft reactions in bullfrog larvae in relation to thymectomy. Transplantation *3,* 446.
13. Cooper, E. L., and Hildemann, W. H. (1965b): The immune response of larval bullfrogs (*Rana catesbeiana*) to diverse antigens. Ann. N. Y. Acad. Sci. *126,* 647.
14. Craddock, C. G. (1965): Bone marrow lymphocytes of the rat as studied by autoradiography. Acta Haemat. *33,* 19.
15. Defendi, V., and Metcalf, D. (1964): The Thymus. Philadelphia, The Wistar Institute Press, 144 pp.
16. Dustin, A. P. (1913): Recherches d'histologie normale et expérimentale sur le thymus des amphibiens anoures. Arch. Biol. *28,* 1.
17. Dustin, A. P. (1920): Recherches d'histologie normale et expérimentale sur le thymus des amphibiens anoures. Arch. Biol. *30,* 601.
18. Fleische, E. (1868): On the construction of the so-called thyroid gland of the frog. Sitzungsbericht der koeniglichen Akademie der Wissenschaften in Wien, Math. Naturwiss. Kl. 57.
19. Gaupp, E. (1896): Anatomisches des Frosches. Braunschweig, A. Ecker and R. Wiedersheim.
20. Good, R. A., and Gabrielsen, A. E. (1964): The Thymus in Immuno-biology. Structure, Function, and Role in Disease. Hoeber Medical Division. New York, Harper and Row, 778 pp.
21. Good, R. A., and Papermaster, B. W. (1964): Ontogeny and phylogeny of adaptive immunity. Adv. Immunol. *4,* 1.
22. Goss, R. J. (1961): Regeneration of vertebrate appendages, in Advances in Morphogenesis, pp. 103-52. New York, Academic Press. M. Abercrombie, J. Brachet. vol. 1.
23. Graetzer, M. A., Wolfe, H. R., Aspinall, R. L., and Meyer, R. K. (1963): Effect of thymectomy and bursectomy on precipitin and natural hemagglutin production in the chicken. J. Immun. *90,* 878.
24. Hammar, J. (1905): Ist die Thymusdruse beim Frosch ein lebenswichtiges Organ? Arch. Ges. Physiol. (Bonn) *110,* 337.
25. Hays, Esther (1966): Personal communication.
26. Hildemann, W. H., and Haas, R. (1959): Homotransplantation immunity and tolerance in the bullfrog. J. Immun. *83,* 478.
27. Kent, S. P., Evans, E. E., and Attleberger, M. H. (1964): Comparative immunology: lymph nodes in the amphibian, *Bufo marinus.* Proc. Soc. Exp. Biol. Med. *116,* 456.
28. Krause, R. (1923): Microscopic anatomy individually presented. III. Amphibia. Berlin, Leipzig.
29. Maurer, F. (1888): Schilddrüse, Thymus, und Keimenreste der Amphibien. Morph. Jahrb. 13.

30. Maximov, A. (1912 [1]), Untersuchungen über Blut und Bindegewebe 4. Ueber die Histogenese der Thymus bei Amphibien. Arch. der mik. Anat. (Bonn) *79*, 560.

31. Mayer, S. (1888): Zur Lehre von der Schilddrüse und Thymus bei den Amphibien. Anat. Anz. Bd. 3.

32. Miller, J. F. A. P. (1963a): Origins of immunological competence. Brit. Med. Bull. *19*, 214.

33. Miller, J. F. A. P., Doak, S. M. A., and Cross, A. M. (1963b): Role of the thymus in recovery of the immune mechanism in the irradiated adult mouse. Proc. Soc. Exp. Biol. Med. *112*, 785.

34. Miller, J. F. A. P. (1964): The thymus and the development of immunologic responsiveness. Science *144*, 1544.

35. Noble, G. K. (1931): The Biology of the Amphibia, New York, Dover Publications, Inc., 577 pp.

36. Nusbaum, J., and Machowski, J. (1902): Die Bildung der concentrischen Körperchen und die phagocytischen Vorgänge bei der Involution der Amphibien Thymus. Anat. Anz. *21*, 110.

37. Regal, P. (1965): Personal communication.

38. Simon, I. (1845): A physiological essay on the thymus gland. London (see Gaupp).

39. Stearner, S. P. (1950): The effects of x-irradiation on *Rana pipiens* (Leopard frog), with special reference to survival and to the response of the peripheral blood. J. Exp. Zool. *115*, 251.

40. Thorbecke, G. J., and Benacerraf, B. (1962): The reticulo-endothelial system and immunological phenomena. Progr. Allergy *6*, 559.

41. Toldt, C. (1868): On the lymphoid organs in amphibians. Sitzungsbericht der königlichen Akademie der Wissenschaften in Wien. Math. Naturwiss. Kl. 58.

42. Witschi, E. (1956): Development of Vertebrates. Philadelphia, W. B. Saunders Company, 588 pp.

43. Yoffey, J. M., and Courtice, F. C. (1956): Biological Significance of Lymphoid Tissue in Lymphatics, Lymph and Lymphoid Tissue. Cambridge, Mass., Harvard University Press, p. 252.

44. Yoffey, J. M. (1960): The Lymphomyeloid Complex in Ciba Foundation Symposium on Haemopoiesis Cell Production and its Regulation, London, J. and A. Churchill Ltd. p. 1.

DISCUSSION

AUERBACH: It seems that your findings on the effect of bone marrow are not unique; after all, the neonatally thymectomized mouse has been shown to be restored by injection of bone marrow cells even without the thymus.

COOPER: I believe Miller suggested in a 1963 paper that in order for the immune response to be restored the bone marrow had to fall under the influence of the thymus.

GOOD: These experiments address themselves to the question of whether or not traffic through the thymus is necessary for the direction of the differentiation toward immunological competence. In Cooper's experiments bone marrow is the only source of new cells after heavy doses of irradiation, and the thymus appears unnecessary. This point needs to be clarified. Data from several sources indicate that such a traffic through the thymus is necessary for bone marrow to become functional.

AUERBACH: Do you know what happens to the lymphoid tissues in thymectomized irradiated animals? Consider for example, that in mice you may get differing effects depending on the dose you use. For example: with 500 r you may get complete lymphoid recovery without the thymus, whereas at a dose of 900 r the thymus is necessary.

COOPER: I have not yet examined the lymphoid tissues during radiation recovery.

HILDEMANN: 3,000 r is an LD^{99} dose for amphibians.

MITCHISON: Can you tell us why the frogs die after irradiation? Is it comparable to the death of mice?

COOPER: Yes. There is a syndrome associated with radiation disease in these animals very much like that in mammals. Skin lesions are produced, their feeding reactions stop completely, and they have muscle spasms.

MITCHISON: After big doses of radiation can they be restored by marrow?

COOPER: Yes, marrow restores, given by injection or protected by shielding.

BLOCK: Have you controlled the temperature? This is important in amphibia.

COOPER: The animals were kept constant at 25° C.

BLOCK: Is it not true in amphibia that if the temperature is lowered, they are less sensitive to radiation?

COOPER: That is true.

BLOCK: You mentioned lympho-epithelial cells in lymph nodes. There has been discussion of epithelium in the formation of lymphocytes in the thymus and perhaps of epithelium in the blood formation in the liver. This is the first time that anyone has postulated that there are epithelial cells in lymph nodes.

COOPER: The cells described look like lympho-epithelial cells found in thymic primordia. Von Braunmühl's terminology is the basis of calling these lympho-epithelial cells.

GOOD: The lymph glands described in the bullfrog must be considered to be very different organs from the lymph nodes of mammals. The structure described many years ago by Braunmühl lies near the gills; during development its stroma appears to be truly epithelial and not mesenchymal reticulum like the lymph nodes of mammals. The so-called lymphocytes are very different in this location from the lymphocytes of mammals and even from the lymphocytes of the thymus of the frog itself. I quite agree, however, that the many different hemopoietic sites in the amphibia as well as in the primitive and more recent fishes contain lymphocytes and demand further functional analysis.

COOPER: There is no cortex and medulla here as in the lymph nodes of mammals. It is a homogeneous structure with packets of so-called lympho-epithelial cells.

BLOCK: We may conclude then that these organs are neither homologous nor analogous to lymph nodes in mammals?

COOPER: We must conclude this for now.

GOOD: The most important implication of these data in amphibians is that multiple sources of cells have the same function that the thymus does in mammals. Among these sources may be the lympho-epithelial lymph glands developing in juxtaposition with the gill.

COOPER: Within the germinal centers of mammalian lymph nodes, there is a group of cells smaller than the lymphoid cells with desmosomal bridges ultrastructurally. This is considered to be an epithelial characteristic.

GOOD: It would be revolutionary at present to accept the presence of true epithelial cells in the mammalian lymph node.

HILDEMANN: This work ought to be appreciated in the context that thymectomy alone of the tadpoles up to an age of 20 to 30 days posthatching leads not only to a profound impairment of the capacity to reject skin allografts but a general impairment of the capacity to produce serum antibodies to a variety of antigens. However, beyond about 30 days posthatching in the bullfrog, thymectomy no longer has this role.

Thus one can visualize the tadpole at about 30 days posthatching as being roughly equivalent to a newborn mouse or rat. The "master organ" role of the thymus as defined in mammals seems to hold in amphibians early in development. Beyond 30 days, there is evidently migration of cells and some takeover of this function elsewhere.

GOOD: The early and important work of John Beard in the embryonic ray showed evidence that the thymus as in mammals was the first organ to show a lymphoid accumulation. He reasoned from his sequential observations that the direction of development was from thymus to the other foci of lymphoid tissues such as in the gonadal tissue and the anterior kidney region. The same sequential events appear to occur in amphibians.

13

CHARLES B. KIMMEL

The response of lysosomes in the chick embryo spleen in the graft-versus-host reaction

THE DEVELOPMENT AND FUNCTION of phagocytic cells and their digestive organelles, the lysosomes (13, 24), present to embryologists and immunologists alike many interesting and perplexing problems. Populations of neutrophil granulocytes (9), eosinophil granulocytes (1), and mononuclear phagocytes or macrophages (10) have been successfully obtained for study, and it is clear that each cell type is active in phagocytosis and rich in lysosomes.

Although the specificity of the phagocytic process and that of intracellular digestion of ingested material is only beginning to be understood, it is clear that it can be quite different depending on the type of cell under study. Neutrophils, the major mediators of the inflammatory response, ingest and digest materials relatively indiscriminately (17, 18), whereas eosinophils may require a specific antibody in order to ingest a given antigen (2, 23), and complement may be necessary for its intracellular digestion by lysosomes (2). The degree of "foreignness" of a given antigen may determine in part the extent to which it will undergo phagocytosis by macrophages (25) and indeed several lines of evidence suggest the macrophage as the site of the initial reactions leading to the antibody response (14, 15, 26). Specificity also is found in the intracellular digestive processes of macrophages, for although ingested bacteria are killed and degraded by macrophages, bacterial immunogens remain in the cells (6, 7, 16), whereas, if neutrophils are studied under similar conditions (6, 7), immunogens cannot be detected.

The maturation in vitro of macrophages has been the object of study of several laboratories—notably in that of Cohn and his coworkers (8). These investigators have shown that, as a result of an unknown stimulus, not necessarily that of phagocytosis, monocyte-like cells differentiate into mature macrophages. This transformation occurs without DNA synthesis, and involves considerable growth of the cell, including the formation of mitochondria, and especially lysosomes.

The embryonic development of phagocytic cells has been studied on the morphological level (11), yet little is known with respect to the emergence of their phagocytic functions and their metabolic activities. Recently, Karthigasu and Jenkin have reported on the development of reticulo-endothelial function in both avian and mammalian embryos (21, 22). Their observations reveal that clearance of bacteria and carbon is accomplished in embryos, and that this capacity increases markedly throughout the latter part of development.

The studies of DeLanney, Ebert, and their coworkers (11) indicated a major role of these cells in the graft-versus-host reaction. As a part of the dramatic splenomegaly occurring as a consequence of the reaction, the production of granulocytes is greatly enhanced. Huge clusters of neutrophils appear in association with pocks or "foci" which develop in the enlarged spleens. These foci, according to the view of Burnet and others, are initiated as clones of the donor cells which are implanted into the embryo (4, 5, 28). So-called giant cells, perhaps macrophages, later are found in and around the foci which then become extremely cystic and necrotic.

With the view that a more complete study of the phagocytic cells during the graft-versus-host reaction would lead to a better understanding of the reaction itself, and especially of the role of the host in it, I have undertaken a biochemical and cytological study of the chick embryo spleen.

Initially, we may ask: Are lysosomes, using the several criteria which operationally define them (12), present in the cells of the embryonic spleen? Although the data will not be shown extensively here,* the answer to this question is a clear yes. The criteria employed include the properties of latency and sedimentability of marker lysosomal enzymes, the distribution of these enzymes among subcellular fractions, in sucrose gradients, and finally the cytochemical localization of marker enzymes in cell particles. The studies were carried out on spleens from normal embryos incubated 17 days. With respect to latency, the activities of six marker hydrolases in carefully prepared Dounce homogenates of pooled embryonic spleens are found to be low when compared to those found when the homogenate is treated to disrupt lysosomes. These activities, designated "free activities," are thought to represent that fraction of the lysosomal enzymes which are found not associated with the lysosomes, but soluble and available to substrates (13). Table 1 presents the results of an experiment in which the free activities of lysosomal enzymes are compared with a typical mitochondrial enzyme, cytochrome oxidase, and a cell-sap enzyme, lactic dehydrogenase (LDH). Whereas LDH is almost completely freely active in the untreated homogenate, cytochrome oxidase is almost completely latent: its activity is only 1% of that found after the homogenate is treated to disrupt the mitochondrial membranes. Similarly, free activity of the lysosomal enzymes is low; about 10-20%

TABLE 1.—FREE ACTIVITIES OF ENZYMES IN HOMOGENATES OF DAY-17 EMBRYONIC SPLEENS

Enzyme Location	Enzyme	Free Activity*
Cell Sap	LDH	82%
Mitochondria	Cytochrome Oxidase	1%
Lysosomes	Acid Phosphatase	22%
	β-Glucuronidase	18%
	Aryl Sulfatase	17%
	Acid DNase	6%
	Acid RNase	13%
	Cathepsin	11%

*Free Activity: Per cent of that found after freezing and thawing plus sonication of the homogenate.

of that found after treatment, in agreement with the results of other investigators.

The distribution of lysosomal enzymes in cell fractions was studied using the differential centrifugation scheme shown in Fig. 1. Homogenates were centrifuged serially to obtain a nuclear fraction, containing primarily nuclei and unbroken cells; a large granule fraction, in which is found the majority of the specific granules of the neutrophil; a classical mitochondrial fraction; and a light mitochondrial fraction. Analysis of marker enzymes is shown in Fig. 2. The activities found in each fraction are presented as columns. The height of the

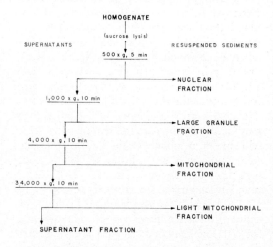

FIG. 1. Scheme for fractionation of sucrose (0.25 M) homogenates of embryonic spleens by differential centrifugation.

*The data which are presented are part of the author's doctoral dissertation. They will be published in a more complete form elsewhere.

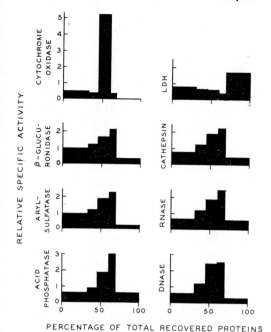

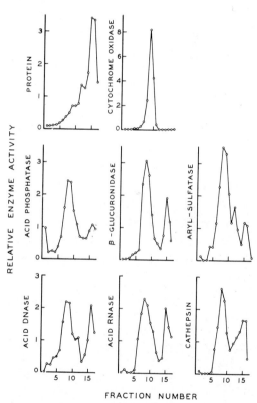

FIG. 2. Intracellular distribution of enzymes in homogenates of day-17 spleens. Pooled spleens were homogenized and fractionated according to the scheme in Fig. 1. Fractions, from left to right, are nuclear, large granule, mitochondrial, light mitochondrial, and supernatant. The relative specific activity (ordinate) is the ratio of the specific activity (units/mg protein) of given fraction to that recovered from all fractions. The abscissa shows the percentage of total protein recovered in a given fraction.

found associated with cell particles of a wide variety of sizes. Furthermore, each of the enzymes reflects this heterogeneity, i.e., one enzyme is *not* found to be primarily associated with the larger granules and another with the smaller.

Analysis of fractions rich in lysosomal enzymes by sucrose density gradient centrifugation has also proved useful in the definition of lysosomes in this system. In the experiment shown in Fig. 3, a homogenate was prepared and centrifuged at 1,000 x g for 10 minutes. 0.5 ml of the supernatant, containing most of the lysosomes and mitochondria as well as cell-sap components, was layered on a 4.0 ml sucrose gradient. The tube was centrifuged,

column shows the specific activity of the enzyme in the fraction; the area of the column shows the total activity found in that fraction. It may be seen that cytochrome oxidase shows a clear localization in the mitochondrial fraction while LDH is predominantly found in the supernatant fraction. Lysosomal enzymes are distributed in each of the particulate fractions, and also a portion of the total activity of each, corresponding to the free activity, is found in the supernatant. Comparison of the lysosomal enzymes in the particulate fractions reveals a distribution pattern common to each of them. The specific activity and total activity is lowest in the large granule fraction, the total activity is highest in the mitochondrial fraction, and the specific activity is highest in the light mitochondrial fraction. We may conclude that embryonic spleen lysosomes are very heterogeneous with respect to size; activity is

FIG. 3. Distribution of enzymes from day-17 spleens after centrifugation through a linear sucrose gradient (0.5 M to 2.25 M.) Centrifugation was for 2 hours at 35,000 rpm in a Spinco model L₂ ultracentrifuge. Fractions were collected as drops from a hole punched in the bottom of the tube. The relative activity (ordinate) is the ratio of the observed activity to that which would have been found if the enzyme had been homogeneously distributed throughout the gradient.

105

fractions collected and assayed for protein and marker enzymes. Most of the protein did not move from the original load volume at the top of the gradient corresponding to fractions 15, 16, and 17; whereas cytochrome oxidase moved into the gradient as a narrow band with a well-defined peak in fraction 9. The activities of the lysosomal markers each have a broader band than cytochrome oxidase, with a peak in fraction 8. Thus lysosomes have a higher density and are more heterogeneous in their density than mitochondria in this system. Also, activity corresponding to the free enzymes is found in the load volume.

Cytochemical localization of a marker enzyme, acid phosphatase, has been carried out using the azo dye method of Barka and Anderson (3) on smears and formalin-fixed frozen sections of the spleen. As may be seen in Fig. 4, the reaction product is found to be distinctly particulate in the cells. Freezing and thawing of the tissue without prior fixation results in a loss of its localization in particles. Here again, this treatment may be thought to act in breaking the lysosomal membrane, permitting the enzyme to diffuse into the cytoplasm.

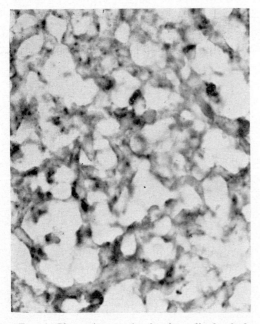

FIG. 4. Photomicrograph of a formalin-fixed, 6μ frozen section of a day-17 spleen, stained (1 hour, 37°) for acid phosphatase. x 1,000

Finally, measurements of the total activity of lysosomal enzymes in spleen homogenates compare favorably with those found in other tissues, including adult rat liver and spleen, which are known to be high in lysosomal enzymes.

These data permit us to say that the cells in the spleen of the 17-day embryo are rich in lysosomes. Furthermore, they serve as a yardstick, with which we can compare normal spleens with those from embryos undergoing the graft-versus-host reaction. To produce the graft-versus-host reaction, embryos were injected intravenously at 12 days of incubation with one-half to two million buffy coat leucocytes from adult donor cockerels. The recipient embryos were killed at various intervals and compared with those which were uninjected, or inoculated with saline only. The interval most commonly used was 5 days: on day 17 the degree of splenomegaly was of the order of tenfold, and the production of foci in these spleens was grossly evident (27).

A most striking change was that of the total activity of lysosomal enzymes in the enlarged spleens. A dramatic increase in the levels of all of these enzymes was found when the spleens were compared on day 17. When the increase was based on the wet weight of the tissue, it was seen that the total increase was at least as much as, and in several cases significantly greater than, the increase in wet weight. The time course of this change is presented for three of the enzymes in Fig. 5. The wet weight increases logarithmically in the experimental group and is significantly greater than the controls by day 15, three days after inoculation. The enzymatic activity increases at least as rapidly as does wet weight (aryl sulfatase), or more rapidly (acid phosphatase and β-glucuronidase).

The free activity of lysosomal enzymes is also increased in the experimental group, as may be seen in Table 2, in which the significance of the increase for two enzymes, β-glucuronidase and aryl sulfatase, is tested. For each, the increase is significant at the 5% level, indicating that in the enlarged spleens more lysosomal enzymes are found *not* associated with lysosomes, perhaps freely active within the cell.

This change is also seen in the fractionation studies, summarized in Fig. 6. The activity

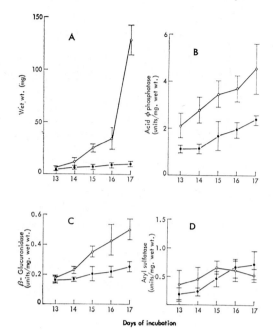

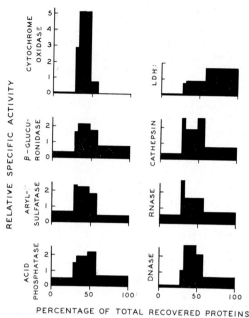

FIG. 5. Lysosomal enzyme activities in developing chick spleens: changes induced by inoculation of adult blood leucocytes on day 12. A: changes in wet weight with development. B, C, and D: changes in enzymatic specific activity with development. Each point is the mean of five determinations, and the length of the vertical line through the mean corresponds to a 95% confidence interval (t test). Closed circles, uninjected control spleens; open circles, spleens from embryos injected intravenously with 5 x 10⁵ cells.

FIG. 6. Intracellular distribution of enzymes in homogenates of day-17 spleens from embryos injected on day 12 with adult blood leucocytes. Otherwise, as in Fig. 2.

TABLE 2.—FREE ACTIVITIES OF β-GLUCURONIDASE AND ARYL SULFATASE IN DAY-17 CONTROL AND EXPERIMENTAL CHICK SPLEENS

Enzyme	Free Activity* in Homogenates (mean ± S.E.)		Probability (t test)
	Control†	Experimental‡	
β-Glucu-ronidase	20.5±2.0	28.3±2.1	0.05> P>0.025
Aryl Sulfatase	5.1±0.5	10.0±0.6	P<0.001

*Free Activity: Per cent of that found after treatment of the homogenate with Triton X-100 (0.05%).

†Determinations on five groups of six pooled spleens.

‡Determinations on five spleens enlarged about sixfold.

found in the supernatant is reproducibly higher for each enzyme in the tenfold enlarged spleens than in the normal spleens (Fig. 2). Also characteristically there is an increase in heterogeneity of distribution among the different lysosomal enzymes in the particulate fractions; they no longer conform to the more simple pattern shown by the normal spleens.

No change was detected in the density of the lysosomes, as analyzed by sucrose gradients. The data shown in Fig. 7, from experimental spleens enlarged about eightfold, conform closely with those shown for normal spleens (Fig. 3): no significant differences are found when comparing the two groups.

Cytochemical studies have complemented the results obtained above with spleen homogenates. Spleens from embryos killed at varying intervals after injection on day 12 were formalin fixed, serially cut at 6μ with the freezing microtome, and stained for acid phosphatase. The first major change was found within two to three days after injection and had the appearance of clusters of more highly reactive cells, found throughout the spleen, as shown in Fig. 8. A higher magnification (Fig.

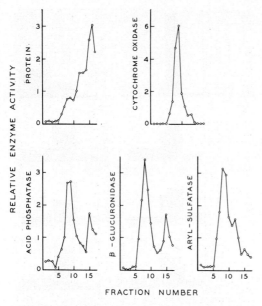

FIG. 7. Distribution in a sucrose gradient of enzymes from day-17 spleens of embryos injected on day 12 with adult blood leucocytes. Otherwise, as in Fig. 3.

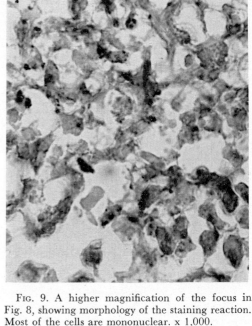

FIG. 9. A higher magnification of the focus in Fig. 8, showing morphology of the staining reaction. Most of the cells are mononuclear. x 1,000.

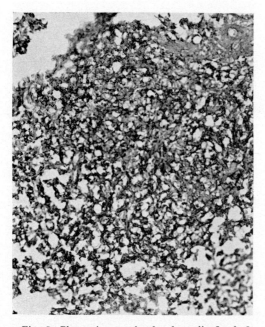

Fig. 8. Photomicrograph of a formalin-fixed, 6μ frozen section of a day-15 embryonic spleen from an embryo inoculated on day 12 with adult blood leucocytes. The section was stained for acid phosphatase (1 hour) by the method of Barka and Anderson, and counterstained with methyl green. A focus of more reactive cells is in the center of the field. x 200

9) indicates that the enzyme is primarily localized in particles. In another two to three days, when foci become evident, there is a dramatic increase in the activity of cells in and especially surrounding these foci (Fig. 10). Both granulocytes and macrophages contribute to this increase of activity. Also now many of the cells show reaction product throughout their cytoplasm; perhaps indicating release of the enzyme from the lysosomes and activation, as shown in a higher magnification of cells in this area (Fig. 11).

These data then indicate a striking involvement of the phagocytic cells, presumably derived from the embryonic host (11, 20, 27), in the graft-versus-host reaction. Weiss and Aisenberg (29) have recently carried a study of the reaction in neonatal rats using the electron microscope; and with minor variation, perhaps attributable to species and age differences, our data and interpretation are in agreement. Howard, using F_1 hosts injected with parental cells, has demonstrated increased phagocytic capacity in older animals undergoing the reaction (19). Many interesting and important questions must now be answered regarding the nature of the involve-

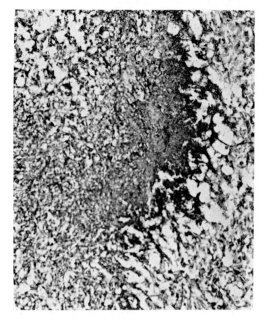

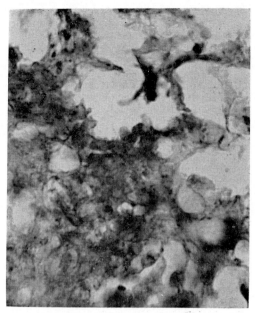

FIG. 10. Photomicrograph of a section of a day-18 spleen from an inoculated embryo, stained for acid phosphatase. A focus takes up most of the field. x 200

FIG. 11. A higher magnification of the border of the focus in Fig. 10. x 1,000

ment. Do these cells, indeed, derive from the embryo? What is the stimulus which marshalls their production, and indeed is it the same stimulus which initiates splenomegaly? Are these cells active in the phagocytosis of host antigen? or donor? or both donor and host? Experiments designed to answer some of these questions are now in progress.

REFERENCES

1. Archer, G. T., and Hirsch, J. G. (1963): Isolation of granules from eosinophil leucocytes and study of their enzyme content. J. Exp. Med. *118*, 277.
2. Archer, G. T., and Hirsch, J. G. (1963): Motion picture studies on degranulation of horse eosinophils during phagocytosis. J. Exp. Med. *118*, 287.
3. Barka, T., and Anderson, P. J. (1962): Histochemical methods for acid phosphatase using hexazonium pararosanilin as coupler. J. Histochem. Cytochem. *10*, 741.
4. Boyer, G. (1960): Chorioallantoic membrane lesions produced by the inoculation of adult fowl leucocytes. Nature *185*, 327.
5. Burnet, F. M., and Burnet, D. (1960): Graft versus host reactions on the chorioallantoic membrane of the embryo. Nature *188*, 376.
6. Cohn, Z. A. (1962): Influence of rabbit polymorphonuclear leucocytes and macrophages on the immunogenicity of *Escherichia coli*. Nature *196*, 1066.
7. Cohn, Z. A. (1964): The fate of bacteria within phagocytic cells. III. Destruction of an *Escherichia coli* agglutinogen within polymorphonuclear leucocytes and macrophages. J. Exp. Med. *120*, 869.
8. Cohn, Z. A., and Benson, B. (1965): The differentiation of mononuclear phagocytes. J. Exp. Med. *121*, 153.
9. Cohn, Z. A., and Hirsch, J. G. (1960): The isolation and properties of the specific cytoplasmic granules of rabbit polymorphonuclear leucocytes. J. Exp. Med. *112*, 983.
10. Cohn, Z. A., and Wiener, E. (1963): The particulate hydrolases of macrophages. I. Comparative enzymology, isolation and properties. J. Exp. Med. *118*, 991.
11. DeLanney, L. E., and Ebert, J. D. (1962): On the chick spleen: origin; patterns of normal development and their experimental modification. Contributions to Embryology, Carnegie Institution of Washington, *34*, 57.
12. de Duve, C. (1959): Lysosomes, a new group of cytoplasmic particles, in: T. Hayashi, ed.: Subcellular Particles. New York, Ronald Press Company, p. 128.

13. de Duve, C. (1963): The lysosome concept, in: de Reuck, A. V. S., and Cameron, M. P., eds.: Lysomes. Boston, Little, Brown and Co., p. 1.

14. Fishman, M. (1961): Antibody formation *in vitro*. J. Exp. Med. *114*, 837.

15. Fishman, M., and Adler, F. L. (1963): Antibody formation initiated *in vitro*. II. Antibody synthesis in x-irradiated recipients of diffusion chambers containing nucleic acid derived from macrophages incubated with antigen. J. Exp. Med. *117*, 595.

16. Gill, F. A., and Cole, R. M. (1965): The fate of a bacterial antigen (streptococcal M protein) after phagocytosis by macrophages. J. Immun. *94*, 898.

17. Hirsch, J. G. (1962): Cinemicrophotographic observations on granule lysis in polymorphonuclear leucocytes during phagocytosis. J. Exp. Med. *115*, 827.

18. Hirsch, J. G., and Cohn, Z. A. (1960): Degranulation of polymorphonuclear leucocytes following phagocytosis of microorganisms. J. Exp. Med. *112*, 1005.

19. Howard, J. G. (1961): Changes in the activity of the reticulo-endothelial system (RES) following the injection of parental spleen cells into F_1 hybrid mice. Brit. J. Exp. Path. *42*, 72.

20. Howard, J. G., Michie, D., and Simonsen, M. (1961): Splenomegaly as a host response in graft-versus-host disease. Brit. J. Exp. Path. *42*, 478.

21. Karthigasu, K., and Jenkin, C. R. (1963): The functional development of the reticulo-endothelial system of the chick embryo. Immunology *6*, 255.

22. Karthigasu, K., Reade, P. C., and Jenkin, C. R. (1965): The functional development of the reticulo-endothelial system. III. The bactericidal capacity of fixed macrophages of foetal and neonatal chicks and rats. Immunology *9*, 67.

23. Litt, M. (1964): Studies in eosinophilia. VI. Uptake of immune complexes by eosinophils. J. Cell. Biol. *23*, 355.

24. Novikoff, A. B. (1963): Lysosomes in the physiology and pathology of cells: contributions of staining methods, in: de Reuck, A. V. S., and Cameron, M. P., eds.: Lysosomes. Boston, Little, Brown and Company, p. 36.

25. Perkins, E. H., and Leonard, M. R. (1963): Specificity of phagocytosis as it may relate to antibody formation. J. Immun. *90*, 228.

26. Schoenberg, M. D., Mumaw, V. R., Moore, R. D., and Weisberger, A. S. (1964): Cytoplasmic interaction between macrophages and lymphocytic cells in antibody synthesis. Science *143*, 964.

27. Seto, F., and Albright, J. F. (1965): An analysis of host and donor contributions to splenic enlargement in chick embryos inoculated with adult spleen cells. Develop. Biol. *11*, 1.

28. Simonsen, M. (1965) Recent experiments on the graft-versus-host reaction in the chick embryo. Brit. Med. Bull. *21*, 129.

29. Weiss, L., and Aisenberg, A. C. (1965): An electron microscope study of lymphatic tissue in runt disease. J. Cell Biol. *25*, 149.

DISCUSSION

HIRSCHHORN: I am quite satisfied that what you are showing on the seventh and eighth days represents some form of phagocytic cell that is gathering around these foci and is most likely host-derived. But the early foci that you show on the third day were not typical of classical granulocytes and macrophages. They looked like transformed lymphocytes.

KIMMEL: Many of the cells are granulocytes. Unfortunately, however, in the embryonic spleen of the bird, histiocytes are very small, and difficult to distinguish from large lymphocytes.

HIRSCHHORN: With this in mind, I would like to mention the observations in the Möller's and the Hellstrom's laboratories in Stockholm, and more recently our own work, that lymphocytes from one individual overlaid on fibroblasts from another individual produces striking changes in the target fibroblasts, perhaps representing a graft-versus-host response *in vitro*. The phenomena are more commonly referred to as allogeneic inhibition, or syngeneic preference when tumor cells are employed. With human tissues, the fibroblasts are destroyed in seven or eight days and the lymphocytes have transformed into large basophilic cells. Addition of phytohemagglutinin to this system speeds up this destruction. The lymphocytes transform more rapidly than they do in the presence of phytohemagglutinin alone. Cell-to-cell adherence is also increased.

The Möller experiments show that F-1 hybrid lymphocytes overlaid on parental fibroblasts does not result in destruction of the fibroblasts unless phytohemagglutinin was also added.

AUERBACH: In our tissue culture system, we obtain reactions such as Hirschhorn describes across millipore filters, therefore, we know what is host and what is donor. If this is a "host response to the graft" *in vitro,* it occurs within three days.

There is a difference between this and the splenomegaly reaction. The host splenomegaly reaction may be looked upon as an embryonic amplification system. The labelling experiments of Fox and others suggest a host component. Our fibroblast system obviously does not. Here the destruction of the cell is the only end point; the splenomegaly system is more complex.

HIRSCHHORN: I am not inferring that splenomegaly is entirely related to the mechanism that has just been proposed. I am only wondering whether the graft aspects of this may also be occurring in the spleen and may be analogous to the isolated fibroblast system.

GOOD: Could the host component in this reaction be a consequence of surface recognition rather than a real immunological reaction?

AUERBACH: Would you accept "surface recognition" which follows transplantation rules?

GOOD: Clearly not. Allogeneic inhibition does not follow classical transplantation rules; the graft-versus-host reaction does.

AUERBACH: In our system the "host" response does.

GOOD: You mean that the cells do not proliferate?

AUERBACH: F-1 cells do not stimulate splenomegaly.

GOOD: That is critical, if true.

MITCHISON: Billingham described a weak effect of the type you are looking for, when he injected F-1 cells of the mouse into parent and produced detectable splenomegaly.

KIMMEL: The question in that system is specificity. Non-specific damage to the system due to injection such as occurs after endotoxin or carbon stimulation might yield some increase in spleen weight.

MAGE: Could you therefore clarify your controls? Do you use controls which are injected with adult radiation-inactivated leucocytes?

KIMMEL: No, nor have I worked with inbred strains.

MAGE: Do you think the injection of adult leucocyte antigen might make a contribution to your phenomenon which you could pick up by this type of control?

KIMMEL: I have some experiments with endotoxin which indicate that these same changes may occur on a much smaller scale. Whether it is specific for an immune reaction directed against the host, I am not willing to say.

EBERT: Evidence is available to answer your question. Several laboratories (for example Mun, Kosin and Sato) have shown that irradiated spleen cells do not elicit a graft-versus-host reaction.

HIRSCHHORN: That is not true in the Möller experiments. The target cell response *in vitro* is initiated with irradiated lymphocytes.

AUERBACH: In our *in vitro* system cells irradiated at 300 are one-quarter as efficient; at 600 r, there is no effect. These surface reactions are not, in my opinion, the same as the reactions you get in the graft-versus-host system.

The host responses we measure with splenomegaly may have a non-specific surface component. The major component of the reaction, however, follows all the rules of the immune system. Otherwise it would work neither with the F-1 to parent test nor after irradiation.

14

WILLIAM H. HILDEMANN

Mechanisms and ontogenetic implications of transplantation (allogeneic) disease

IT IS NOW WELL KNOWN that when immunologically competent cells in substantial numbers are inoculated into infant, juvenile, or even adult allogeneic animals incapable of destroying these cells, a syndrome called runt disease, homologous disease, allogeneic disease, or now more generally "transplantation disease" usually ensues. More severe or accelerated disease is regularly observed if lymphoid cells are obtained from preimmunized donors rather than normal donors. The early, initiation phase of such disease is clearly attributable to graft-versus-host reactions. Put in more precise immunogenetic terms, when two individuals or inbred strains differ with respect to one or more strong histocompatibility genes and antigens, transfer of adult (mature) lymphoid cells from one strain to perinatal recipients of another strain (or F_1 hybrids of the two strains) commonly leads to fatal runting disease. There are several qualifications attached to this generalization that warrant further scrutiny. Among other experimental variables which may be considered in detail, the course and severity of transplantation disease are substantially affected by the species-strain combination tested, by the age of the hosts, and by the type and number of donor cells. The acute forms of transplantation disease in various mammalian and avian species are associated with numerous pathologic features, including inhibition of growth, emaciation, diarrhea, hepatomegaly, splenomegaly, and atrophy of lymphoid tissue (13, 14). A definitive review of the earlier work in this field up to 1961 has been written by Simonsen (23). Although the manifestations of graft-versus-host reactions have been extensively described, the sequential mechanisms involved remain obscure. Some newer findings tend at least to clarify the problems of interpretation of diverse experimental "models."

COMPLEXITY OF DEVELOPMENTAL AND IMMUNOGENETIC VARIABLES

There appear to be only three essential requirements for the induction of transplantation disease: (a) the host cells must possess one or more histocompatibility antigens absent from the donor cells; (b) the donor cells must be immunologically competent or reactive; (c) the host must be incapable of rapid rejection of the donor cells. Theoretically, the least complicated situation fulfilling these requirements involves injection of adult lymphoid cells from an inbred parent strain into infant F_1 hybrids derived from the same parent strain and another inbred strain. Since a "one dominant allele—one histocompatibility antigen" relationship is well established, F_1 hybrids, regardless of their age, should be genetically incapable of reacting against parent strain cells. Actually, F_1 hybrids become increasingly resistant to runt disease induction beyond the first few days after birth. If allogeneic, adult lymphoid cells are injected into embryonic or newborn recipients, the development of transplantation disease has been thought to depend upon concurrent induction of host tolerance. However, the capacity of such immature recipients to develop immunity rapidly in response to low dosages of donor cells (4) raises the definite possibility that host-versus-graft reactions complicate this interpretation of results. Regardless of the test system employed, certain major variables should be considered or controlled as follows:

1. Strength of histocompatibility disparity
2. Type(s) and numbers of donor cells inoculated
3. Route of donor cell administration
4. Ages of hosts
5. Ages of donors
6. Sex of donors and hosts.

Extensive studies with inbred and congenic strains of mice reveal that adult donor-host differences at the H-2 locus on the 9th chromosome almost invariably lead either to acute graft rejection or acute transplantation disease. H-2 differences then constitute a "strong" histocompatibility disparity. Genetic differences restricted to other mouse histocompatibility loci, such as H-1, commonly lead to chronic allograft rejection, or weak graft-versus-host reactions which fail to produce the usual manifestations of runt disease (31). These weak histoincompatibilities then have led to definition of so-called "weak histocompatibility loci." This viewpoint is an oversimplification, however, since recent work clearly shows that the allelic (congenic strain) combination, rather than the gene locus as such, determines the relative strength of the observed histoincompatibility (Snell and Hildemann, to be published). Moreover, multiple weak histocompatibility antigens may have additive or augmentative effects leading to heightened alloimmune reactions. Conspicuous disparities in the severity of infant runt disease have been observed in strain combinations of mice differing at the strong H-2 locus (2). One may now suspect that other non-H-2 genetic differences distinguishing these strains account for the wide spectrum of mortality observed. There have been relatively few studies of graft-versus-host reactions involving single or multiple weak histocompatibility differences thus far. Optimal control of immunogenetic variability may best be achieved by use of congenic strains differing only with respect to a single histocompatibility gene. Studies necessarily involving genetically heterogeneous donor-recipient combinations, such as human beings, now show promise of more meaningful evaluation through application of leucocyte typing techniques (15).

From a developmental standpoint, attention has been focused primarily on host age as a determinative variable. Although embryonic and newborn animals of numerous species are most vulnerable to transplantation disease, there is marked variation among species usually attributed to differences in the normal ontogenesis of alloimmune responsiveness. Recent evidence indicates that immunological reactivity, including the capacity to vigorously reject allogeneic tissue, may appear in very immature individuals soon after appropriate stimulation (4, 22). Indeed, mammalian fetuses of diverse species have been shown to form antibodies and to develop delayed hypersensitivity. Even 13- to 15-day-old chick embryos may be capable of alloimmune responses if exposed to foreign cells at low dosage (25). Hence, the usually assumed absence of host-versus-graft reactions in presumably tolerant juveniles manifesting transplantation disease is doubtful. As might be expected, donor cells capable of reacting against host cells are obtainable from young chicks or mice within a few days after birth. The ability of chicken spleen cells to evoke hepatomegaly and splenomegaly in embryo hosts was found to increase with age to a peak after 21 weeks of age (24). Comparable data for mammalian donor cells are not at hand. It appears that both host age and donor cell age are important variables, perhaps affecting host homeostasis as well as immune interactions.

INITIATION OF DELETERIOUS REACTIONS: INVOLVEMENT OF CIRCULATING LYMPHOCYTES AND OTHER CELL TYPES

Most transplantation disease studies have involved the inoculation of mixed populations of adult lymphoid cells. It has thus been demonstrated that immunologically competent cells are present in the spleen, lymph nodes, blood, bone marrow, thoracic duct lymph, skin—indeed, probably in all tissues where lymphocytes are prevalent. Purified small lymphocytes from peripheral blood (14) or from thoracic duct lymph (8) are capable of producing acute runt disease in rodents. Purified small blood lymphocytes from adult chickens similarly produce splenomegaly in embryonic hosts (25). Szenberg and Warner (27) have claimed that large and medium rather than small lymphocytes are responsible for CAM pock production. Our own unpublished observations of this system clearly support the contrary assertion (25), especially with respect to the splenomegaly reaction. Isogenic adult populations of small lymphocytes also possess the capacity to protect infant mice against fatal transplantation disease provided they are injected within 48 hours after administration of allogeneic lymphocytes (12). However, much evidence peripheral to the present topic indicates that small lymphocytes constitute a functionally heterogeneous population of cells. At least one subpopulation of small lymphocytes is certainly a principal, though not necessarily the sole, source of cells mediating transplantation immunity. Immune peritoneal macrophages also appear to be able to induce acute allogeneic disease in mice (32). However, this conclusion is open to the objection that the macrophage preparations employed included substantial numbers of lymphocytes. The claim that large blood lymphocytes of mice are also immunologically reactive (5) has not yet been confirmed.

Apart from questions of cell purification, the real problem of identifying the cell type responsible for graft-versus-host reactions hinges on the occurrence and kinetics of cell transformation. Many small lymphocytes transform upon antigenic stimulation into large pyroninophilic cells. These pyroninophilic cells in turn are supposed by some investigators to develop into mature plasmacytes elaborating serum antibodies or alternatively into "committed" small lymphocytes responsible for cellular immunity. Thymidine labelling experiments suggest that the pyroninophilic cells are derived directly from small lymphocytes and many subsequently appear to transform back into small (committed?) lymphocytes (9). The interpretation of such experiments involves inferences about protracted developmental sequences of cells from the distribution of isotopic labels and this is not altogether convincing because of apparent re-utilization. The functional role of the large

pyroninophilic cells is still a mystery. These cells have not yet been demonstrated to generate the lymphocytes implicated as effectors of transplantation immunity.

Whether macrophages may function as actively immune cells, or whether they merely process antigens or provide informational RNA codons for lymphoid cells, or whether they transform into other cell types following antigenic stimulation is still unresolved. In my own tentative view, small lymphocytes initiate deleterious alloimmune reactions, but other cell types including histiocytes (macrophages) may be essential participants in sequential stages of transplantation immunity. If circulating small lymphocytes indeed include multipotential stem cells, the sequence and kinetics of cell transformations become the dominant consideration, rather than possibly misleading morphological cell identities.

SPECIFICITY OF PATHOLOGIC CHANGES: PROBLEMS OF CAUSE AND EFFECT

Our recent studies revealed that small lymphocytes from adult C57BL/6 (H-2^b) mice promptly attack neonatal A/J (H-2^a) or (A/J x C57BL/6) F$_1$ hosts. The injected cells rapidly spent themselves within 2 days, leaving few or no descendants with the *donor* antigenic constitution (12). In similar experimental situations involving inoculation of mixed populations of cells, donor cells or their descendants are usually found to persist in hosts for prolonged periods. That the purified lymphocytes in the above combination rapidly disappeared was surprising, since overt symptoms of runt disease are not evident until 8 days of age or later. The apparently long latent period between the initial damage presumably done by these lymphocytes and discernible disease suggested a study of very early changes in host lymphoid tissues. In the light of compelling evidence that the thymus is a "master organ" of immunologic responsiveness during early development, our findings could be explained if injected small lymphocytes attacked the newborn thymus directly or if an assault on the spleen and lymph nodes indirectly led to rapid thymic depletion.

The concept of an early "immunologic thymectomy" as a primary cause of acute transplantation disease was supported by the interdependent changes found in lymphoid tissues of neonatal hosts (13). The weight of the thymus declined in association with spleen and lymph node enlargement prior to the onset of clinical manifestations. A consistent pattern of thymic atrophy in conjunction with hypertrophy of spleen and lymph nodes emerged with respect to donor inoculums of both spleen cells and purified small lymphocytes as early as 1 to 2 days after injection. Relative to control animals, the normal growth of thymus and spleen was altered in opposite directions. The progressive disappearance of lymphoid cells from thymus, spleen, and lymph nodes was associated with a histiocytoid conversion of these tissues. While this process was so extensive in spleen and nodes as to produce organ weight gains, it was insufficient to offset persistent weight loss in the thymus. The final histologic pattern was essentially the same in mice given spleen cells as compared with those receiving peripheral lymphocytes, albeit some differences were apparent during the early period preceding runting. Splenic enlargement tended to be more severe in spleen cell-injected mice, perhaps reflecting the effects of donor hematopoietic cells, whereas lymph node changes were consistently more severe in recipients of small blood lymphocytes.

The question arises whether these lymphoid tissue changes were merely a nonspecific consequence of "stress." A single injection of hydrocortisone acetate into neonatal mice is sufficient to induce a wasting syndrome grossly similar to runt disease and the postthymectomy syndrome (20). Marked reductions in the weights of *both* thymus and spleen were found within a day after injection of hydrocortisone. Although general lymphoid tissue atrophy may be produced by excessive doses of adrenal corticosteroids, the spleen and lymph node hypertrophy in transplantation disease appears to be distinctive. Juvenile runting as such can be caused by various deleterious agents. The susceptibility of infant mice to runting induced by polyoma virus is one example. Similarly, splenomegaly is often associated with infections, notably so in infection of susceptible mouse genotypes by Friend leukemia virus. However, infections and other host insults do not mimic the spectrum of lymphoid tissue changes observed in early, acute transplantation disease in mammals.

If lymphocytes mediate a functional thymectomy in vulnerable allogeneic hosts, the localization of the inoculated cells should be demonstrably correlated with the early pathologic changes. The distribution of adenosine-labelled small lymphocytes injected into the blood of isogenic rats is revealing in this connection. The labelled lymphocytes "homed" rapidly and in large numbers into the lymph nodes, splenic white pulp, and Peyer's patches of the intestine. Few such cells were found in other host tissues. No labelled small lymphocytes were detected in the thymus of adult recipients, but adult donor cells did pass in small numbers into the deep thymic cortex of newborn hosts (10). Since this evidence is germane to allogeneic situations as well, I would suggest that the host thymus is depleted in the process of restitution of rapid damage to peripheral lymphoid tissue by donor cells. The possibility of a direct immunologic attack on the neonatal host thymus remains conjectural.

Among other manifestations of immunologic impairment, lymphoid cells from neonatally thymectomized mice are less capable of producing transplantation disease in appropriate recipients than the same quantity of lymphoid cells from normal mice (17). Until recently, the similarities between transplantation disease and the wasting syndrome following neonatal thymectomy alone have suggested a common pathogenesis in both conditions. Experiments with gnotobiotic, thymectomized mice reveal that they do not develop the characteristic wasting syndrome unless subsequently exposed to microorganisms. However, both germ-free mice and mice raised under normal laboratory conditions are equally vulnerable to allogeneic disease after neonatal injection with adult spleen cells (gnotobiotic donors in the case of gnotobiotic recipients) (18, 33). Thus transplantation disease is evidently a direct consequence of alloimmune reactions, whereas postthymectomy wasting is attributable to the effects of infectious agents or their products in immunologically impaired animals. In the late stages of either disease, generalized lymphoid tissue atrophy regularly occurs. It is noteworthy that nearly all deaths from acute transplantation disease in mice occur before 30 days of age; in contrast, almost all wasting deaths following neonatal thymectomy occur after the first month of postnatal life. This conspicuous difference in timing may be interpreted as evidence that destruction of the thymus alone does not lead to the earlier deaths in transplantation disease. Since even gnotobiotic animals are not necessarily virus- and rickettsia-free, the possible involvement, especially of viral disease, in the terminal phases of transplantation disease deserves further investigation. Finally, I would re-emphasize the possibility that the effective adult graft-versus-neonatal host attack may be concluded within 1-2 days in situations characterized by strong histoincompatibility. Subsequent pathologic changes may then reflect only host reactions and derangement consequent upon the initial damage. Late disease manifestations may commonly have an infectious or toxemic etiology.

Unresolved Relationships: Age Dependence and Strength of Histoincompatibility

We now know that animals of any age or stage of development, including fully mature adults, may manifest transplantation disease if exposed to a sufficient inoculum of suitable donor cells. In general, very much higher doses of donor cells are required to produce typical manifestations of allogeneic disease in normal adult hosts as compared with juvenile hosts. Although this line of evidence is consistent with the assumption that effective graft-verus-host reactions require induction of host tolerance or unresponsiveness, other evidence indicates that substantial host tolerance is neither a necessary nor sufficient condition for vulnerability. An inoculum of as few as 50,000 adult spleen cells, far fewer than the million or more cells required to induce skin allograft tolerance, may cause acute transplantation disease in neonates. On the other hand, F_1 hybrids which theoretically should be tolerant of parent strain grafts at all ages, nevertheless become markedly resistant to attack by parental lymphoid cells even in high dosages at one to two weeks after birth. The reasons for this resistance of F_1 hybrids are unknown. Host homeostatic mechanisms may be decisive. If donor cells must first find niches in host lymphoid tissue in order to kill host cells, it is likely that more mature hosts would provide less of the required *Lebensraum*. However, the occurrence of "hybrid resistance" to parental cells as a consequence of gene interaction or allelic suppression in F_1 hybrids may often be significant when there is heterozygosity at H-2 or similarly complex loci (6).

Given the same dosage, the intravenous or intracardiac route for donor cell inoculation is generally more effective than the intraperitoneal route, while the subcutaneous route is ineffective for induction of transplantation disease in neonatal mice. These differences presumably reflect for the most part the rapid immunological maturation of the newborn: the less rapidly the cell inoculum becomes systemically dispersed, the better able is the host to reject the foreign cells. In the case of F_1 hybrid hosts, differences in access to critical target cells rather than immune elimination of donor parent cells may be invoked to account for route differences. However, early elimination of reactive donor cells through "allergic injury" may well be a factor in this connection. Apparent tolerance of host antigens by persistent donor spleen cells (7) could be attributable to uncommitted lymphocytes or hematopoietic cells in the inoculum, even though immunologically reactive donor cells rapidly expired.

Contrary to earlier assumptions, sex-associated histocompatibility antigens may also be important to the outcome of parent $\rightarrow F_1$ hybrid experiments. Unless a female donor $\rightarrow$ female recipient design is employed, either X- or Y-linked antigenic disparity (1) may implement rejection of donor cells by postneonatal F_1 recipients (16). Although runt disease has not been observed as a consequence of weak, sex-associated histoincompatibility alone, chronic immune reactions have been apparent (3) and deserve further investigation.

As stated earlier, there have been few detailed studies of graft-versus-host reactions referable to single or multiple weak histocompatibility differences. Simple distinctions between "strong" and "weak" histocompatibility genes or loci have proved misleading. Actually, a complete spectrum of allograft incompatibilities is evident among congenic strains of mice ranging from quite strong to exceedingly weak reactions (11). The non-H-2 incompatibilities depend upon the products of particular alleles rather than the gene locus involved. Since prolonged skin or tumor allograft rejection is the rule among the many non-H-2 combinations tested, it is probable that chronic graft-versus-host reactions would also obtain in these combinations. The typical features of more acute transplantation disease should accordingly be subdued or wholly absent in the weaker incompatibilities.

Implications of Transplantation Disease with Respect to Cancer and Aging

Association of subtle, chronic reactions with weak antigenic disparities or with more resistant adult hosts has recently been suggested as a theoretical mechanism in development of cancer and of aging (21, 31). Several "autoimmune" diseases in man show clinical features analogous to transplantation disease as produced in experimental animals. The lesions of disorders such as systemic lupus erythematosus, acquired hemolytic anemia, scleroderma, and rheumatoid arthritis of man have pathological counterparts in experimental transplantation disease, especially in the more chronic disease in adult animals. Cutaneous lesions induced in adult rats (26) and hematologic abnormalities produced in adult mice (19) by inoculation of immunocompetent cells have been considered as models of similar human disease thought to have an autoimmune basis. In our study involving strong histocompatibility differences that led to acute runt disease in juvenile hosts, no histologic evidence for processes resembling the human disorders was discerned (13), such as connective tissue changes similar to those encountered in "collagen diseases" in the heart, kidney, joints, or elsewhere. Such changes might require a more chronic disease process which may in turn depend upon a less vulnerable victim or weaker histoincompatibility.

It is generally presumed that autoimmune disease involving tissues naturally exposed to circulating lymphocytes is the result of reactions of mutant or aberrant lymphoid cells against normal tissue macromolecules. For such lymphoid cells to react against self-constituents, a loss or mutation of a histocompatibility gene in a clone of lymphoid cells may be required. Tyler (28) has proposed that spontaneous cancer arises from single cells that suffer loss or inactivation of histocompatibility genes. Such cells are assumed to react against normal cells possessing the relevant antigen(s) as in experimental graft-versus-host reactions. The precancer cell is supposed to respond to the proliferative stimulus of the new, foreign "host" antigen with the result that cancer cells gradually destroy and replace normal ones. If this hypothesis has validity, one would expect that animals which escape acute transplantation disease should later show a significantly higher incidence of tumors. Walford (29) has advanced a similar theory of aging. In this context, aging may be essentially regarded as the result of prolonged histoincompatibility reactions among immunologically diversifying cells within an individual. Spontaneous somatic mutation of "weak" histocompatibility genes in immunocompetent cells could lead to chronic "autoimmune" reactions that are pathogenetically associated with the aging process. In essence then, both theories invoke immunogenetic mutation leading to subsequent deleterious reactions among somatic cell populations.

Several lines of recent evidence lend experimental support to these theories. A long-term study of the fate of parabiotic Syrian hamsters differing only at very weak histocompatibility loci revealed chronic immunopathologic reactions typical of transplantation disease. Moreover, amyloidosis morphologically identical to the senile type was found in chronologically young to middle-aged animals in parabiosis (30). It appears then that the major disease of aging in hamsters is substantially accelerated in the face of weak parabiotic incompatibility. Newborn mice injected with adult spleen cells from a congenic strain differing only for a single, weak histocompatibility gene (H-1^b → H-1^a) did not manifest acute disease, but did show significant life shortening compared with control animals inoculated with isogenic spleen cells (H-1^a → H-1^a). These experimental mice showed a higher incidence of lymphomas during mid-adult life which also appeared much earlier than in control animals. Both C3H mouse strains employed normally manifest only a negligible incidence of lymphoma or leukemia.

Experiments with inbred strains of mice differing at both H-2 and non-H-2 loci also reveal that malignant lymphomas may be produced in association with chronic transplantation disease (21). In this study, 6-week-old male (C57BL/6 x DBA/2) F_1 mice were given four weekly injections each of about 80×10^6 male C57BL/6 spleen cells. The long-term survivors of this immunologic assault developed lymphoid neoplasms of host origin which resembled Hodgkin's disease and lymphosarcoma. These provocative findings, though not yet sufficient to allow conclusive interpretation, suggest escalation from an immunologic to a neoplastic disease.

The ubiquitous manifestations of transplantation disease as an experimental "model"

have obviously complicated determination of sequential cause-and-effect relationships. The early phase of initiation of deleterious reactions in terms of immunogenetic disparities and lymphoid tissue changes is now better understood than later phases yielding acute disease. Very much less may be confidently deduced about chronic disease processes necessarily involving a substantial part of the total life span.

Acknowledgment.—Aided by grant from the U.S. Public Health Service HD-01252.

REFERENCES

1. Bailey, D. W. (1964): Genetically modified survival time of grafts from mice bearing X-linked histoincompatibility. Transplantation 2, 203.
2. Billingham, R. E., and Brent, L. (1959): Quantitative studies of tissue transplantation immunity. IV. Induction of tolerance in newborn mice and studies on the phenomenon of runt disease. Phil. Trans. Roy. Soc. B 242, 439.
3. Billingham, R. E., Silvers, W. K., and Wilson, D. B. (1965): A second study on the H-Y transplantation antigen in mice. Proc. Roy. Soc. (Biol.) 163, 61.
4. Boraker, D. K., and Hildemann, W. H. (1965): Maturation of alloimmune responsiveness in mice. Transplantation 3, 202.
5. Cole, L. J. and Garver, R. M. (1961): Homograft-reactive large mononuclear leukocytes in peripheral blood and peritoneal exudates. Amer. J. Physiol. 200, 147.
6. Cudkowicz, G. (1965): The immunogenetic basis of hybrid resistance to parental marrow grafts, in: Isoantigens and Cell Interactions, Wistar Institute Symp. Monogr. No. 3, Wistar Institute Press, Phila., p. 37.
7. Fox, M. (1966): Lymphoid repopulation by donor cells in the graft-versus-host reaction. Transplantation 4, 11.
8. Gowans, J. L. (1962): The fate of parental strain small lymphocytes in F_1 hybrid rats. Ann. N. Y. Acad. Sci. 99, 432.
9. Gowans, J. L. (1965): The role of lymphocytes in the destruction of homografts. Brit. Med. Bull. 21, 106.
10. Gowans, J. L., and Knight, E. J. (1964): The route of recirculation of lymphocytes in the rat. Proc. Roy. Soc. (Biol.) 159, 257.
11. Graff, R. J., Hildemann, W. H., and Snell, G. D. (1966): Histocompatibility genes of mice. VI. Allografts in mice congenic at various non-H-2 histocompatibility loci. Transplantation 4, 425.
12. Hildemann, W. H. (1964): Immunological properties of small blood lymphocytes in the graft-versus-host reaction in mice. Transplantation 2, 38.
13. Hildemann, W. H., Gallagher, R. E., and Walford, R. L. (1964): Pathologic changes in lymphoid tissues in early transplantation (runt) disease in mice. Amer. J. Path. 45, 481.
14. Hildemann, W. H., Linscott, W. D., and Morlino, M. J. (1962): Immunological Competence of Small Lymphocytes in the Graft-versus-Host Reaction in Mice; Ciba Found. Symp. Transplantation, London, J. and A. Churchill, Ltd., p. 236.
15. Histocompatibility Testing (1965): Publ. 1229, National Academy of Sciences — National Research Council, Washington, D.C. 192 pp.
16. Howard, J. G. (1961): The development and course of graft-versus-host reaction as modified by the Eichwald-Silmser phenomenon. Transpl. Bull. 28, 115.
17. Miller, J. F. A. P. (1963): Origins of immunological competence. Brit. Med. Bull. 19, 214.
18. Miller, J. F. A. P., McIntire, K. R., and Sell, S. (1964): The role of the thymus in the development of immunological competence, in: Experimental Hematology No. 7, Biology Division, Oak Ridge National Laboratory, p. 28.
19. Oliner, H., Schwartz, R., and Dameshek, W. (1961): Studies in experimental autoimmune disorders. I. Clinical and laboratory features of au-

toimmunization (runt disease) in the mouse. Blood *17*, 20.

20. Schlesinger, M., and Mark, R. (1964): Wasting disease induced in young mice by administration of cortisol acetate. Science *143*, 965.

21. Schwartz, R. S., and Beldotti, L. (1965): Malignant lymphomas following allogenic disease: transition from an immunological to a neoplastic disorder. Science *149*, 1511.

22. Silverstein, A. M. (1964): Ontogeny of the immune response. Science *144*, 1423.

23. Simonsen, M. (1962): Graft-versus-host reactions. Their natural history and applicability as tools of research. Progr. Allergy *6*, 349.

24. Solomon, J. B. (1961): The onset and maturation of the graft-versus-host reaction in chickens. J. Embryol. Exp. Morph. *9*, 355.

25. Solomon, J. B. (1964): The onset of immunological competence in the chicken. Folia Biol. (Praha) *10*, 268.

26. Stastny, O., Stembridge, V. A., and Ziff, M. (1963): Homologous disease in the adult rat, a model for autoimmune disease. I. General features and cutaneous lesions. J. Exp. Med. *118*, 635.

27. Szenberg, A., and Warner, N. L. (1962): Quantitative aspects of the Simonsen phenomenon. I. The role of the large lymphocyte. Brit. J. Exp. Path. *43*, 123.

28. Tyler, A. (1962): A developmental immunogenetic analysis of cancer, in: Henry Ford Hospital Internatl. Symp.: Biological Interactions in Normal and Neoplastic Growth, Little, Brown and Co., p. 533.

29. Walford, R. L. (1962): Autoimmunity and aging. J. Geront. *17*, 281.

30. Walford, R. L., and Hildemann, W. H. (1964): Chronic and subacute parabiotic reactions in the Syrian hamster: significance with regard to transplantation immunology, experimental amyloidosis, and an immunologic theory of aging. Transplantation *2*, 87.

31. Walford, R. L., and Hildemann, W. H. (1965): Life span and lymphoma-incidence of mice injected at birth with spleen cells across a weak histocompatibility locus. Amer. J. Path. *47*, 713.

32. Weiser, R. S., Granger, G. A., Brown, W., Baker, P., Jutila, J., and Holmes, B. (1965): Production of acute allogeneic disease in mice. Transplantation *3*, 10.

33. Wilson, R., Sjodin, K., and Bealmer, M. (1964): Thymus studies in germfree (axenic) mice, in: The Thymus, Wistar Institute Symp. Monogr. No. 2, p. 89.

DISCUSSION

Good: I agree with Dr. Hildemann that one of the paradoxes of runt disease has been the behavior of the thymus. Let me state the paradox and then offer experimental evidence from our laboratory which, we believe, sheds light on the conflict. When one injects parental strain lymphoid cells intraperitoneally or intravenously in young F1 recipients these recipients show lymph node enlargement, spleen enlargement, followed ultimately by lymph node involution and later by splenic involution and atrophy. From the outset the thymus undergoes progressive involution and atrophy. These observations have given rise to the concept expressed here by Hildemann of immunological thymectomy associated with the graft-versus-host reaction. An aspect of this which always puzzled us was the observation of Gowans that the thymus is specifically excluded from the recirculation pathways for immunologically competent cells. In contradistinction to the observations of Ford, Barnes, Harris, and Micklem, the thymus seems to be in the direct path for cells from the marrow and may provide an environment wherein uncommitted bone marrow cells gain immunological competence.

Lyle Heim, a degree candidate working with Professor Martinez, studied the effect of adrenal extirpation on homologous disease. He found that the peripheral lymphoid tissue such as spleen and lymph node went through all the organ changes described here and the animals developed wasting and died earlier and more frequently. The thymus was, however, spared. The apparent wasting of the thymus in transplantation disease is mediated, then, through the pituitary-adrenal axis and not as a consequence of direct immunological assault on the organ. This observation appears to resolve the paradox of "immunological thymectomy" when immunologically competent cells do not recirculate through the thymus.

We are intrigued with the ideas of Walford and Hildemann concerning a possible immunological contribution to aging. It must be pointed out, however, that observations on the development of malignancy of the lymphoid system may be a function of a low-grade immunological process which in turn interferes with the general immunological competence. Some years ago Howard and Woodruff and Blaese, Martinez, and I showed that a vigorous graft-versus-host reaction results in profound inhibition of host responsiveness to unrelated antigens. In parabiotic intoxication even of a low-grade type the ability to resist endogenous or exogenous infection is adversely affected. If such is the case, the agents responsible for development of certain malignancies might be resisted imperfectly and malignant disease of the lymphoid tissue might result.

That ability to resist infection in humans may indeed be correlated with development of malignancies of the lymphoreticular system has been suggested. Mongoloid children, for example, show a high frequency of lymphatic leukemia at the same time they seem inordinately prone to infection. Children with the sex-linked recessive type of hypogammaglobulinemia develop leukemias with unusual frequency.

The Chediak-Hagashi disease is characterized both by recurrent infections and by malignancy. All of the children studied in the past with this strange autosomal recessive disease anomaly have died early in life with infection. With careful attention to treatment of their infections most now live longer but die of lymphoreticular malignancy. This particular form of malignancy of the lymphoid system seems to begin as a general infiltrative process involving mononuclear cells in nerves, kidneys, and lymphoid organs. It later distorts and destroys the architecture of the lymphoid organs and thus has all characteristics of lymphosarcoma. When Peter Dent and I cultured these cells in tissue culture we could show that here too they behaved as malignant cells having lost capacity for contact inhibition and like malignant cells they produced tumors upon injection into the hamster cheek pouch. White, working with our cases, showed that in the blood cells and tumor cells of these patients could be found many virus-like particles, on the order of 10,000 per cell.

Increased susceptibility to infection in these patients appears to be due to an abnormality of their lysosomal structure and presumably their lysosomal function as well. The lysosomes in these patients are abnormal in size. Even the pigmentary anomaly is due to the large size of the melanosomes.

In this disease neither aging nor malfunction of the immunological apparatus is responsible for the regular development of malignancy but rather another anomaly rendering the patient unable to resist infection.

Such studies of patients with immunological deficiency diseases offer increasing support for Lewis Thomas' concept of immunological surveillance as the primary defense against neoplasia. The concept may conceivably be broadened to include non-immunological processes involved in resistance to infection including the lysosomal function.

HILDEMANN: You recall that we have been very careful to point out the possibility that viral infection may be involved in increased incidence of tumors presumably initiated by chronic graft-versus-host reactions. This is very difficult to disprove.

I would like any specific suggestions as to how one might utilize immunologically competent cells in such a way as to rule out virus etiology. Congenic strains, differing by a single histocompatible locus, ought to be carrying similar viruses, but this has not been established.

Part of the burden of my argument is that there are sufficient differences in detail between runting induced by hydrocortisone injection, the wasting in the postthymectomy syndrome, and typical transplantation disease to warrant a meaningful distinction among these different processes.

The adrenalectomy experiment Good describes augments the complications of interpretation. The effects of the corticosteroids are ubiquitous and it is impossible for me to circumscribe their various effects in interpreting the pathology of transplantation disease. In attempts to assess the role of infection we have tried to culture bacteria from acutely ill animals in the late stage of transplantation disease and usually failed to do so. Trying to rule out viral disease in this way is more difficult. The presence of virus-like particles does not constitute critical proof of viral etiology, I know you agree.

The one experiment that stands as a strong argument against the infectious agent role in transplantation disease was reported by MacIntyre and Miller. Germ-free neonates injected with adult cells from germ-free donors developed typical transplantation disease.

Germ-free animals were not vulnerable to postthymectomy syndrome. This argues against infectious etiology although these mice were not necessarily virus- and rickettsia-free.

FELDMAN: In your experiments on the effect of allogeneic cells in increasing the incidence of leukemia, your controls also showed a high incidence of neoplasms. The difference between the two groups was that the experimental animals developed leukemia earlier than in the control ones. Since your controls were treated by addition of isogeneic cells what is the incidence of leukemia in non-treated animals?

HILDEMANN: It is low. The main difference between the two groups is the timing.

FELDMAN: Are the cell types of the leukemia those of the donor or of the host?

HILDEMANN: We do not know for sure whether they are of host or donor type. Transplantation tests of malignant tumor cells may be misleading with very weak antigens unless the hosts are suitably preimmunized.

FELDMAN: That is an interesting point, because you may remember that some years ago Uphoff and Law published results of treating irradiated F_1 hybrids with parental strain cells. They got a relatively high incidence of leukemia, 66% of which were of the donor type, i.e., the type of cell expected to react against the isoantigens of the host. The idea was that the donor type cells which undergo a high rate of replication are the ones which are transformed to leukemic cells.

15

MAX D. COOPER, ANN E. GABRIELSEN, and
ROBERT A. GOOD

The development, differentiation, and function
of the immunoglobulin production system

At the first Immunology Workshop we presented experimental evidence indicating a sharp division of the avian lymphoid system into two separate cell systems having distinct morphology and function (21). The thymus was shown to be necessary for the development and function of a population of lymphoid cells, mainly small lymphocytes, in peripheral lymphoid tissues. As in mammals, the avian thymus system of cells effects delayed allergic reactions, graft-versus-host reactivity, and at least the major portion of homograft rejection, immunologic functions that are collectively termed cellular immunity. On the other hand, plasma cell and germinal center development was demonstrated to be dependent on the bursa of Fabricius. The bursa system of cells is responsible for the synthesis of immunoglobulins. The observations (20, 22) leading to this concept confirm the thesis that the avian thymus and bursa of Fabricius play different roles in immune responsiveness and strongly support the contention that cellular immune functions can be sharply separated from those immunologic functions associated with circulating antibodies (7, 8, 10, 40, 42, 44, 45, 47, 69-72).

Three lines of evidence led us to propose that the mammalian lymphoid system is similarly composed of a bursal cell system, or immunoglobulin production system, as well as a thymus system of cells. Small lymphocytes and cellular immunity as well as plasma cells and humoral immunity are found in early ver-

tebrates long before the evolutionary emergence of birds and mammals (35, 63). Experimentally, the roles of the avian thymus and mammalian thymus proved parallel (7, 8, 10, 20-22, 38, 44, 47, 50, 52, 53, 70) and neither seems to affect plasma cell differentiation or immunoglobulin synthesis directly (7, 10, 20-22, 34, 42, 44, 47). Finally, nature has neatly separated the thymus system and the immunoglobulin production system in several immune deficiency diseases in man which closely parallel the experimental division achieved in chickens (12, 29, 33, 37, 57).

The chicken provides a valid model for the study of plasma cell differentiation and immunoglobulin synthesis. Accordingly, we will consider here the beginning steps in understanding the development, differentiation, and function of this cell system.

Removal of the bursa of Fabricius in newly hatched chicks prevents development of normal antibody-producing capability. This observation, originally made by Glick et al. (36), has been repeatedly confirmed (15, 16, 22, 40, 42, 55, 56). The means by which the bursa controls antibody responsiveness was unclear as plasma cell differentiation and immunoglobulin synthesis were observed even in bursectomized birds producing no detectable antibody. The levels of immunoglobulins are definitely reduced in bursectomized birds and plasma cells may be reduced as well according to some (13, 22, 42, 49, 61, 69, 71, 72).

Subsequently, it has been shown that antibody responsiveness can be augmented in bursectomized birds by implantation of bursal tissue within a cell impenetrable diffusion chamber (46, 67). These observations suggest that a diffusible factor may be produced by the bursa which is essential for the development of normal antibody-producing capacity in chickens.

By insuring complete removal of the bursa in newly hatched chickens, Ortega and Der were able to produce chicks capable of γM-type immunoglobulin synthesis but unable to synthesize γG-type immunoglobulin (61). We have confirmed this observation and shown that the γM-type immunoglobulin level of such chickens is strikingly elevated although germinal center and plasma cell development appears normal even in these γG-type agammaglobulinemic birds (22). None of these γG agammaglobulinemic chicks has produced detectable circulating antibody to several antigens in our hands. One possible explanation of these observations is that a diffusible bursal factor is required for the maturation of capacity to make the immunoglobulin synthesis shift from γM- to γG-immunoglobulins.

Since the effects of early thymectomy can be correlated with the stage of peripheral lymphoid development at the time of thymectomy and since this development is considerable in the newly hatched chick we added near lethal x-irradiation to bursectomy to test the lymphopoietic role of the bursa (20-22). Seven-week-old chicks bursectomized and heavily irradiated in the newly hatched period have no germinal center and plasma cell development, are γM and γG agamma-globulinemic, and are incapable of circulating antibody production. These bursectomized and irradiated birds fully recover their thymus system of cells and exhibit intact cellular immunity. Chickens thymectomized and irradiated in the newly hatched period fail to recover their small lymphocyte population and cellular immunity but their germinal center and plasma cell development as well as immunoglobulin synthesis appear normal. Irradiated control birds exhibit complete recovery of lymphoid tissues and immunologic competence when tested at age 7 weeks. Serial evaluation of spleen tissues after bursectomy and irradiation at hatching reveals plasmablasts and plasma cells in the early weeks of life. The subsequent absence of these cellular elements suggests that stem cells necessary for survival of this cell line are lacking following these treatments.

These observations suggested to us that germinal center cells and plasma cells derive from bursal lymphoid cells. After bursal removal and irradiation in newly hatched chicks we have put back autologous bursal lymphoid cells as one means of testing this hypothesis (23). Bursectomized and irradiated chickens receiving bursal lymphoid cells by the intracoelomic route exhibit near normal germinal center and plasma cell development and γM- and γG-immunoglobulin synthesis while untreated bursectomized-irradiated birds do not (Table 1). It seems likely that we did not provide the bursal diffusible factor by this

TABLE 1.—RESTORATION OF γ-GLOBULIN PRODUCTION IN AGAMMAGLOBULINEMIC CHICKENS*

| Experimental Group | Germinal Centers | Plasma Cells | γ-Globulins | | BSA Agglutinins Mean Titer (Log₂) | Brucella Agglutinins Mean Titer (Log₂) |
			γM	γG		
Control-irradiated	6/6	6/6	6/6	6/6	7.2	6.2
Bursectomized-irradiated	0/6	0/6	0/6	0/6	0	0
Bursectomized-irradiated, injected with autologous bursal cell suspension	7/7	7/7	7/7	7/7	0	0

*After bursectomy on the day of hatching, all birds were given a skin dose of 740 r x-irradiation. Autologous and unirradiated bursal cells were injected into the coelomic cavity of each bursectomized and irradiated bird in one group. All animals were immunized with 20 mg of BSA and 10^9 Brucella abortus organisms at age 40 days and bled and killed 9 days later.

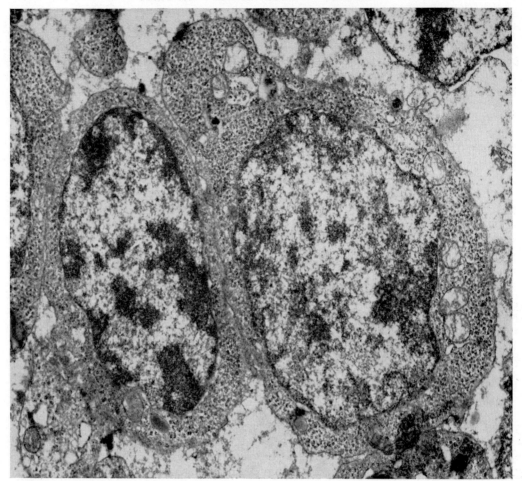

Fig. 1. Electron micrograph of typical lymphoid cells within a bursal follicle of a two-month-old chicken. The cytoplasm of these cells contains many ribosomal clusters. Each cluster consists of 4-7 ribosomes in close conformation. Formation of endoplasmic reticulum is not seen in the illustrated cells. (Orig. mag. x 15,500) Electron microscopy performed by Dr. C. C. Clawson.

means of treatment as this restoration of the immunoglobulin producing cells was not accompanied by detectable circulating antibody responsiveness. Also, the treated bursectomized-irradiated chickens usually die at about two months of age as do untreated bursectomized-irradiated agammaglobulinemic birds. Although these observations provide support for the concept of non-antibody γ-globulin or "non-sense" γ-globulin other interpretations are possible. Perhaps with the fully dispersed bursal cells we have reconstituted the chicks with few of many potential clones of bursal cells and plasma cells and with the antigens used in our tests have not assayed for those few antigens to which these chickens can respond. Or as seems even more likely to us,

we may have reconstituted these animals with a limited number of committable cells that promptly became directionalized by exposure to antigens in the environment precluding a possible response to the antigens used in our assay of responsiveness 6 or 7 weeks later. It appears most likely then that in the chicken at least plasma cells do not arise from primitive reticular cells throughout the lymphoreticular tissues of the body but rather begin this type of differentiation in a special gut epithelium related site.

The lymphoid cells within the bursal follicles vary from small lymphocytes (approximate diameter of 4μ) with densely clumped nuclear chromatin and scant faintly pyroninophilic cytoplasm to larger lymphoid cells (ap-

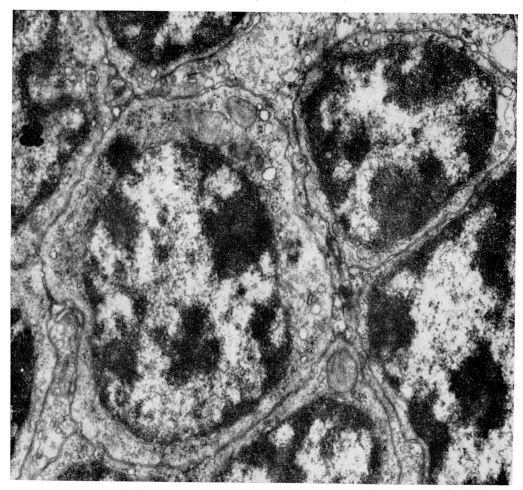

Fig. 2. Electron micrograph of typical thymus lymphocytes of a two-month-old chicken. Note that ribosomes are randomly distributed in the cytoplasm of these thymus lymphocytes in marked contrast to the ribosomal clustering in the cytoplasm of bursal lymphocytes. (Orig. mag. x 24,300)

proximate diameter of 8μ) with large nuclei having a reticular chromatin pattern and often a prominent nucleolus. These larger lymphocytes have more cytoplasm which is also faintly pyroninophilic. Rather uniformly the bursal lymphoid cells exhibit cytoplasmic ribosomal organization into a cluster conformation with approximately 4-7 ribosomes per cluster or rosette (Fig. 1). These cells occasionally may contain sparse islets of endoplasmic reticulum. Plasma cells and preplasma cells are not seen in the bursal follicles but are found in bursal interstitial tissue (lamina propria) between follicles, particularly just beneath the secretory epithelial lining. The lymphoid cells within the germinal centers of the spleen vary from cells indistinguishable from bursal lymphocytes to large transitional cells or plasmablasts with fairly intense cytoplasmic pyroninophilia. The latter cell type, seen most regularly near the periphery of the germinal center, often are well along a plasma cell line of differentiation with substantial development of rough endoplasmic reticulum. Many preplasma and plasma cells are found in spleen areas adjacent to germinal centers. It is our interpretation then that the morphology of these cells is consistent with a differentiation of bursal lymphoid cells to plasma cells with cells of the germinal centers representing an intermediate stage in this pathway of differentiation (17, 18).

In contrast to bursal lymphoid cells, the thymus lymphocytes are smaller, more uniform in cell size, and lacking in ribosomal organization into cytoplasmic clusters (Fig. 2) (17, 18). These structural differences between thymus and bursal lymphocytes provide further evidence of a different influence on differentiation by the thymus on the system of cells dependent upon it.

Dent and Good (30) have shown that bursal lymphoid cells do not synthesize either sheep erythrocyte lysins or agglutinins after intravenous immunization although cells of the spleen produce both. Bursal lymphocytes fail to stain with fluorescein-tagged rabbit antibody directed at chicken γ-globulin. Finally, bursal explants produce little γ-globulin by comparison to spleen explants. In a system based on incorporation of C_{14} labelled amino acid into γ-globulin, the spleen can be shown to produce considerable amounts of this protein. By contrast, under the same conditions the bursa produces little γ-globulin (31).

It is well known that cells of both mammalian and avian germinal centers contain immunoglobulins having antibody specificity (17, 59, 73, 74). These observations are consonant with the observations made of the fine structural features of some germinal center cells. It will be of interest to see whether all the germinal center cells have this capacity since one might doubt synthesis of a specific secretory product by those cells with tight ribosomal clusters and lacking significant endoplasmic reticulum in their cytoplasm.

On the basis of over-all morphology and histochemical staining characteristics of the developing bursa, it has been concluded that local epithelial cells are induced to become lymphoid (1-3). This conclusion has been contested on both morphologic and theoretic grounds (9, 60). Recently, Moore and Owen (54) have provided convincing evidence of origin of bursal lymphocyte precursors from blood cells by employing karyotypic analysis of bursal lymphocytes in embryos mismatched with respect to sex. In these experiments, cells clearly of female karyotype turn up in the bursa of the male birds. Similar observations have been made after parobiotic union of chicken and turkey embryos (43). The appearance and origin of this blood borne bursal lymphocyte precursor is as yet unknown.

Another area demanding analysis is the mechanism involved in induction for lymphoid differentiation within the bursa. Perhaps the best clues available at present lie in the observations of situations in which this type of lymphoid differentiation has been altered.

For example, it has been shown by Meyer et al. (51) that testosterone interferes with bursal lymphoid differentiation if given in adequate dosage in the early embryonic period. Chickens treated in this manner fail to develop normal antibody-producing capability (51, 55, 56, 62, 69, 71, 72). Testosterone treatment begun after birth appears to stop further follicular differentiation within the bursa but the lymphoid cells present at the onset of treatment appear unaltered by testosterone treatment and bursal lymphoid follicles persist for several weeks after initiation of testosterone administration (Fig. 3). However, when testosterone treatment is begun after the bursal lymphoid cells are destroyed by x-irradiation in the newly hatched period (Fig. 4), lymphoid regeneration does not occur (Fig. 5) although this regeneration occurs rapidly following irradiation alone (Fig. 6). The combination of posthatching irradiation and testosterone treatment prevents development of normal antibody-producing capability while neither treatment alone is effective at this age (27). These observations suggest that testosterone is not toxic to the cells of the bursal system but instead interferes with the induction of lymphoid differentiation. Since testosterone inhibits alkaline phosphatase activity within the bursa it has been suggested that this enzyme may play an inductive role in local lymphoid differentiation (3).

Another example of abnormal bursal lymphocyte differentiation is observed in the virus-induced lymphoid malignancy of chickens, lymphoid leukosis. The first evidence that this was a malignancy of the bursal cell system, in contrast to lymphoid malignancies of mice involving the thymus system, was the observation that bursectomy prevented development of lymphoid leukosis whereas thymectomy did not (64, 66). In current studies (24) we have shown that this malignant lymphoid transformation occurs first in the bursa well before malignant cells are seen in germinal center distribution in the periphery. The peripherally distributed malignant cells appear similar to plasmablasts by ordinary light microscopy but mature plasma cells are extremely

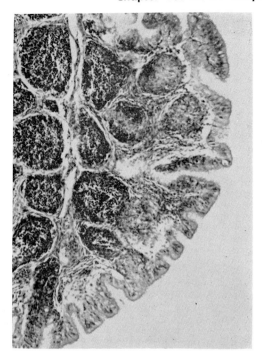

FIG. 3. Bursal plicae from a 14-day chicken that was treated with 19 nor-testosterone (3 injections of 6 mg/week) since hatching. Note the persistence of deep lymphoid follicles with the formation of epithelial crypts and lack of morphologic evidence for ongoing lymphoid follicle formation in association with epithelium. (H & E x 40)

Recently, however, Di George (32, 33) has observed a child who exhibited failure of differentiation of the 3d and 4th pharyngeal pouch epithelium. Although this boy lacked a thymus and its dependent peripheral lymphocyte population and also lacked parathyroid glands, he had plasma cells and circulating immunoglobulins. Even though plasma cell differentiation and γ-globulin synthesis may proceed without an intact thymus system in both clinical and experimental circumstances this developmental relationship precludes normal specific antibody production (4, 10, 20-22, 32-34, 38, 41, 44, 53, 70). The thymus system in some way then appears necessary for the initiation of specific antibody synthesis in response to stimulation with certain antigens. The thymus system apparently does not participate in the anamnestic antibody response (11, 48). It appears that the collaborative role of the thymus system is limited to the initial induction of specific antibody synthesis.

rare or are not found in the neighborhood of the malignant follicles. Consistent with this evidence of "arrested" differentiation is the lack of ribosomal organization into rosettes and lack of endoplasmic reticulum formation in the cytoplasm of these malignant cells. In addition, the malignant cells do not synthesize detectable amounts of γ-globulin. The earliest recognizable malignant stage in lymphoid leukosis features focal follicular lymphoid transformation within the bursa itself. Indeed, one malignant bursal follicle may be surrounded by more than 500 normal follicles. On the basis of these observations we believe that this malignancy represents an abnormal differentiation of bursal lymphocytes and that an abnormal induction process is more likely the basis than a virus-induced abnormality of the cells precursor to the bursal lymphocytes.

At one time we considered the possibility that the thymus system cells play a critical role in initiating bursal lymphoid differentiation.

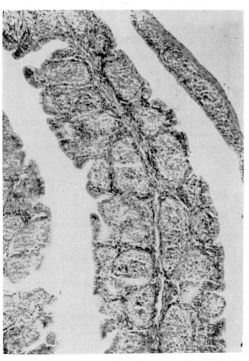

FIG. 4. Section of a bursa from a 2-day chick that was given 650 r whole body x-irradiation 24 hours earlier. The bursal follicles are essentially devoid of intact lymphoid cells. (H & E x 40)

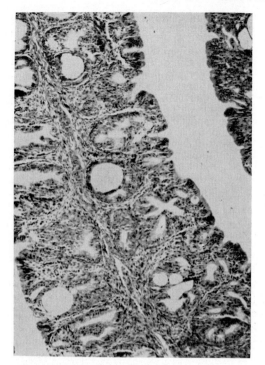

Fig. 5. Section of a bursa from a 6-day chick that was x-irradiated at hatching and then treated with 19 nor-testosterone. There are no lymphoid follicles, formation of epithelial crypts and cystic degeneration are prominent. (H & E x 40)

A further pressing question is what, if any, mammalian tissue is equivalent to the avian bursa of Fabricius. An analogous site of induction of differentiation toward the immunoglobulin-synthesizing plasma cell seems most probable. Criteria gained from the chicken model aid in this search: (a) this site should have follicular or germinal center type of lymphoid structure; (b) follicular organization should appear earlier than peripheral germinal centers prior to and independent of antigenic stimulation; (c) this tissue should be associated with gut epithelium and exhibit a lympho-epithelial relationship; (d) it should exhibit maximal growth in early life probably succeeding shortly the thymus in development and differentiation and probably should show some involution later in life following sexual maturation; (e) this bursa-equivalent tissue should be "central" in type, lacking or relatively lacking in immunological potential itself; and (f) such tissue or organ should be absent in patients congenitally lacking germi-

nal centers and plasma cells in peripheral lymphoid tissues.

Earlier, we considered the palatine tonsils a likely candidate for the bursal role. Experimentally we could not demonstrate an effect on antibody-synthesizing capacity in rabbits after neonatal tonsillectomy even in combination with total body irradiation (28). On the basis of the similarities by the above criteria and by older observations of Carlens (14) and more recent observations of Cornes (28) on the development of Peyer's patches, we chose to look again (5, 6, 68) experimentally at the Peyer's patch type of tissue in mammals.

The lymphoid tissues as seen in mammalian Peyer's patches and the appendix and sacculus rotundus of the rabbit appear to fulfill all of these criteria. Morphologically, these tissues exhibit a lympho-epithelial association with related follicular lymphoid organization (Figs. 7a and 7b). In man, Peyer's patch follicular development is apparent by 20 to 24 weeks of gestation long before germinal center development appears in lymph nodes and spleen and

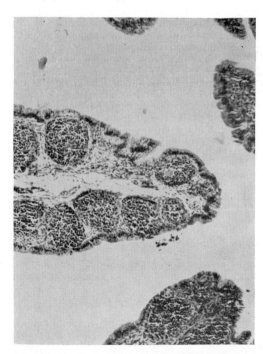

Fig. 6. By 6 days the lymphoid follicles of the bursa have completely regenerated in this chick that was given 650 r x-irradiation at hatching. (H & E x 40)

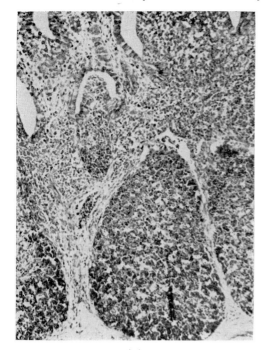

(a)

Fig. 7. (*a*) Section of the appendix of a young adult rabbit. Note the follicular organization of the lymphoid tissue and its association with the intestinal epithelium. (H & E x 100) (*b*) Higher magnification of the rabbit appendix illustrating the lympho-epithelial relationship which is found in the areas of epithelium overlying lymphoid follicles. (H & E x 250)

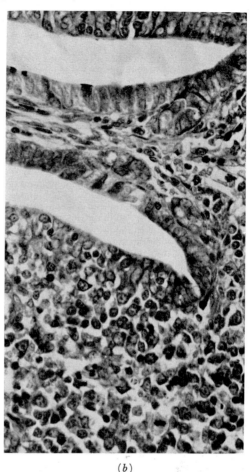

(b)

prior to known antigenic exposure (28). Peyer's patch development appears normal in both germ-free mice and rats when compared with conventional animals (58) and these structures fail to develop in congenital sex-linked agammaglobulinemia (39). Further, the follicular component of Peyer's patches appears to involute beginning soon after sexual maturation in man. Our preliminary experimental results following removal of these intestinal lympho-epithelial structures in rabbits are consistent with a selectively bursectomy-type effect on immunologic development (25). Indeed, a slight defect in antibody synthesis following neonatal appendectomy in rabbits was shown some time ago in this laboratory (24). These experiments were carried out on the basis of morphologic similarity of the rabbit appendix and sacculus rotundus to the avian bursa (5, 6). Since these observations were made before the delineation of the thymus and bursal systems in the chicken, this effect was considered a thymectomy type of effect. It seems more likely now that these observations parallel more closely a partial bursectomy effect. At any rate, we are optimistic that a clear-cut bursal role for these intestinal lympho-epithelium associated tissues will be supported by solid experimental results in the near future.

Acknowledgments.—Original clinical and experimental studies from these laboratories cited were aided by grants from the U.S. Public Health Service (NB-02042, AI-00798, HE-02085, HE-06314), National Foundation, American Cancer Society, American Heart Association, Graduate School of the University of Minnesota, Minnesota Heart Association, and Minnesota Chapter of the Arthritis Foundation.

PART III — EDITOR: ROBERT AUERBACH

REFERENCES

1. Ackerman, G. A., and Knouff, R. A. (1959): Lymphocytopoiesis in the bursa of Fabricius. Amer. J. Anat. *104*, 163.
2. Ackerman, G. A. (1962): Electron microscopy of the bursa of Fabricius of the embryonic chick with particular reference to the lymphoepithelial nodules. J. Cell Biol. *13*, 127.
3. Ackerman, G. A., and Knouff, R. A. (1964): Lymphocytopoietic activity in the bursa of Fabricius, in: Good, R. A., and Gabrielsen, A. E., eds.: The Thymus in Immunobiology. New York, Hoeber-Harper.
4. Archer, O., and Pierce, J. C. (1961): Role of thymus in development of immune response. Fed. Proc. *20*, 26.
5. Archer, O. K., Sutherland, D. E. R., and Good, R. A. (1963): Appendix of the rabbit: A homologue of the bursa in the chicken? Nature *200*, 337.
6. Archer, O. K., Sutherland, D. E. R., and Good, R. A. (1964): The developmental biology of the lymphoid tissue of the rabbit: Consideration of the role of the thymus and appendix. Lab. Invest. *13*, 259.
7. Arnason, B. G., Janković, B. D., Waksman, B. H., and Wennersten, C. (1962): Role of the thymus in immune reactions in rats. II. Suppressive effect of thymectomy at birth on reactions of delayed (cellular) hypersensitivity and the circulating small lymphocyte. J. Exp. Med. *116*, 177.
8. Aspinall, R. L., Meyer, R. K., Graetzer, M. A., and Wolfe, H. R. (1963): Effect of thymectomy and bursectomy on the survival of skin homografts in chickens. J. Immun. *90*, 872.
9. Auerbach, R. (1964): In discussion of paper by Ackerman, G. A., and Knouff, R. A., in: Good, R. A., and Gabrielsen, A. E., eds.: The Thymus in Immunobiology. New York, Hoeber-Harper.
10. Azar, H. A., Snyder, R. W., and Williams, J. (1963): Dissociation between serum gamma globulin and precipitin antibody in rats thymectomized at birth. Fed. Proc. *22*, 600.
11. Barr, M., and Fairley, G. H. (1961): Circulating antibodies in reticuloses. Lancet *1*, 1305.
12. Bruton, O. C. (1952): Agammaglobulinemia. Peds. *9*, 722.
13. Carey, J., and Warner, N. L. (1964): Gamma globulin synthesis in hormonally bursectomized chickens. Nature *203*, 198.
14. Carlens, O. (1928): Studien über das lymphatische Gewebe des Darmkanals bei einigen Haustieren, mit besonderer Berücksichtigung der embryonalen Entwicklung, der Mengenverhältnisse und der Altersinvolution dieses Gewebes im Dünndarm des Rindes. Z. Anat. Entwicklungsgesch. *86*, 393.
15. Chang, T. S., Rheims, M. S., and Winter, A. R. (1957): The significance of the bursa of Fabricius in antibody production in chickens. 1. Age of chickens. Poult. Sci. *36*, 735.
16. Chang, T. S., Rheims, M. S., and Winter, A. R. (1958): The significance of the bursa of Fabricius of chickens in antibody production. 2. Spleen relationship. Poult. Sci. *37*, 1091.
17. Clawson, C. C., Cooper, M. D., and Good, R. A. (1966): Comparison of the fine structure of the bursa of Fabricius, the thymus and the germinal center. Fed. Proc. *25*, 309.
18. Clawson, C. C., Cooper, M. D., and Good, R. A.; Lymphocyte fine structure in the bursa of Fabricius, thymus and the germinal center. Lab. Invest. [In press]
19. Coons, A. H., Leduc, E. H., and Connolly, J. M. 1955): Studies on antibody production. I. A method for the histochemical demonstration of specific antibody and its application to a study of the hyperimmune rabbit. J. Exp. Med. *102*, 49.
20. Cooper, M. D., Peterson, R. D. A., and Good, R. A. (1965): Delineation of the thymic and bursal lymphoid systems in the chicken. Nature *205*, 143.
21. Cooper, M. D., Peterson, R. D. A., and Good, R. A. (1965): The development of the immune system in the chicken, in: Phylogeny of Immunity. Gainesville, University of Florida Press, p. 243.
22. Cooper, M. D., Peterson, R. D. A., South, M. A., and Good, R. A. (1966): The functions of the thymus system and the bursa system in the chicken. J. Exp. Med. *123*, 75.
23. Cooper, M. D., Schwartz, M. L., and Good, R. A. (1966): Restoration of gamma globulin production in agammaglobulinemic chickens. Science *151*, 471.
24. Cooper, M. D., Payne, L. N., Dent, P. B., Clawson, C. C., Peterson, R. D. A., Burmester, B. R., and Good, R. A. (1966): The role of the bursa in avian lymphoid leukosis. Fed. Proc. *25*, 310.
25. Cooper, M. D., Perey, D. Y., McKneally, M., Gabrielsen, A. E., Sutherland, D. E. R., and Good, R. A. (1966): A mammalian equivalent to the bursa of Fabricius. Lancet *1*, 1388.
26. Cooper, M. D., Peterson, R. D. A., and Good, R. A.: Unpublished observations.
27. Cooper, M. D., Schwartz, M. L., and Good, R. A.: Unpublished observations.
28. Cornes, J. S. (1965): Number, size and distribution of Peyer's patches in the human small intestine. Gut *6*, 225.
29. Craig, J. M., Gitlin, J. M., and Jewett, T. C. (1954): The response of lymph nodes of normal and congenitally agammaglobulinemic children to antigenic stimulation. Amer. J. Dis. Child. *88*, 626.
30. Dent, P. B., and Good, R. A. (1965): Absence of antibody production in the bursa of Fabricius. Nature *207*, 491.
31. Dent, P. B., and Peterson, R. D. A. (1966): Immunoglobulin production and the bursa of Fabricius. Fed. Proc. *25*, 474.
32. Di George, A. M.: Personal communication.

33. Di George, A. M. (1965): In discussion of paper by M. D. Cooper, *et al.* J. Pediat. *67,* 907.
34. Fahey, J. L., Barth, W., and Law, L. W. (1964): Investigations on mechanisms of normal and defective immunity. J. Clin. Invest. *43,* 1239.
35. Finstad, J., Papermaster, B. W., and Good, R. A. (1964): Evolution of the immune response. II. Morphologic studies on the origin of the thymus and organized lymphoid tissue. Lab. Invest. *13,* 490.
36. Glick, B., Chang, T. S., and Jaap, R. G. (1956): The bursa of Fabricius and antibody production. Poult. Sci. *35,* 224.
37. Good, R. A. (1954): Agammaglobulinemia: An experimental study. Amer. J. Dis. Child. *88,* 626.
38. Good, R. A., Dalmasso, A. P., Martinez, C., Archer, O. K., Pierce, J. C., and Papermaster, B. W. (1962): The role of the thymus in development of immunologic capacity in rabbits and mice. J. Exp. Med. *116,* 773.
39. Good, R. A., Kelly, W. D., Rötstein, J., and Varco, R. L. (1962): Immunological deficiency diseases. Progr. Allergy *6,* 187.
40. Graetzer, M. A., Wolfe, H. R., Aspinall, R. L., and Meyer, R. K. (1963): Effect of thymectomy and bursectomy on precipitin and natural hemagglutinin production in the chicken. J. Immun. *90,* 878.
41. Humphrey, J. H., Parrott, D. M. V., and East, J. (1964): Studies on globulin and antibody production in mice thymectomized at birth. Immunol. *7,* 419.
42. Isaković, K., and Janković, B. D. (1964): Role of the thymus and bursa of Fabricius in immune reactions in chickens. II. Cellular changes in lymphoid tissues of thymectomized, bursectomized and normal chickens in the course of first antibody response. Int. Arch. Allerg. and Appl. Immunol. *24,* 296.
43. Jaffe, P. (1965): Personal communication.
44. Janković, B. D., Waksman, B. H., and Arnason, B. G. (1962): Role of the thymus in immune reactions in rats. I. The immunologic response to bovine serum albumin (antibody formation, Arthus reactivity, and delayed hypersensitivity) in rats thymectomized or splenectomized at various times after birth. J. Exptl. Med. *116,* 159.
45. Janković, B. D., and Išvaneski, M. (1963): Experimental allergic encephalomyelitis in thymectomized, bursectomized and normal chickens. Int. Arch. Allerg. Appl. Immunol. *23,* 188.
46. Janković, B. D., and Leskowitz, S. (1965): Restoration of antibody producing capacity in bursectomized chickens by bursal grafts in millipore ® chambers. Proc. Soc. Exp. Biol. Med. *118,* 1164.
47. Janković, B. D., and Isaković, K. (1964): Role of the thymus and the bursa of Fabricius in immune reactions in chickens. I. Changes in lymphoid tissues of chickens surgically thymectomized at hatching. Int. Arch. Allerg. Appl. Immunol. *24,* 278.
48. Leuchars, E., Cross, A. M., and Davies, A. J. S. (1964): Retention of immunological information by thymectomized syngeneic radiation chimaeras. Nature *203,* 1042.
49. Long, P. L., and Pierce, A. E. (1963): Role of cellular factors in the mediation of immunity to avian coccidiosis (Emeria Tenella). Nature *200,* 426.
50. Martinez, C., Kersey, J., Papermaster, B. W., and Good, R. A. (1962): Skin homograft survival in thymectomized mice. Proc. Soc. Exp. Biol. Med. *109,* 193.
51. Meyer, R. K., Rao, M. A., and Aspinall, R. L. (1959): Inhibition of the development of the bursa of Fabricius in embryos of the common fowl by 19-nor-testosterone. Endocrinology *64,* 890.
52. Miller, J. A. F. P. (1961): Immunologic function of the thymus. Lancet *2,* 748.
53. Miller, J. A. F. P. (1962): Effect of neonatal thymectomy on the immunological responsiveness of the mouse. Proc. Roy. Soc. (London) Ser. B. *156,* 415.
54. Moore, M. A. S., and Owen, J. J. T. (1965): Chromosome marker studies on the development of the hemopoietic system in the chick embryo. Nature *208,* 956.
55. Mueller, A. P., Wolfe, H. R., and Meyer, R. K. (1960): Precipitin production in chickens. XXI. Antibody production in bursectomized chickens and in chickens injected with 19 nor-testosterone on the fifth day of incubation. J. Immun. *85,* 172.
56. Mueller, A. P., Wolfe, H. R., Meyer, R. K., and Aspinall, R. L. (1962): Further studies on the role of the bursa of Fabricius in antibody production. J. Immun. *88,* 354.
57. Nezelof, C., Jammet, M. L., Lertholary, P., Labrune, B., and Lamy, M. L. (1964): L'hypoplasia héréditaire du thymus: sa place et sa responsabilité dans une observation d'aplasie lymphocytaire normoplasmocytaire et normoglobulinémique du nourrisson. Arch. Franc. Pediat. *21,* 897.
58. Olson, G. B., Cooper, M. D., and Good, R. A.: The development of Peyer's patches in mice and rats raised in germfree or conventional environments. [In preparation]
59. Ortega, L. G., and Mellors, R. C. (1957): Cellular sites of formation of gamma globulin. J. Exp. Med. *106,* 627.
60. Ortega, L. G., Kattine, A. A., and Spurlock, B. O. (1965): Lympho-epithelial interactions in the developing bursa of Fabricius. Fed. Proc. *24,* 160.
61. Ortega, L. G., and Der, B. K. (1964): Studies of agammaglobulinemia induced by ablation of the bursa of Fabricius. Fed. Proc. *23,* 546.
62. Papermaster, B. W., Friedman, D. I., and Good, R. A. (1962): Relationship of the bursa of Fabricius to immunological responsiveness and homograft immunity in the chicken. Proc. Soc. Exp. Biol. Med. *110,* 62.
63. Papermaster, B. W., Condie, R. M., Finstad, J., and Good, R. A. (1964): Evolution of the immune response. I. The phylogenetic development of adaptive immunologic responsiveness in vertebrates. J. Exp. Med. *119,* 105.

64. Peterson, R. D. A., Burmester, B. R., Fredrickson, T. N., Purchase, H. G., and Good, R. A. (1964): Effect of bursectomy and thymectomy on the development of visceral lymphomatosis in the chicken. J. Nat. Cancer Inst. *32*, 1343.

65. Peterson, R. D. A., Cooper, M. D., and Good, R. A. (1965): The pathogenesis of immunologic deficiency diseases, Amer. J. Med. *38*, 579.

66. Peterson, R. D. A., Purchase, H. G., Burmester, B. R., Cooper, M. D., and Good, R. A. (1966): The relationship among visceral lymphomatosis, the bursa of Fabricius and the bursa-dependent lymphoid tissue of the chicken. J. Nat. Cancer Inst. *36*, 585.

67. St. Pierre, R. L., and Ackerman, G. A. (1965): Bursa of Fabricius in chickens: Possible humoral factor. Science *147*, 1307.

68. Sutherland, D. E. R., Archer, O. K., and Good, R. A. (1964): The role of the appendix in development of immunologic capacity. Proc. Soc. Exp. Biol. Med. *115*, 673.

69. Szenberg, A., and Warner, N. L. (1962): Dissociation of immunological responsiveness in fowls with a hormonally arrested development of lymphoid tissues. Nature *194*, 146.

70. Waksman, B. H., Arnason, B. G., and Janković, B. D. (1962): Role of the thymus in immune reactions in rats. III. Changes in the lymphoid organs of thymectomized rats. J. Exp. Med. *116*, 187.

71. Warner, N. L., and Szenberg, A. (1964): Immunologic studies on hormonally bursectomized and surgically thymectomized chickens: Dissociation of immunologic responsiveness, in: Good, R. A., and Gabrielsen, A. E., eds.: The Thymus in Immunobiology. New York, Hoeber-Harper.

72. Warner, N. L., Szenberg, A., and Burnet, F. M. (1962): The immunological role of different lymphoid organs in the chicken. I. Dissociation of immunological responsiveness. Aust. J. Exp. Biol. Med. Sc. *40*, 373.

73. White, R. G., Coons, A. H., and Connolly, J. M. (1955): Studies on antibody production. III. The alum granuloma. J. Exp. Med. *102*, 73.

74. White, R. G. (1963): Functional recognition of immunologically competent cells by means of the fluorescent antibody technique, in: Wolstenholme, G. E. W., and Knight, J. eds.: Ciba Foundation Study Group on the Immunologically Competent Cell. Boston, Little, Brown and Company. p. 6.

DISCUSSION

FELDMAN: I found interest in your demonstration that transformed neoplastic cells appear in the bursa following inoculation with the leukemia virus. It appears that lymphomatosis, when progressing within the chicken, does not generally involve the bursa. When foci of transformed cells appear in the bursa, do they appear as progressively growing tumors within the bursa or do the cells migrate out of the bursa and replicate in other lymphoid tissue?

A second question: Since bursectomy reduces the incidence of virus leukemia in chicken, and since the leukemia virus can induce other types of neoplasms, does bursectomy affect the incidence of the other types of tumors produced by the lymphomatosis virus?

M. COOPER: When the bursa was removed as late as 5 months of age, the development of malignancy was affected. As early as 12 weeks, before any evidence of malignancy is found in the peripheral lymphoid tissues, liver and pancreas, and other affected sites, malignant follicles are seen in the bursa. With a large sample 6 out of 10 positives are seen at 16 weeks.

At 5-9 months peripheral manifestations are evident and most birds die. The point is that peripheral involvement lags several weeks that in the bursa. We have no direct evidence that the peripheral cells are derived from bursa. The sequence of development is compatible with seeding.

GOOD: Removal of the bursa any time before the disease is present in the periphery blocks the disease. This is additional circumstantial evidence of the distribution of the malignancy from the bursa.

FELDMAN: Under these conditions, have transformed cells already appeared in the bursa?

GOOD: Yes.

M. COOPER: In answer to Feldman's second question, bursectomy increases the incidence of osteopetrosis. We need to watch bursectomized birds sufficiently long to develop other disorders such as myeloid leukemia.

EBERT: What do you suspect is the origin of bursal lymphoid cells, accepting the data of Moore and Owen at face value?

M. COOPER: I don't know.

GOOD: That question is a critical one in our thinking. We are not satisfied with Ackerman and Knouff's evidence that the bursa cells originate directly from the bursal epithelium. In embryonic as well as adult animals, cells can enter the bursa from the blood. We postulate that they are then induced by the environment of the bursa to differentiate with characteristics that ultimately produce germinal centers and plasma cells in the periphery.

EBERT: What is the timing at which one first sees the lymphoid elements of the chick in the various organs? Is it possible that the thymus in a sense is equivalent to a neural crest; that everything ultimately comes from the thymus, seeds out, with one group of cells stopping temporarily in the bursa?

M. COOPER: The thymus becomes lymphoid 2 or 3 days before the bursa.

EBERT: Perhaps we ought to be thinking of true primordial cells equivalent of the neural crest or primordial germinal center cells. What about the yolk sac?

GOOD: The best hint of the origin of this population of cells is from Auerbach's work with the thymus *in vitro*. The question regarding his model is whether cells that originated elsewhere penetrated the epithelial primordium *prior* to the time he removed it and induced its differentiation with mesenchyme. Observations later in life indicate that there is traffic into this site; perhaps *before* the lymphoid differentiation.

AUERBACH: First the fact that something may occur in the absence of the thymus may be misleading, since the thymus may have had some effect before it was removed.

Concerning the origin of the lymphoid cells of the thymus, it is high time that facts are separated from speculation. It has been demonstrated by many workers that lymphoid cells may travel to and from the thymus in adult animals. No such demonstration has been forthcoming for embryonic thymus. On the other hand there is excellent evidence that in the embryonic thymus of the mouse and chicken no cell migration takes place during the period of lymphopoiesis. Thus, tissue explants of 12-day mouse thymus mature into lymphoid organs. In this process most of the original cells (epithelial) participate as judged by experiments involving tritiated thymidine. Thus the transformation from epithelial to lymphoid cells does not involve just a few precursor cells which might have slipped in undetected.

Similarly, grafting experiments involving transplantation of thymus rudiments into irradiated mice indicate that lymphopoiesis in the thymus is intrinsic. In the chicken embryo,

the same type of results are suggested by the experiments described earlier today of Moore and Owen. In those experiments, involving parabiosis, a circulatory transfer of cells between bone marrow, spleen, and bursa was seen. In these same experiments *no* significant transfer of thymus cells between parabionts was detected.

The point raised by Dr. Ebert, concerning a possible yolk sac origin of immunocompetent cells, is a real possibility but entirely speculative. The one convincing experiment supporting non-thymic origin of immunocompetent cells in mammals is that of Taylor. It indicated that 12-day mouse embryonic cells other than those from thymus or liver were capable of some restoration of immunocompetence in irradiated mice.

We have tried to obtain lymphoid development *in vitro* from explants of embryonic spleen, liver, and yolk sac, but have not been successful. We were also unable to obtain bursal lymphoid development when the initial explant was comprised of 9-day (prelymphoid) bursal tissue. From this standpoint I would like to ask Dr. Cooper whether he was able to get bursal lymphoid cells to survive in tissue culture.

COOPER: The tissue cultured bursal cells survived during the few days they were observed. More work is necessary on this.

Lymphoid differentiation does occur when an explant of bursal primordium or non-lymphoid bursa is placed upon the chorioallantoic membrane.

AUERBACH: In that case you cannot exclude the possibility that cells from the circulation enter the bursa. The experiment, as I recall it, was that a 9-day old bursal rudiment was taken out of one embryo and placed upon the chorio-allantoic membrane of another 9-day embryo. Thus whatever controlled bursa development could conceivably enter the graft as well as the host bursa.

MITCHISON: Fetal liver cells will do the same things—as judged by karyological markers—as bone marrow. These marker experiments have intrinsic problems, but there is evidence from Ford's work that seeding of thymus takes place during parabiosis without transplantation or irradiation. This is the basis of Taylor's ideas that fetal liver cells may seed the thymus.

AUERBACH: In one experiment, he eliminated the fetal liver cells, and got the same result as when fetal liver cells were present. In other words, anything seems to work.

It cannot be ignored that during early development cells may do many things. Thus, early embryonic cells may upon injection act like blast cells. This does not mean, however, that these are the cells that would normally give rise to the primordial blast cells of the thymus or of the immune system.

GOOD (to Auerbach): Is it not incongruous that in the thymus lymphoid cells develop from epithelium, but from other primordial cells in other locations?

AUERBACH: Let me put it this way: The fact that cells can migrate does not mean that they always do. Similarly, the fact that cells may be produced *in situ* does not mean that that is the only way they are produced.

With regard to the thymus there are two critical experiments which appear now mutually incompatible but which in fact are quite compatible. The first is that during embryonic development, non-lymphoid cells from the thymic anlagen can become lymphoid. This is well established. The second is that in later development lymphoid cells from outside the thymus move into it. This is also established. Two items of evidence indicate that once the lymphoid system has evolved the thymus acts in a different fashion from the way it acts during embryonic development.

We cannot exclude the possibility that cells migrate into the thymus before it becomes a recognizable rudiment. We must also recognize that even if this were true the cells which might enter the thymic rudiment are not lymphoid cells but cells which may be precursors to lymphoid differentiation. If the cells that migrate into the bursa are lymphoid cells, then the only obvious source of these cells is the thymus because this is the only organ which precedes the bursa in lymphoid development. On the other hand, if cells migrate into the bursa as non-lymphoid precursor cells, then their source cannot as yet be deduced.

E. COOPER: Can we generalize on structures analogous to the bursa or is this organ specific for gallinaceous birds?

M. COOPER: The bursa functions similarly in all those birds which have been studied including the duck, turkey, and chicken.

GOOD: The literature indicates, where a thorough search has been made, that all young birds have a bursa. It will be very important to study in detail the differences in development of the peripheral lymphoid tissue in the various groups of birds. For example, some water birds are said to have well-developed lymph nodes. Finstad and I with the Minnesota ornithologist Warner plan to examine the central and peripheral lymphoid tissue of representatives of each order of birds newly hatched, adult and aged populations.

E. COOPER (to Good): What is the status of the lymphoid tissue in monotremes?

GOOD: We recently had the opportunity to carry out extensive dissections of the Australian monotreme, Echidna. Diener of the Hall Institute, Melbourne, also has carried out morphological and immunological studies of these animals. We found a non-involuted mammalian type thymus, no evidence of a bursa or even a site suggestive of an involuted bursa. The lymphatic tissue was of great interest. These animals have lymph nodes, but each lymph node is a single follicle with a single germinal center. The spleen contained well-developed red pulp and white pulp and plasma cells are abundant. Further, the monotremes have a well-developed lamina propria of the intestine and plasma cells. These structures have been associated by Crabbé *et al.* with γA production in mammals. The Echidna has beautiful, well-developed Peyer's patches and appendiceal Peyer's patch-type tissue like the rabbit. Here the lymphoid tissue is in intimate relation to epithelium.

Finstad and I studied the lymphoid tissues of all of the derivatives of the primitive reptiles (Cotylosaurs) in an effort to define in each derivative form, germinal center type of development and the plasma cell line. Thus far it is clear that all derivatives of the Cotylosaurs have plasma cells and at least some development of the germinal centers in their peripheral lymphoid tissue.

The marsupials have well-developed germinal centers in their spleens, lymph nodes, and Peyer's patches. The crocodilians have what appears to us to be primitive follicular tonsils.

These morphological studies provide good guidelines for the experimental studies, but morphology without experimental analysis can as often be misleading as revealing.

16

N. A. MITCHISON

Immunological paralysis as a problem of cellular differentiation

FOR THE STUDENT of cellular differentiation the immunologically competent cell has long had a special interest, on account of the extraordinary sensitivity of this cell to stimulation by minute amounts of inducer and because the response is modulated with great precision by inducer structure. For these reasons a situation in which the cell responds in an unusual way has a very special interest. In the induction of immunological paralysis we seem to be able to detect a response on the part of the reactive cell which parallels the normal immune response in sensitivity and degree of specificity but takes another form. It is the purpose of this communication to examine some of the details of this second type of inductive response.

Before doing so, however, it is perhaps worth while pointing out a special merit of paralysis for the study of induction. In the process of immunization the response appears normally to be initiated in a fairly small number of cells even if a very large number of antibody-forming cells are finally produced. A remarkable example of this restriction can be found in the recent work of Ceppellini (personal communication) and his collaborators on the response of rabbits to an "O" antigen obtained from *Salmonella enteritides,* where the number of plasma cell precursors falls in the 10-20 range. This may be something of an exception, but in general it seems that the fraction of the "lymphon" that participates initially in any one immune response is quite

small. For this reason the prospects for examining the molecular details of induction are poor since the events that matter occur so infrequently. In paralysis, on the other hand, induction must take place in the entire cellular population at risk for complete suppression of the immune response.

In arriving at this conclusion the assumption has been made that paralysis comes about through an alteration in the responsive cell rather than through a mechanism whereby a response induced in a small fraction of the total cellular population manages to inhibit other cells. That the immune response is subject to inhibition by the product of a restricted number of cells has been known for some time in the context of "enhancement." This phenomenon, as originally described, is the suppression of the homograft reaction by soluble antibody; antiserum can be administered from an external source or produced within the "lymphon" of an enhanced animal with the consequence that rejection of homografts is delayed or prevented. Apparently the antibody sets a screen between the graft and the reactive cell or its product. It now appears that antibody can also suppress immunological responses to classical antigens such as foreign erythrocytes or bacteriophages. Rowley and Fitch (10) even argue that this is the mechanism underlying immunological tolerance in general. In my opinion that is unlikely, principally because of the evidence that comes from experiments on cell transfer. A population of

135

paralysed cells remains so upon isolation and transfer to a second host, and normal cells transferred into a paralysed recipient retain their capacity to react immunologically (6).

The problems concerning immunological tolerance to be discussed here are:

1. In what cell is paralysis induced; i.e. in cellular terms, what is the target for antigen?

2. How long does the process take?

3. How is the inducer recognized; i.e., what sort of receptor, if any, exists for antigen in the immunologically virgin cell?

To take the matter of the target first. It has been established, mainly through the work of Gowans (6) and his collaborators, that paralysis once established is a property of the small lymphocyte, for thoracic duct lymphocytes collected from paralysed rats display a specific failure of response, and this property has not been found in any other type of cell.

Some question arose about the function of macrophages in paralysed animals, but the claim that the paralysed animal displays abnormal localization has not been confirmed, and it seems probable that the original observations of Nossal and Ada (9) can be ascribed to the presence of small amounts of antibody in their otherwise tolerant rats. The experiments of Gowans do not throw light directly on the means by which the lymphocyte becomes tolerant nor do they exclude the participation of another cell such as the macrophage in this process. It is worth while therefore examining the role that the macrophage might play. There is considerable evidence of an indirect nature which indicates that phagocytosis favours immunization rather than paralysis.

Dresser (3) has shown that the inductive properties of bovine γ-globulin in mice can be altered by removal of aggregated material by centrifugation. The supernatant fraction of BGG will not immunize adult mice of certain strains but will induce paralysis even when administered in minute doses. Much the same holds true of BSA in rabbits. Frei, Benacerraf, and Thorbecke (5) have removed material subject to phagocytosis from solutions of BSA by passage in the circulation. The antigen that has been cleaned up in this way will still paralyse but has lost the power to immunize. As these authors point out, it seems likely that the well-known efficiency of the oral and mesenteric vein routes for inducing drug tolerance is due to screening out of aggregated or denatured material by the liver. The most satisfactory way of answering the question would be to induce paralysis by the direct exposure of lymphocytes to antigen in vitro. Such an experiment presents no obvious difficulty. Cells from spleen, lymph node, or peripheral blood can be collected and treated in this way with an antigen such as BSA in concentrations that would certainly induce paralysis in an animal. The cells can then be washed and transferred back into a histocompatible host that has been rendered unresponsive by irradiation or by the prior induction of paralysis. Dr. Jeanette Thorbecke and Dr. Richard Smith have attempted to paralyse cells in this way and so have I. None of us has succeeded. I wonder why? Perhaps we do not know how to keep lymphocytes sufficiently happy outside the body, and there are manoeuvres to improve things that could be tried. This is a matter that ought to take a high place on our agenda.

In the meanwhile it seemed worth while to expose lymphocytes to a brief pulse of antigen in vivo and then to isolate and wash them so that their reactivity could be tested upon transfer into a non-reactive recipient. This I have done and I find that lymphocytes collected from the peripheral blood of mice that were injected with human or bovine serum albumin 2 hours previously have already become unresponsive. This then sets an upper limit to the time required for uptake of inducer and serves, provisionally at least, to identify the target cell as the small lymphocyte.

Turning now to the question of recognition. I have attempted to pursue the procedure introduced by Dutton and Bulman (4) of hapten inhibition. In the original experiments cells from the lymph nodes of rabbits primed with dinitrophenol conjugates were found to increase the rate of DNA synthesis (as judged by incorporation of tritiated thymidine) upon stimulation in vitro by the conjugate. In collaboration with Dr. Rosalind Pitt-Rivers and Mr. Alan Brownstone (2) I have found that a somewhat similar effect can be produced with conjugates of an iodine-containing hapten, termed NIP (4-hydroxy-3-iodo-5-nitrophenylacetic acid). Dutton and Bulman (4) found that DNP-lysine could inhibit stimulation by the complete conjugate and in an analogous way we find that NIP-aminocaproic acid inhibits synthesis of NIP-binding antibody. From this inhibition the conclusion can be drawn that the primed cell bears a receptor for the conjugate, and that binding of the inducer to this receptor can be competitively inhibited by the free hapten. Here in the context of the secondary response the receptor in question is likely to be antibody. If not antibody with precisely the same binding properties as that which is found in the circulation, it is at least likely to be antibody with a somewhat similar binding site.

The detection of antibody, or at least of an antibody-like site on primed cells, should come as no surprise. What is of much greater interest is whether this method can be used to detect similar receptors on the cells of untreated animals. We are asking, in fact, whether the primary response to conjugates or the induction of paralysis is also subject to inhibition by free hapten. There are certain obvious difficulties in this approach. So far as tolerance is concerned the difficulty lies in finding a suitable concentration of antigen. High concentrations induce rapidly, as in the foregoing experiment where the albumin doses were in the range 10-100 mg. This sort of dose may be too high to be subject to inhibition by the concentration of free hapten that can be attained without killing the mice. The *in vitro* experiments with NIP suggest that concentrations of conjugate up to about 1 μg/ml can be inhibited, but above this the free hapten that is needed becomes toxic. Concentrations of a conjugate in the μg/ml range have been found to paralyse, but do so only very slowly. After a month of treatment the mice are still only partially unresponsive. Obviously to maintain the concentration of a rapidly excreted small molecule so long a time presents serious difficulties.

There is another difficulty with conjugates —the Weigle (11) effect. Mice that one would expect to have been very adequately paralysed by prolonged treatment with NIP-BSA fail to respond in the expected way to the NIP group when administered in conjugation with chicken globulin, but the failure of response is quite transient, and within 3 weeks of the challenge immunization large amounts of NIP-binding antibody begin to be made.

For inhibition of primary immunization the phenomenon of inhibition by free hapten may be easier to demonstrate but its interpretation is less sure. Let us suppose that a mouse is immunized for the first time with a NIP conjugate and that free hapten is then kept in the circulation for T hours. As a consequence the mouse fails to mount a normal primary response. Can we conclude that NIP receptor was there beforehand? We can do so only by assuming that NIP-binding antibody is not synthesized during the T hours, or that the antibody produced by such synthesis plays no part in the further development of the primary response. When T is very small these assumptions may be justified, but they certainly introduce an element of uncertainty into any interpretation.

In spite of all these objections I have, nevertheless, looked for these sorts of inhibition by hapten in the NIP system. For paralysis, cells from normal mice were exposed to milligram quantities of NIP conjugate *in vivo* with or without the presence of NIP-aminocaproic acid and then transferred for test into irradiated recipients where they were challenged with NIP on a second carrier protein. The results of these experiments have been confused and unsatisfactory; either no unresponsiveness was found in the absence of hapten, or something else went wrong. Nevertheless, there is a hint of the expected kind of inhibition. Adopting the alternative stratagem, μg amounts of NIP conjugate were administered with or without NIP-aminocaproic acid 3 times a week for 10 weeks, and the mice then challenged with NIP on another conjugate. So far as the main purpose was concerned the results were completely negative. But one interesting fact emerged. Control mice injected only with μ moles of NIP-aminocaproic acid 3 times a week for 10 weeks then became somewhat unresponsive to immunization with a NIP mouse serum albumin conjugate.

Does this mean that the free hapten succeeded partially at least in blocking the naturally-occurring cross-stimulation that would otherwise give rise to naturally-occurring NIP-receptors? Or does it mean only that our preparation of NIP-aminocaproic acid formed small amounts of conjugate with body protein and so induced drug unresponsiveness of the classical type?

By far the most exciting results were obtained with the primary response. Mice were immunized with 80 μg of NIP chicken globulin absorbed on to alum and mixed with pertussis, and were bled after 10, 20, and 40 days. Nine injections at 8-hour intervals, each of 2 μ moles of NIP-aminocaproic acid reduced the titre of NIP-binding antibody by one-half. Furthermore, the same schedule of hapten injections could inhibit primary immunization by NIP chicken globulin which had been taken up by macrophages transferred from syngeneic donors. Any interpretation of these findings is open to doubts about the partially secondary character of the response that had been raised. Nevertheless, it is exciting to find provisional evidence of naturally-occurring NIP receptors.

The final question that requires discussion is how closely the cellular receptor resembles the binding site of normal serum antibody. Here the available evidence is incomplete and inconclusive. Until very recently there were strong grounds for believing that the cellular receptor differed markedly in its binding properties, being directed towards a relatively wide area of antigen and not recognizing minor differences in haptenic structure (8). Thus, for example, in both adult hypersensitivity and the secondary response carrier protein plays an important part in determining the activity of a conjugate in eliciting the response, whereas purified antibody appears to combine efficiently with a given hapten on a variety of carriers. The Weigle effect points in the same direction. The recent work of Leskowitz (7) and Benacerraf (1) suggests that this difference may have been overemphasized. On the one hand carrier specificity is largely lacking in adult hypersensitivity to arsenyl conjugates, and on the other purified anti-DNP antibody shows a certain degree of carrier specificity towards a polylysine carrier. Perhaps the chief interest in this distinction lies in the hope that an assay can be found for cellular receptor as distinct from normal antibody. Without such a differential assay the search for receptor and attempts at its isolation would be almost hopeless. My own feeling is that if ever receptor is isolated much of the present discussion will prove redundant, and in the meanwhile an assay for the purpose of isolation is the most practical aim to bear in mind.

REFERENCES

1. Benacerraf, B. (1966), in: Regulation of the Antibody Response, Toronto, February, 1966. Charles C. Thomas, Illinois.
2. Brownstone, A., Mitchison, N. A., and Pitt-Rivers, R. (1966): Biological studies with a synthetic immunological determinant 4-hydroxy-3-iodo-5-nitrophenylacetic acid (NIP) and related compounds. Immunology 10, 481.
3. Dresser, D. W. (1963): Specific inhibition of antibody production. III. Apparent changes in the half-life of bovine gamma globulin in paralysed mice. Immunology 6, 345.
4. Dutton, R. W., and Bulman, H. N. (1964): The significance of the protein carrier in the stimulation of DNA synthesis by hapten-protein conjugates in the secondary response. Immunology 7, 54.
5. Frei, P. C., Benacerraf, B., and Thorbecke, G. J. (1965): Phagocytosis of the antigen, a crucial step in the induction of the primary response. Proc. Nat. Acad. Sci., Wash. 53, 20.
6. Gowans, J. L., and McGregor, D. D. (1965): The immunological activities of lymphocytes. Progr. Allergy 9, 1.
7. Leskowitz, S. (1963): Immunochemical study of antigenic specificity in delayed hypersensitivity. II. Delayed hypersensitivity to polytyrosine-azobenzene arsonate and its suppression by haptens. J. Exp. Med. 117, 909.
8. Mitchison, N. A. (1966): Recognition of antigen by cells. Progr. Biophys. 16, 1.
9. Nossal, G. J. V., and Ada, G. L. (1964): Recognition of foreignness in immune and tolerant animals. Nature, Lond. 201, 580.
10. Rowley, D. A., and Fitch, F. W. (1964): Homeostasis of antibody formation in the adult rat. J. Exp. Med. 120, 987.
11. Weigle, W. O. (1961): The immune response of rabbits tolerant to BSA to the injection of other heterologous serum albumins. J. Exp. Med. 114, 111.

DISCUSSION

MIESCHER: In transfer experiments where you used peripheral blood to induce the immunization, do you think it is a lymphocyte and not the macrophage which did the job?

MITCHISON: Yes. I didn't describe how the lymphocytes are prepared. They are collected by a procedure comparable with that used by Dr. Hildemann. I cannot say they are uncontaminated with macrophages, but such contamination is of a low order.

HILDEMANN: How do you explain that small lymphocytes from sensitized animals either failed to transfer adoptive antibody production, or did so poorly, unless they are restimulated with the antigen in the new donor?

MITCHISON: If syngeneic lymphocytes are put into an irradiated recipient and the cells are stimulated by BSA after the transfer or, indeed, during the transfer, then there is a response. If BSA isn't given, then there is no detectable response.

This means to me that the lymphocyte in this kind of experiment, serves as a primed cell, but not as a producer. A lymphocyte isn't a plasma cell.

HILDEMANN: Does this require an irradiated recipient?

MITCHISON: It is a great deal more efficient in such an animal.

MIESCHER: What cellular mechanism is conceivable to explain what the lymphocyte does within the short period of two hours after the donor animal has been injected?

MITCHISON: This is the essential question of induction. How does antigen work at the cellular level?

What our experiments with hapten inhibition indicate to me is as follows: if we conceive that antigen in a macrophage stimulates a lymphocyte, a blocking macromolecule with the same structure as the antigen which is placed in this pathway would block stimulation of the lymphocyte. This implies that the lymphocyte has on it a recognition site for the antigen. In immunization then, the antigen may be reaching the lymphocyte from the macrophages either with a label attached to it or perhaps because the macrophage feeds it in the right way. And this stimulates the cell. But if the antigen reaches the combining site, there are two possibilities, it seems to me:

either this site is destroyed or it is irreversibly blocked. A lymphocyte can live for 8 years. Thus, because irreversibility is of such long duration, I am reluctant to accept the idea of a block. And if an individual cell never recovers from paralysis, as I think, then an irreversible block is a most unattractive idea. The second idea, that it smashes the receptor machinery or the whole cell, therefore seems to me easier to visualize.

BRAUN: Could the requirement for more antigen in the production of unresponsiveness in the secondary response be due to an ability of antibody, in the process of secretion, to act as an additional recognition site on the lymphocyte?

MITCHISON: That is exactly what I was trying to express—that antibody competes with this recognition site.

GOOD: How do you deal with the observation in guinea pigs that tolerance can be broadened in its scope to include antigens not used in inducing tolerance? Why is it that you cannot induce tolerance in adult mice with antigens like lysozyme, ovalbumin, or diphtheria toxoid if you use a sufficiently small dose of antigen given over a long enough period?

MITCHISON: The broadening effect you refer to operates only during the induction of what I call high dose paralysis and does not operate once the paralysis has been established.

I am confident that this effect has nothing to do with the establishment of tolerance in guinea pigs. Large doses of antigen induce concomitant immunization as in the high zone paralysis we demonstrate with bovine serum albumin. Competition of antigen is taking place and the high and immunizing dose eventually results in an unresponsive guinea pig.

The point that I want to emphasize is that there is a concentration of antigen below which lymphocytes don't notice it, and we establish this threshold at about 10^{-8}M. Even if this amount of antigen is enough to get into any appreciable number of the macrophages and produce an immunogenic form of antigen, there will be no low dose tolerance detectable.

MIESCHER: You produce paralysis with large doses then, because you circumvent the macrophages that block the lymphocytes?

MITCHISON: The details get fairly complicated; some competition must be involved.

CEBRA: If low dose tolerance is due to the elimination of a group of cells with specific recognition site could one enhance tolerance by a "double pulse" treatment? Animals could be given a low dose of antigen followed at a later, perhaps critical, time by a low dose of antibody specific for the antigen and homologous for the animal. Perhaps then the animal's scavenger system might eliminate the group of cells in question and so result in tolerance.

PART IV

PRE- AND POSTNATAL FUNCTION OF THE LYMPHORETICULAR SYSTEM

EDITOR: ARTHUR M. SILVERSTEIN

A. M. SILVERSTEIN, C. J. PARSHALL, and R. A. PRENDERGAST: Studies on the nature of immunologic immaturity

DISCUSSION

M. BLOCK: The "fetal" opossum as an experimental tool in ontogeny of immunologic competence

DISCUSSION

W. H. ADLER, J. H. CURRY, and R. T. SMITH: Quantitative aspects of early postnatal immunoglobulin peptide chain synthesis in the rabbit

DISCUSSION

G. J. THORBECKE and R. VAN FURTH: Ontogeny of immunoglobulin synthesis in various mammalian species

DISCUSSION

A. J. L. STRAUSS, P. G. KEMP, and S. D. DOUGLAS: An immunohistological delineation of striated muscle cells in the thymus

DISCUSSION

A. G. JOHNSON and G. HOEKSTRA: Acceleration of the primary antibody response

W. BRAUN and M. NAKANO: The reinforcement of immunological stimuli by oligodeoxyribonucleotides

DISCUSSION
(Johnson and Hoekstra's and Braun and Nakano's papers)

17

ARTHUR M. SILVERSTEIN, CHARLES J. PARSHALL, and ROBERT A. PRENDERGAST

Studies on the nature of immunologic immaturity

So LONG AS it appeared that the mammalian fetus was incapable of any form of immunologic response in utero and that the earliest antibody responses of the newborn animal were initially halting and feeble, the concept of immunologic immaturity appeared to be not only valid but also quite reasonable. By analogy with other systems in developmental biology, the concept of immunologic immaturity was considered to include a slow transition from a state of complete immunologic incompetence (the so-called immunologic "null" period) and then a gradual maturation of the several mechanisms until they reached normal adult levels—a sort of "tooling up" process presumably representing the immunologic requirement that the animal learn to crawl before it could walk and run.

The study of the ontogenesis of the immune response during recent years has furnished data which appear to demand a re-examination of the concept of immunologic immaturity. One pertinent line of evidence was the demonstration that the earliest immune responses of neonates might be suppressed or completely abolished by the presence of antibody passively acquired from the mother, and that in the absence of maternal antibody the neonatal response might be quite respectable (18). Another significant line of evidence lies in the recent frequent observation that the mammalian fetus of a number of species in utero is capable of immunologic responses of one type or another (for recent reviews cf. 2,

10, 17). Especially interesting along these lines was the demonstration that the developing fetus does not achieve immunological competence simultaneously to all antigens, but rather possesses the ability to respond to some quite early in gestation, to others only later in gestation, and to several only some time after birth (15).

The purpose of this paper is to review some of these data and a number of experiments designed to test the concept of immunologic immaturity and to ascertain whether the earliest responses of the developing fetus are truly halting attempts by the immature animal only slowly developing full competence—or rather, as we shall attempt to indicate, the apparently de novo responses of a precociously mature immunologic apparatus.

THE APPEARANCE OF IMMUNOLOGIC COMPETENCE

The early notion that the mammalian fetus was immunologically incompetent was supported by evidence on the inability of neonates to form antibodies, and on their susceptibility to the induction of immunologic tolerance (3, 16) and to the inhibition of immunogenesis as a result of thymectomy (1) (primarily in small laboratory rodents). However, other evidence began to accumulate as early as 1904 that in at least certain species the fetus was able to respond to antigenic stimulus in utero (6). Such evidence has accumulated quite rapidly in the last few years and has been extended to cover a variety of species (cf. 2, 10, 17). These studies indicate that developing animals, still immature from other points of view, are able to demonstrate immunological reactivity. Thus the fetal lamb and fetal Rhesus monkey *in utero* are able to form antibody during the first half of gestation (11, 15), while the very immature opossum in the pouch forms antibody as early as the fifth day (8), at a time when its lymphoid tissues are still relatively immature. At the present time, however, we are unable to equate the ability of a developing animal to form antibody with the full maturation of its immunologic capabilities. Thus the fetal lamb *in utero* is able to form antibodies to bacteriophage ϕX174 as early in gestation as it has been technically feasible to immunize and bleed the small fetus (38-40 days gestation of a total of 150 days); at this time it appeared unable to respond specifically to antigenic stimulus by any other antigens tried. Only later in gestation (at about 66 days) did the fetus show an initial ability to form circulating antibodies against ferritin. At 120 days it first became able to form antibodies against crystalline egg albumin, while only after birth was active antibody formation found to diphtheria toxoid or *Salmonella typhosa* (15). The ability to reject orthotopic skin homografts developed in the fetal lamb only at about 80 days gestation. The development of immunologic competence against different antigens at different stages of gestation appears also to be true of the fetal Rhesus monkey, and may prove to represent a general immunobiologic phenomenon.

It becomes evident, then, that any evaluation of the immunologic competence of a developing animal can be made only in terms of one or another antigen, and not in terms of the over-all immunologic capability of the animal. For any given species and at any developmental stage, the animal may be "competent" with respect to one or more antigens while remaining "incompetent" to other antigens.

The basis for this sequential development of competence to different antigens at different developmental stages is currently unclear. It may on the one hand represent a true immunologic maturation, reflecting perhaps the initial appearance of clones of cells specific for different antigens at different stages of development; on the other hand it may represent an essentially non-immunologic maturation. Although competence for all antigens may conceivably appear very early in gestation, we may in fact be measuring the ontogenetic sequence of development of enzyme systems required to degrade suitably any given antigen so that it will be available in a form able to stimulate the immunologic apparatus. A preliminary test of the latter possibility was performed by studying the catabolic rate of egg albumin in fetal lambs *in utero* both before and after the age at which they were able to develop circulating antibodies in response to ovalbumin stimulus. In this instance no significant difference in the ability of the animal to catabolize the antigen either early or late in gestation was observed (5).

HOMOGRAFT REJECTION IN THE FETAL LAMB

The fact that the fetal animal *in utero* is able to reject specifically a skin homograft was first reported by Schinkel and Ferguson in 1953 (9). More recent reports have verified these findings and have shown that the fetal lamb first develops immunologic competence in this respect at about 85 days gestation (13). Orthotopic skin homografts applied prior to this age not only fail to be rejected but may in fact induce immunologic tolerance specific for the donor, as evidenced by the fact that second set grafts from the same donor applied subsequent to the 85th day of gestation in such animals are also not rejected, although grafts from unrelated donors are rejected in the usual fashion.

Of interest in the present discussion is a comparison of the manner in which the fetus rejects a graft immediately after competence has been attained, as compared with the way in which the adult rejects a graft. In the adult sheep, orthotopic split thickness skin grafts are rejected within 7 to 9 days in a manner quite typical of homograft rejection in other species, as outlined in detail in the original report of Medawar (7). When skin grafts of the same type are applied onto the fetal lamb, an animal which has to the best of our knowledge never responded to any form of antigenic stimulus, it is found that the grafts are specifically rejected in a manner apparently identical to that observed in the adult. Thus the timing of graft rejection at 7 to 9 days is the same, as is the typical histologic picture of graft rejection involving perivascular cuffing by round cells, lymphocytic and monocytic infiltration, and a typical pattern of vascular thrombosis and hemorrhage, death of epithelial cells, and disorganization of the normal collagen pattern. The same course of rejection was observed with grafts from unrelated adult sheep, from the mother, and with fetal and even sibling skin.

As judged, then, by the normal temporal and histologic criteria applied in the study of homograft rejection, the fetal animal appears to manifest a full capacity for homograft rejection once it becomes competent to do so at about 85 days gestation. At no time does one see in any respect a hesitant or "immature" attempt at graft rejection—the fetus either cannot perform the graft rejection function at all prior to this stage of development, or thereafter can accomplish the rejection in a typical adult manner.

IMMUNE ELIMINATION OF ANTIGEN IN THE FETAL LAMB

We have studied the response of the fetal lamb to bacteriophage ϕX174 in collaboration with Dr. Jonathan Uhr. In earlier reports (11, 15), it was indicated that the fetal lamb was capable of forming circulating antibody to this antigen during the first trimester of gestation, as early as was technically possible to accomplish the immunization and bleeding of the animal. Since earlier reports had indicated that the kinetics of the earliest antibody response could be studied and assayed employing the immune elimination of bacteriophage antigen (19), this approach was used in studies of the fetal lamb in utero, taking advantage of a newly developed technique permitting the implantation of a permanent indwelling catheter into the circulation of the fetus, thus giving continuous access to the fetal blood through the catheter emerging outside the mother's body.

Previous reports of studies in the adults of other species made it clear that with the small doses of bacteriophage antigen which could be employed, the onset of immune elimination of antigen could be detected as early as 40 to 48 hours following intravenous injection. Once the antigen had been eliminated, and depending to a certain extent on the original dosage employed, first γM antibody and then γG antibody was found in the circulation of the animal.

The results of these kinetic studies of immune elimination of antigen and subsequent appearance of circulating antibody in the "immunologically virgin" fetal lamb proved to be similar in all respects to those reported for adults (12). After an initial equilibration of the antigen in the fetal animal, bleedings made through the catheter at 3- to 4-hour intervals showed the antigen to be only relatively slowly catabolized for the first 41 to 47 hours. At a point near the end of the second day following immunization, the slope of the antigen clearance curve changed sharply and the antigen disappeared very rapidly thereafter, yielding a typical straight line on the plot of log antigen versus time. Continued bleeding of these animals showed that during the next day or so γM antibody appeared and increased in titer for the ensuing several days. Only some days after the first appearance of γM antibody was γG antibody detected in the circulation, and it too increased in titer.

These data demonstrate by yet another approach that the apparently immature fetal lamb, possessing only a relatively immature set of lymphoid tissues (by morphologic standards), is able to respond to immunologic stimulus with a mature set of responses worthy of an adult animal with much broader experience in immunologic affairs.

CELLULAR KINETICS OF THE ANTIBODY RESPONSE IN THE FETAL MONKEY

A new dimension in the estimation of immunologic competence appeared with the introduction by Jerne et al. (4) of their hemolytic plaque assay technique for the estimation of numbers of antibody-forming cells in response to antigenic stimulus during the primary and secondary response. These investigators showed in the mouse that within 24 to 48 hours of intravenous administration of sheep erythrocytes, hemolytic plaque formers could be found among the lymphoid cells of the spleen. The subsequent expansion of this population of antibody-producing cells was very rapid, reaching a peak at about 4 days and then falling off in numbers. Restimulation with the same antigen some time later resulted in a new expansion of the population of antibody-forming cells as part of the anamnestic booster response. The general nature of these results has been confirmed repeatedly in a variety of species, with only slight variation in the time of peak numbers of antibody-forming cells and in the proportion of antibody formers per million lymphoid cells in the spleen of the recipient animal. The ability to screen large numbers of spleen cells and to express the results in terms of antibody producers per million lymphoid cells provides a powerful tool for the study of the nature of the antibody response mechanism, and permits a more precise comparison of the kinetics of the antibody response than is provided by the assay of circulating antibody.

We have taken advantage of this approach to compare the kinetics of hemolytic antibody response in the fetal Rhesus monkey with those observed in the adult Rhesus. This comparison is simplified by the ability to express the antibody response in terms of numbers of plaque formers per million lymphoid cells, furnishing a convenient built-in control for the markedly different size and blood volume of the fetus as compared with the adult, and for the marked difference in the amount and general level of maturity of the lymphoid tissue between the fetus and the adult.

Once again it was found (14) that the fetal response was similar to that of the adult both qualitatively and quantitatively. Both showed the same early appearance of antibody-forming cells in response to injection of sheep erythrocytes, the same expansion of this population to a maximum on the 6th day after immunization, and a subsequent decline in numbers which could be boosted on the 8th day with a second injection of antigen. In fact, the kinetic curve of this antibody response in the fetal monkey was, within the limits of experimental error, identical to that found in the mature adult. It may be pointed out again that in this situation the fetal animal had, to the best of our knowledge, not previously responded to antigenic stimulus, and was found to have morphologically a quite immature and sparsely populated lymphoid tissue, and a relatively low peripheral white blood count. Yet the fetus showed no signs of immaturity in the form of its primary antibody response to this antigenic stimulus.

DISCUSSION AND CONCLUSIONS

We have tested the concept of the immunologic immaturity of the developing mammalian fetus *in utero,* employing three different immunologic test systems in two mammalian species: the fetal lamb and fetal Rhesus monkey. The immunologic responses studied were the rejection of orthotopic skin homografts, the kinetics of antigen elimination and early appearance of circulating antibody, and the cellular kinetics of the primary response to erythrocyte antigens. It was found in each instance that the earliest response by the fetus shows no hesitancy, no faltering, no presently detectable qualitative or quantitative difference from the response expected of the adult, such that we could say that the fetal response observed was "immature." With the antigens and immunologic systems employed in this study and with the species used, we must conclude that once the developing fetus is capable of a given immunologic response, it demonstrates this response in a highly mature fashion. To return to the analogy mentioned earlier, the developing fetus does not appear to crawl first and then learn to walk, but leaves the immunologic gate running in response to the first appropriate antigenic stimulus.

The only form of immunologic immaturity that we have observed with certainty in our studies of the ontogenesis of the immune response is that associated with the apparent inability of the developing organism to respond to certain antigens until an apparently fixed and critical stage of gestation is reached. This critical age of development appears to be different for each different antigen in the given species. Prior to this age the animal seems not to recognize a substance as antigenic and not to respond to it; after this age the earliest response appears to be quite mature. If this in fact represents immunologic immaturity, then it must be pointed out that while the animal may be "immature" with respect to any one antigen at a given stage of gestation, it simultaneously can be fully mature, as indicated above, to respond to a number of other antigens. The data discussed in this review thus raise the question of the fundamental significance and current utility of the term "immunologic immaturity."

Acknowledgments.—Supported by Contract No. DA49-193-MD-2640 from the United States Army Research and Development Command, Washington, D.C.; by Grant No. A106713 from NIAID, the National Institutes of Health, Bethesda, Maryland; by an unrestricted grant from the Alcon Laboratories, Inc.; and by an International Order of Odd Fellows Research Professorship.

REFERENCES

1. Good, R. A., and Gabrielson, A. E. (eds.) (1964): The Thymus in Immunobiology, Hoeber-Harper, New York.
2. Good, R. A., and Papermaster, B. W. (1964): Ontogeny and phylogeny of adaptive immunity. Adv. Immunol. *4*, 1.
3. Hašek, M., Lengerová, A., and Hraba, T. (1961): Transplantation immunity and tolerance. Adv. Immunol. *1*, 1.
4. Jerne, N. K., Nordin, A. A., and Henry, C. (1963): The agar plaque technique for recognizing antibody-producing cells, in: Amos, B., ed.: Cell-Bound Antibodies, Philadelphia, Wistar Inst. Press, p. 109.
5. Kaplan, J., Parshall, C. J., and Silverstein, A. M. (1966): Unpublished observations.
6. Kreidl, A., and Mandl, L. (1904): Ueber den Uebergang der Immunohämolysine von der Frucht auf die Mutter. Wien. Klin. Wschr. *18*, 611.
7. Medawar, P. B. (1944): The behavior and fate of skin autografts and skin homografts in rabbits. J. Anat. *78*, 176.
8. Rowlands, D. T., LaVia, M. F., and Block, M. H. (1964): Studies of the blood and blood-forming tissues of the newborn opossum II. J. Immun. *93*, 157.
9. Schinkel, P. G., and Ferguson, K. A. (1953): Skin transplantation in the fetal lamb. Aust. J. Exp. Biol. Med. Sc. *6*, 533.
10. Silverstein, A. M. (1964): Ontogeny of the immune response. Science *144*, 1423.
11. Silverstein, A. M., and Kraner, K. L. (1965): Studies on the ontogenesis of the immune response; in, Molecular and Cellular Basis of Antibody Formation. Czech. Acad. Sci., Prague, p. 341.
12. Silverstein, A. M., Parshall, C. J., and Uhr, J. W. (1966): In preparation.
13. Silverstein, A. M., Prendergast, R. A., and Kraner, K. L. (1964): Fetal response to antigenic stimulus. IV. The rejection of skin homografts by the fetal lamb. J. Exp. Med. *119*, 955.
14. Silverstein, A. M., Prendergast, R. A., and Parshall, C. J. (1966): In preparation.
15. Silverstein, A. M., Uhr, J. W., Kraner, K. L., and Lukes, R. J. (1963): Fetal response to antigenic stimulus. II. Antibody production by the fetal lamb. J. Exp. Med. *117*, 799.
16. Smith, R. T. (1961): Immunological tolerance of non-living antigens. Adv. Immunol. *1*, 67.
17. Šterzl, J., and Silverstein, A. M. (1966): Developmental Aspects of Immunity. Adv. Immunol. 6. [In press]
18. Uhr, J. W., and Baumann, J. B. (1961): Antibody formation. I. The suppression of antibody formation by passively administered antibody. J. Exp. Med. *113*, 935.
19. Uhr, J. W., Finkelstein, M. S., and Baumann, J. B. (1962): Antibody formation. III. The primary and secondary antibody response to bacteriophage φX174 in guinea pigs. J. Exp. Med. *115*, 655.

DISCUSSION

BLOCK: Can we anticipate that mesenchymal cells in the embryo, even at the yolk stage, are able to give rise to immunologically competent cells and that their failure to do so is due to a lack of stimulus? Normally, the rat yolk sac makes almost exclusively eosinophil megaloblasts; by altering the environment of the yolk by intraocular transplantation to adult rats, their yolk sac can be made to form large numbers of erythroblasts, granulocytes, and megakaryocytes. Why, then, cannot the failure of yolk sac mesenchymal cells to give rise to immunologically competent cells be due, not to an inability to do so, but to the lack of proper stimulation? Proper processing of antigen might represent the missing stimulus.

EBERT: Are you suggesting that lymphocyte differentiation right from the very beginning is dependent on processed antigens.

BLOCK: No; I am bringing out the possibility that these cells, even in such an immature stage as the yolk sac mesenchymal cells, are capable of forming any of the cells subsequently formed by the organism.

147

For example, we don't ordinarily think of a yolk sac as forming megakaryocytes. My argument is that if only the proper method could be attained such as by using macrophages to process the antigen, there would be no reason why even in such a stage as the yolk sac, we couldn't get the development of immunologically competent cells.

EBERT: I think you have raised a fundamental question. We have tended to think of the development of immunologically competent cells as involving at least two steps: a first independent of antigenic stimuli, and a second dependent on antigenic stimulus. Your comment indicated that you believe that immunogenesis is totally dependent on antigenic stimulus. Is that what you mean?

BLOCK: Not necessarily. But the problem may be to set up the environment so that the situation is favorable for mesenchymal cells to form immunologically competent cells. One way to make this environment would be to supply the environment with antigen processed by macrophages.

EBERT: This is a major point from the standpoint of the embryology of this system. It is clear that the environment of any embryonic cell determines to a major degree into what it develops. If your argument turns out to be correct, this would be a major departure in our thinking. We have been talking continuously of a situation where we assume a primordial strain of cells. We raised the possibility that these might possibly come from the yolk sac. In the absence of any information at all, this is pure speculation.

We know something about the thymus, perhaps the original source of such cells. We know of a thymus-to-spleen transfer of cells. And in birds cells go from bursa to spleen. If we take Moore and Owen and other experiments at face value, the bursal cells come from somewhere else, possibly from thymus or from some other primordial site. The so-called virgin cell essentially originated in thymus or elsewhere. It becomes capable by this hypothesis of becoming an antibody-forming cell, a primed cell, under the influence of antigen. Your argument that just supplying antigen at this primordial level will now convert the cell to an antibody-forming cell, is a most interesting one.

MITCHISON: Isn't there a direct method of testing Block's hypothesis—take out the yolk cells, and put them into an environment where they could be expected to react immunologically, for example, into an allogeneic host?

BLOCK: That is what I was trying to bring out—namely, the ability of cells in the yolk sac, which ordinarily don't form erythroblasts, granulocytes, and megakaryocytes, to do so by changing their environment. If these cells form erythroblasts, granulocytes, and megakaryocytes by changing of the environment, why can't appropriate treatment lead to the formation of immunologically mature cells?

EBERT: Changing environment can mean several different sets of things. If by "environment" is meant the presence of processed antigen, that's one thing. If by "environment" is meant the proper interactions with other embryonic tissues apart from antigen, that's another kind of point. We are dealing with two possibly different types of inductive mechanisms. Don't we have some information on the processing of various antigens by the embryo?

BLOCK: We know something about macrophages in embryos. There are macrophages, even in the yolk sac. McBang in 1909 illustrated macrophages in the yolk sac, phagocytizing the eosinophil megaloblasts which are the only cells there phagocytized.

MITCHISON: One experimental observation is that of Simonsen some years ago, which showed that human erythrocytes injected into the chicken on day 14 induced tolerance very nicely. But if injected on day 11, it had no effect at all. The interpretation he put on it, which seems to me sensible, was that there weren't on day 11 any cells susceptible to the induction of tolerance.

KIMMEL: There are some data also on phagocytosis in the chick which I think are relevant. Karthigatsu and Jenkins showed that the embryo can phagocytize bacteria throughout the last half of gestation. However, the ability of these cells to *kill* the bacteria (perhaps a measure of degradation) does not appear concomitantly, but only much later.

SILVERSTEIN: One of the implications of what Mitchison suggests is that if the maturation which we described here is really the non-immunologic maturation of phagocytic abilities, and if the fetus has competent cells at this stage, wouldn't you suspect that prior to what we are calling the assumption of competence, any dose of antigen should be able to induce tolerance? We have looked at this possibility, but find that it is very difficult to induce tolerance of albumin, for instance, under these conditions.

With respect to the interesting fetal protein fetuin, which is produced by many species *in utero,* the fetal lamb produces large amounts during gestation. Production seems to cease about birth. We have tried extensively to immunize adult animals with this protein in adjuvants, but have never been able to stimulate an immune response to it.

Perhaps the adult animals produce subliminal levels all the time, but we cannot detect any. We thus do not see any reason for the maintenance of tolerance, but, in fact, it appears to be maintained. Would you entertain the possibility that there really may be two types of tolerance—that to self and that to non-self?

MITCHISON: If I could comment briefly on that, I would show you another observation which actually runs in exactly the opposite direction. Rabbits which are exposed to the maternal allotypic γ-globulins for a period of at least weeks after birth, you would expect the young rabbit to develop tolerance. Gell and Kelus say that they become responsive. That is an observation running the opposite way.

Has anything been said or has any evidence been presented which would lead one to infer that the macrophage is altered in the induction of tolerance or involved in the induction of tolerance? I am not willing to admit the macrophage to the select family of altered cells in the tolerant animal unless somebody can produce some evidence. And no one seems to have done so. We know that small lymphocytes are tolerant. Perhaps the best experiment is that of Gowans, taking clean lymphocytes out of the thoracic duct of the tolerant animal and showing that they have altered activity. That sort of experiment has never been done so nicely with macrophages. But when it is done, when their functions are tested by any of the available methods of test, they appear perfectly normal.

AUERBACH: Some results of Chaperon need to be taken into account here. A massive dose of BSA injected at hatching of the chicken produces a transient unresponsiveness to BSA. In a thymectomized chicken, this "transient" tolerance is retained. Thus, recovery from immunologic unresponsiveness in this system is thymus-dependent.

18

MATTHEW BLOCK

The "fetal" opossum as an experimental tool in ontogeny of immunologic competence

MAMMALS are divided into three subgroups—protheria, metatheria, and eutheria. Eutheria are the true or common mammals. Metatheria, also known as marsupials, are aplacentate mammals born at a relatively immature stage of development who continue what would be considered fetal development in eutheria in a pouch on the ventral side of the maternal abdomen (Fig. 1). After remaining continuously attached to the maternal teat in the pouch for a variable length of time, the metatherian mammal leaves the pouch in a sort of second birth at a much more advanced stage of development than at true birth. Practically all metatheria reside only in Australia. Protheria, consisting of two species, the duckbilled platypus and the anteater, are the only egg-laying mammals, and are found only in Australia.

The North American opossum, *Didelphis virginiana*, is the only North American marsupial. It is a primitive and ancient mammal dating from the Upper Cretaceous period (8). It has reptilian and avian characteristics, the most obvious of which is intrasinusoidal erythropoiesis. The opossum lacks a bursa of Fabricius. Birth follows a gestation period of only 12.5 days during which time the fetus lies in a fold in the uterus. The average birth weight is 0.1 gm and weight is gained in the pouch at a rate approximating that of a eutherian intrauterine gestation (9, 10). A litter may contain 25 animals; only those attaching to one of the 13 nipples survive (8). The pouch usually contains about 9 "fetuses" in females

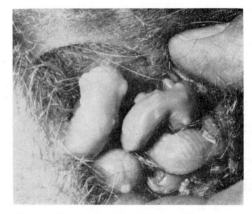

FIG. 1. Pouch containing 12-day-old opossums.

inseminated in the wild and about 5 "fetuses" after insemination in captivity.

The "fetuses" climb into the pouch by a negative geotropism and each remains attached to a nipple for about 60 days at which time it weighs 20-40 gm (Fig. 2). If a "fetus" is removed from the nipple prior to 40 days of age, it will not be able to reattach itself to the nipple and will die. The opossum leaves and returns to the pouch during the 60th through the 90th days and leaves it permanently after 90 days of postnatal life.

During the 12.5 days of intrauterine gestation, nourishment is obtained from the small amount of material in the egg at fertilization and, lacking a placenta, by diffusion of nutrients through fetal membranes. After birth the "fetal" gastrointestinal tract and maternal

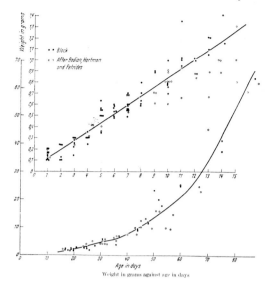

Weight in grams against age in days

FIG. 2. Weight in grams plotted against age in days. Dark circles represent my data, light circles represent data from Bodian, Hartman, and Petrides. Reprinted with permission of editors from Ergebn. Anat. Entwicklungsgesch. *37*:237-366, 1964.

teat are the only connection between "fetal" and maternal tissues and function as a eutherian placenta. Urine and stool are discharged into the pouch and cleared by its mucous membrane.

The opossum is of interest to biologists for several reasons (2). First, being a primitive mammal, it lacks specialized features that many mammals have and so has been studied as a prototype of a primitive mammal and as a link to birds and reptiles. For example, sensory and motor representation in the cerebral cortex of the opossum has been correlated with representation of corresponding functions in the eutherian cerebral cortex (12). The immunologic response of the adult has hardly been investigated (20). In view of its albuminiglobulin ratio of 1:3 to 1:5, one would anticipate differences between the opossum and eutheria. Second, because of its residence in the maternal pouch it is the only mammalian "fetus" directly accessible for experimentation with assurance that experimental procedures will not be modified or diluted by maternal or placental tissues or fetal membranes. Third, being a "fetus" it lacks specialized cells, tissues, and organs common to postnatal mammals. Experiments may therefore be designed to

study the function ascribable to these structures by analyzing the reaction of the "fetal" opossum prior to development of the structure under consideration. The opossum may be regarded as nature's experiment, offering the biologist conditions which, although desirable, are difficult if not impossible to devise in the laboratory.

The opossum has certain practical disadvantages (2). It is a vicious animal capable of inflicting an extremely painful injury by biting. It is a very poor breeder in captivity and with rare exceptions (19) 25 females will produce no more than 10 litters in a breeding season. For larger-scale experiments females must be captured in the wild in the hope that they will be pregnant or contain pouch young. There is no reliable means to determine if females are pregnant. The breeding season begins in the last week in January or first week in February in Texas and Florida and in March in Illinois and Colorado. At the beginning of the breeding season about one of three females with empty pouches caught in the wild will be pregnant. Many not pregnant will have pouch young. The age of the latter may be estimated from the data in Fig. 2. The breeding season is short and a female usually produces only one litter a year.

NORMAL DEVELOPMENT OF THE OPOSSUM

The blood and blood-forming tissues of an opossum at birth correspond in development to an 8-week human, 10-day rat or mouse, and 24-day guinea pig embryo (2), and to the adult hagfish, a primitive cyclostome (17, 18). It lacks lymphatic tissues, bone marrow, plasma cells, and medium or small lymphocytes. Large lymphocytes (stem cells) are found in the liver. The thymus is an unvascularized epithelial sheet, although the presence of mesenchymal cells cannot be excluded (Fig. 3). The spleen contains mesenchymal cells and a few sinusoids (Fig. 4). Myeloid hematopoiesis is restricted to the liver (Fig. 5) and a minute amount in the mediastinal mesenchyme. The circulating blood consists almost entirely of eosinophil megaloblasts originating from the yolk sac prior to birth (Fig. 6). Subsequent development of hematopoietic tissues is listed in Table 1.

Of special interest to immunobiologists are the following elements. In the thymus large

TABLE 1.—THE BLOOD-FORMING TISSUES AND BLOOD OF THE NEWBORN OPOSSUM
NORMAL DEVELOPMENT

	Liver	Thymus	Spleen	Marrow	Lymph node	Connective tissue	Blood
1 day	50% hematopoietic; maturation to basophil erythroblasts; fewer cells in granulocytic lineage but more maturation; megakaryocytoblasts without platelet formation.	Pure epithelial sheet; large lymphocytes bordering capillaries between lobules.	Avascular but mesenchyme more dense than in embryo as a whole; rare transitional form between mesenchymal cell and large lymphocyte.	Endochondral bones solidly cartilaginous; diaphyseal cartilage cells more swollen than in rest of bone; membranous bone irregular bone spicules.		No specialization; rare immature mast cell; rare histioid wandering cells and myelocytes in mediastinum.	Practically all cells are nucleated eosinophil megaloblasts; rare neutrophil myelocytes, megakaryocytes, and platelets.
2 days	Increased concentration of hematopoietic tissue; maturation to polychromatophil erythroblast; fine granulation in megakaryocyte cytoplasm.	Large and a few medium lymphocytes in center; periphery mostly stroma with many transitions between stroma and large lymphocytes; many mitoses and degenerating cells.	Increased mitoses, more closely packed mesenchymal cells, more prominent sinusoids; rare large lymphocyte.	No change except increase in size.		More histioid wandering cells and myelocytes in mediastinum, erythroblasts in mediastinum; collagenous fibers in corium.	Neutrophils and platelets appear, rare erythroblasts; nucleated count falling; platelets increased.
3 days	Erythroblast maturation to eosinophil stage; granulocytopoiesis in capsule and portal connective tissue, neutrophil precursors more frequent than eosinophil; coarse megakaryocytic granulation.	Rapid growth in size; medium lymphocytes in center, large lymphocytes and transitional forms at periphery; further increases in mitoses and karyorrhexis.	More transitional stages between mesenchymal cells and large lymphocytes; still no hematopoiesis; small amount of nuclear debris.	Mesenchyme of membranous bones more vascular and edematous; spicules lined by osteoblast and osteoclasts.	Cervical lymph nodes begin to appear.	More histioid wandering and mast tissue cells; increase in granulocytopoiesis in thorax but less maturation than in liver; increase in collagen.	Continued fall in nucleated count, increase in reticulocytes and red cells, white count (primarily neutrophils) 3,000-12,000; basophils appear; platelets increased.
4 days	Greater increase in erythroblasts than in granulocytes; platelet formation in some megakaryocytes.	Marked increase in size; primarily medium lymphocytes; smaller lymphocyte-poor edge.	Rare small foci of basophil erythroblasts and rare single megakaryocytes; more prominent sinusoids.	Periosteum formed at diaphysis, diaphyseal cartilage cells more swollen.	1 of 7 animals first evidence of node near thymus.	Further increase in histioid wandering and mast tissue cells; hematopoiesis only cranial to diaphragm; islands of granulocytes in mesonephros and between ribs.	Ratio of red cells to nucleated megaloblasts 1:1 to 1:5, reticulocytes at 90%; most white cells in neutrophil lineage, rare basophils; most platelets still contain megakaryocytic nuclei.
5 days	Hematopoiesis more focalized; increased ratio of granulo- to erythropoiesis, eosinophil precursors appear.	Decrease in ratio of large to medium lymphocytes, small lymphocytes at center; very thin lymphocyte-poor growing edge, numerous mitoses and karyorrhexis; primitive Hassall's corpuscles.	Many discrete islands of erythroblasts, myelocytes; less maturation than in liver; arterioles only near hilum.	Diaphysis of endochondral bones in cranial half contain 1° marrow; primary marrow in membranous bone.	Only in mediastinum; consist of mesenchymal network crossing sinusoid with histioid wandering cells and transitions between latter and mesenchymal cells; intrasinusoidal erythroblasts.	Appearance of hematopoiesis in loose mesenchyme caudal to diaphragm, erythropoiesis primarily in adrenal; persistence of granulocytic infiltrates in mesonephros and between ribs.	Red cells outnumber nucleated red cells, 90% reticulocytes, 10 megaloblasts to one erythroblast; increase in eosinophil granulocytes.

TABLE 1 (Continued)

	Liver	Thymus	Spleen	Marrow	Lymph node	Connective tissue	Blood
6 and 7 days	Eosinophils and precursors as numerous as neutrophils and precursors.	Small lymphocytes predominate in center, medium at periphery; thin lymphocyte-poor growing edge persists, more mitoses and karyorrhexis than any other area; Hassall's corpuscles have swollen epithelial cells and nuclear debris.	Marked increase in number, size, and maturation of hematopoietic foci; eosinophils as numerous as neutrophils; less maturation but same distribution of cell lineages as liver; arterial capillaries distributed through red pulp.	Mature eosinophil and neutrophil granulocytes in extravascular mesenchyme in endochondral bones.	Only cranial to diaphragm; small and medium lymphocytes among mesenchymal cells, basophil erythroblasts in sinusoids.	Decrease in granulocytopoiesis, persistence of erythropoiesis especially in adrenal; eosinophils more numerous than neutrophils; adipose tissue in cranial half.	Persistent extreme reticulocytosis; rare large and medium lymphocytes, increase in eosinophils, decrease in basophils; more platelets and fewer megakaryocytes.
8 and 9 days	Beginning decrease in hematopoietic cells and increase in ratio of mature to immature hematopoietic cells.	Center occupied by small lymphocytes, decrease in karyorrhexis and mitoses but still more than in any other area.	Increase in number and size of hematopoietic foci and of mitoses.	Increase in percentage of endochondral bone occupied by marrow.	Found caudal to diaphragm; myeloid cells still as numerous as medium and small lymphocytes.	More mast tissue cells and more collagenous fibers.	Beginning of rapid fall in percentage of reticulocytes and rapid increase in red count; only a few megakaryocytes, platelets otherwise as in mature animal.
10 to 12 days	Continued decrease in concentration of hematopoietic cells especially neutrophil precursors; most of mitoses in erythroblasts; nuclear debris in Kupffer cells.	Thymus except for Hassall's corpuscles filled with small lymphocytes; very small lymphocyte-poor growing edge.	More rapid increase in erythroblasts than in granulocyte precursors; granulocytopoiesis near connective tissue, trabeculae, arterioles and capsule, eosinophils more numerous than neutrophils; perivascular mesenchymal cells separate arterioles from myeloid tissue of red pulp.	Increased number of eosinophil granulocytes separated from cortex by myxoid mesenchyme; a few intravascular large lymphocytes and basophil erythroblasts.	Recognizable cortex with dense diffuse lymphatic tissues; medulla with medullary cords with scattered small and medium lymphocytes; myelocytes, erythroblasts, and megakaryocytes in sinusoids.	Myeloid metaplasia only in loose connective tissue without collagenous fibers; latter present wherever found in postnatal life.	Further decrease in reticulocytes and increase in red cells, occasional hemoglobin deficient red cells; increased percentage of eosinophils, first appearance of small lymphocytes with increase in all lymphocytes; smaller vessels still occluded by erythroblasts.
13 to 16 days	Decrease in number and increase in focalization of hematopoietic cells.	First appearance of medullary lymphatic tissue with fewer lymphocytes than cortex; small lymphocytes fill cortex to capsule; eosinophil droplets in Hassall's corpuscles; decrease in mitoses and karyorrhexis.	Rapid growth of spleen due more to increase in erythroblasts than granulocyte precursors or megakaryocytes; more mitoses than any other organ.	Increase in amount of marrow in endochondral bone.	Decrease in myeloid metaplasia; loss of anterior-posterior gradient of maturation.	Dense collagen in corium, myeloid metaplasia only in prevertebral tissues.	Disappearance of megaloblasts; increase in small and medium lymphocytes; slower rate of increase of red count and of decrease in reticulocytes; up to 15% lymphocytes of small and medium size; megakaryocytes almost entirely in the lung.

Table 1 (Continued)

	Liver	Thymus	Spleen	Marrow	Lymph node	Connective tissue	Blood
17 to 22 days	Decrease in hematopoiesis; erythroblasts in lobules, granulocyte precursors in portal tissue; no change in ratio of immature to mature cells; a few eosinophil precursors persist in lobules, eosinophil lineage outnumbers neutrophil lineage.	Increase in ratio of medullary to cortical tissue; persistence of epithelial lined cysts and formation of eosinophil material in Hassall's corpuscles.	Solidly filled with erythroblasts, lesser increase in granulocytopoiesis and megakaryocytes; first appearance of medium lymphocytes and transitional forms between latter and reticular cells in periarteriolar mesenchyme.	Sinusoids fill with large lymphocytes and erythroblasts; higher ratio of immature to mature cells in sinusoids than in granulocytic tissue outside sinusoids.	Increase in number and size; increased number of small lymphocytes in cortex; decrease in myelocytes and megakaryocytes, to lesser extent in erythroblasts.	Decrease in granulocytopoiesis and granulocytic infiltrates in mesonephros and between ribs.	No change in reticulocyte percentage; white cells equal nucleated red cells, increase in percentage of small lymphocytes and eosinophils.
23 to 32 days	Decrease in amount of hematopoietic tissue; eosinophil lineage no more numerous than neutrophil lineage.	Resembled fully developed thymus.	Decrease in myeloid tissue, especially granulocytopoiesis; white pulp found in all animals, lymphocytes outnumbered by mesenchymal cells.	Endochondral bones filled with marrow except at epiphyses; ratio of intravascular to extravascular hematopoiesis increased.	Clear separation of cortex and medulla; large lymphocytes found in cortex, small lymphocytes in medullary sinusoids and in walls of veins.	Gross decrease in extramedullary hematopoiesis except in prevertebral tissue (myelocytes) and in small intestine (erythroblasts); eosinophil granulocytes increased, especially in GI tract.	Increase in percentage of small lymphocytes and eosinophils.
33 to 45 days	Only occasional hematopoietic foci, no change in ratio of immature to mature cells, cessation of subcapsular granulocytopoiesis.		Decrease in myeloid tissue; increase in amount of white pulp with increase in ratio of lymphocytes to mesenchymal cells.	Increase in ratio of immature to mature granulocytes and of intrasinusoidal erythroblasts and megakaryocytes to extravascular granulocytes and precursors; occasional myelocytes in membraneous bone marrow.	Increase in size due to increased number of lymphocytes.	Further decrease in myeloid metaplasia and increase in granulocytes in GI tract. Peyer's patches beginning to develop. Lymphatic tissue in tonsil.	Red cells tend to be hypochromic, persistence of nucleated red cells.

TABLE 1 (Continued)

	Liver	Thymus	Spleen	Marrow	Lymph node	Connective tissue	Blood
46 to 65 days	One small island of hematopoiesis (usually erythroblasts or megakaryocyte) per 3-4 lobules.		Increased ratio of white to red pulp; decrease in myeloid hematopoiesis in red pulp; white pulp consists of inner densely lymphocytic core and outer less lymphocyte rich rim.	More intrasinusoidal erythropoiesis and megakaryocytopoiesis than extravascular granulocytopoiesis; increase in ratio of mature to immature erythroblasts, and of immature to mature granulocytes.	Diffuse increase in lymphocytes; cortex forms complete crescent separating subcapsular sinus from medulla, islands of large lymphocytes in cortex; increase in large lymphocytes and proplasma cells in medullary cords, rare plasma cells; very slight myeloid metaplasia; nuclear debris in cortex and medulla.	End of extramedullary hematopoiesis except in one animal. Well-developed Peyer's patches.	No significant change.
66 to 100 days	One or two foci of erythroblasts and rare megakaryocyte in each section; no iron by Prussian blue stain.		Differentiation of lymphatic nodules with reactionary and germinal centers.	Similar to marrow of mature animal.	Persistent rapid increase in size due to increase in number of lymphocytes; decrease in area occupied by medullary sinusoids; nodules with reaction and germinal centers in cortex; increase in plasma and proplasma cells.	Similar to mature animals.	Increase in hemoglobin concentration of red cells.

Reprinted with permission of Springer-Verlag from Ergebn. Anat. Entwicklungsgesch. 37, 237 (1964).

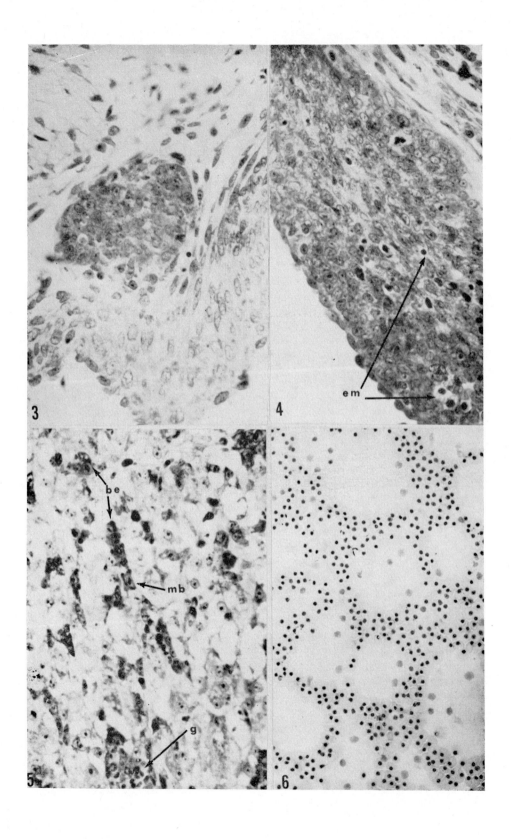

lymphocytes are first seen at the end of the first 24 hours, Hassall's corpuscles on the 5th day, and a differentiated medulla on the 13th day of life. Lymph nodes are recognizable in the neck on the 3d day of life, in the mediastinum on the 5th day of life, and caudal to the diaphragm on the 8th day. In the spleen myeloid hematopoiesis begins on the 5th day and lymphatic tissue is recognizable on about the 16th or 18th day. Endochondral bones are cartilaginous at birth, and the primary marrow of Maximow is recognizable in these bones at the cranial end of the "fetus" at about the 8th day. Peyer's patches are erythroblastic until about the 40th day. The appendix contains very little if any lymphatic tissue throughout the life of the animal. Plasma cells and secondary nodules are first demonstrable at 40-60 days of age. Because of technical difficulties only scattered observations have been made by paper electrophoresis of serum proteins. The latter differ at the beginning and end of life in the pouch.

The "Fetal" Opossum as a Tool for Experimental Analysis of Embryonic Development

The effect of thymectomy.—The relation of the thymus to origin and development of extrathymic lymphatic tissue has been the subject of intense interest in recent years (14, 25). However, none of these experiments pertain to the *origin* of extrathymic lymphatic tissue since in the animals studied extrathymic lymphatic tissue has already developed prior to birth, the earliest time at which thymectomy was possible (2, 15). The opossum is suitable for investigation of this relationship since the thymus is an epithelial rudiment at birth and large lymphocytes appear in it at the end of the first 24 hours of life. Extrathymic lymphocytes are first formed in cervical nodes on the 3d day, in mediastinal nodes on the 5th day, in abdominal nodes on the 7th day, and in spleen by the 16th to 18th days after birth. Opossums were thymectomized to investigate the role played by the thymus in origin of

extrathymic lymphatic tissue (15). For technical reasons (the small size of the animals, delicacy of the tissues, huge blood vessels, bleeding due to thrombocytopenia, and the encirclement of the aortic arch by the thymus) it was impossible to complete thymectomies until about the 5th and usually not until after the 7th day after birth without killing the "fetuses." However, opossums were thymectomized at a much more immature stage of development than feasible in eutherian mammals.

Following thymectomy the spleen grossly enlarged due to an increase in myeloid tissue, especially erythroblasts (compare Fig. 7 with Fig. 8). Furthermore the erythroblastic tissue was anaplastic with a pathologically elevated ratio of immature to mature erythroblasts and often a persistence of granulocytic precursors and megakaryocytes. Lymphatic tissue did not appear during the two weeks that the animals were followed after thymectomy. A similar sequence of events, i.e., failure of disappearance of myeloid tissue and very poor development of lymphatic tissue, was found in lymph nodes. Large number of basophil, polychromatophil, and eosinophil erythroblasts and ruptured lymphocytes were found in the blood.

These results indicate not merely that thymectomy inhibits *origin* of lymphatic tissue in abdominal nodes and spleen but also that the thymus is needed to suppress myeloid tissue. It is probable that the major role of the thymus is first to suppress myeloid tissue in order to allow subsequent development of lymphatic tissue in spleen and lymph nodes. Furthermore, thymectomy seems to remove an inhibitory effect exerted by the thymus on erythropoiesis in lymph nodes and spleen resulting in a hyperplasia and dysplasia of erythropoiesis. A related phenomenon is the increased incidence of myeloid leukemia and decreased incidence of thymic conditioned lymphoma in mice thymectomized after inoculation with leukemogenic virus (7).

An attempt was made in 1965 to extend these preliminary observations on a larger

Fig. 3. Thymus of day-old opossum composed of epithelial (? mesenchymal) cells. x 400; Fig. 4. Spleen of day-old opossum composed of mesenchymal cells and a few sinusoids containing eosinophil megaloblasts (em). x 400; Fig. 5. Liver of day-old opossum. Larger dark cells are basophil erythroblasts (be) or megakaryoblasts (mb); cells with lobed nuclei are granulocytes and precursors (g). x 400; Fig. 6. Blood smear of day-old opossum. All cells are nucleated eosinophil megaloblasts formed in the yolk sac. x 400

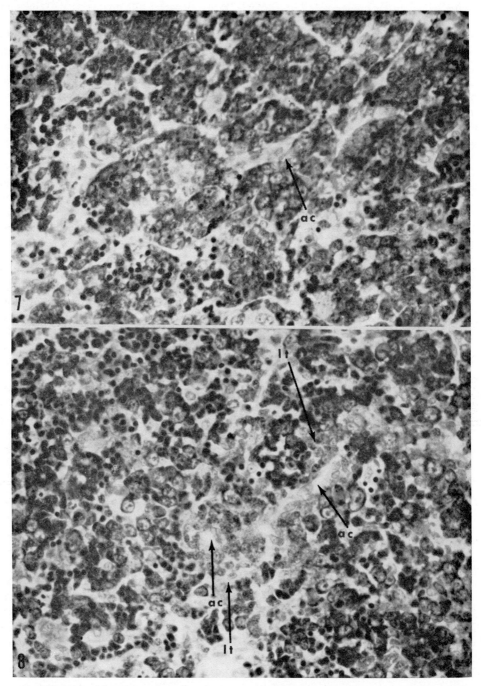

Fig. 7. Spleen of opossum thymectomized at 12 days of age and sacrificed 16 days thereafter. Arterial capillary (ac) lacks lymphatic sheath. Surrounding erythroblasts have a higher ratio of immature to mature erythroblasts than in control litter mate in Fig. 8. x 400; Fig. 8. Normal litter mate of same age as thymectomized animal in Fig. 7; lymphatic tissue sheath (lt) surrounds arterial capillary (ac); lower ratio of immature to mature erythroblasts than in Fig. 7. x 400

series of thymectomized opossums and to compare immunologic competence and serum proteins in thymectomized and non-thymectomized opossums (16). Unfortunately, almost all thymectomized opossums surviving the operation died while being bled to obtain serum for antibody titers and for paper and immunoelectrophoresis.

Because of the lack of suitable eutherian mammals to explore the role played by the thymus in the *origin* of extrathymic lymphatic tissue, and because this problem cannot be investigated in opossums by thymectomy for technical reasons, it is desirable to attack the problem in other ways. The thymus of 2-day-old opossums, prior to appearance of extrathymic lymphatic tissue, contains numerous dividing cells so that H_3-thymidine should be incorporated into these cells by pulse-labelling as well as into any other rapidly dividing cells, myeloid cells in the liver for example, and to a lesser degree into cells in the "fetus" as a whole because of the relatively high percentage of dividing cells in fetal tissues. By counting the number of H_3-thymidine marked lymphocytes in cervical lymph nodes on the 3d or 4th day of life and in mediastinal nodes on the 5th or 6th day of life after pulse-labelling on the 1st or 2d days of life, it should be possible to determine whether these lymphocytes are formed locally or originate by metastasis from the thymus or other areas where cells had been labelled by the H_3-thymidine (23). Fortunately, lymphatic sinusoids in which lymph nodes develop contain practically no dividing cells on the 1st and 2d days of life (4, 13). By repeating the labelling experiments prior to the 16th day of life, it should be possible to investigate the origin of splenic lymphocytes.

Effect of radiation and other agents on development of organs.—Since the opossum is accessible in the maternal pouch, it may be radiated without simultaneously radiating maternal tissue, placenta, or fetal membranes. It is therefore feasible to study the effect of radiation upon origin of a tissue or cell lineage in the fetus by radiating prior to the time that the tissue or lineage of cells normally appears.

Figs. 9 and 10 show the effect of such radiation. Radiation of day-old opossums results in inhibition of appearance of large lymphocytes in the thymus at the end of the 1st day of life, these cells first appearing after a delay of about 4 days (compare Fig. 9 with Fig. 10). When lymphocytes do appear subsequently, their development is highly pathological. Similar observations have been made upon the appearance of lymphatic or myeloid cells in other organs or tissue by radiating the opossum at the appropriate age in the maternal pouch (3). The probable interpretation is that radiation prevented the transformation of precursors (epithelial or mesenchymal cells) into large lymphocytes.

Treatment with cortisone and related corticosteroids will grossly decrease lymphocytopoiesis without significantly affecting myeloid tissue (5). Newborn mice undergo atrophy of lymphatic tissue leading to a wasting syndrome following a single injection of corticosteroids (21). The younger the mice and the larger the dose the more profound is the lymphatic atrophy. Since a day-old opossum is obviously more immature than a day-old mouse, injection of corticosteroids in adequate dosage on the 1st day of life should result in animals without lymphatic tissue and presumably lacking in the functions ascribed to this tissue and to lymphocytes and plasma cells formed by this tissue. By injecting corticosteroids into newborn "fetal" opossums rather than treating with radiation or radiomimetic drugs, development of myeloid tissue should not be inhibited and therefore neutropenia, anemia, and thrombocytopenia should not cause premature death of the animals. This experiment is now in progress (23).

The "Fetal" Opossum as a Tool for Analysis of Function of Cells, Tissues, or Organs

Development of immunologic capacity.— The fertilized egg is immunologically incompetent (22). Until recently it was believed that in mammals plasma cells, secondary nodules, and immunologic competence developed only after birth (2, 26). However, plasma cells, secondary nodules, and some types of antibodies are demonstrable in eutherian embryos subjected to specific types of antigenic stimulation (6, 22). Furthermore, immunologic response is not an all-or-none phenomenon, antibody response to some antigens developing earlier than to others, macroglobulins being the first type of antibody to develop (24). Because of technical difficulties it is impossible

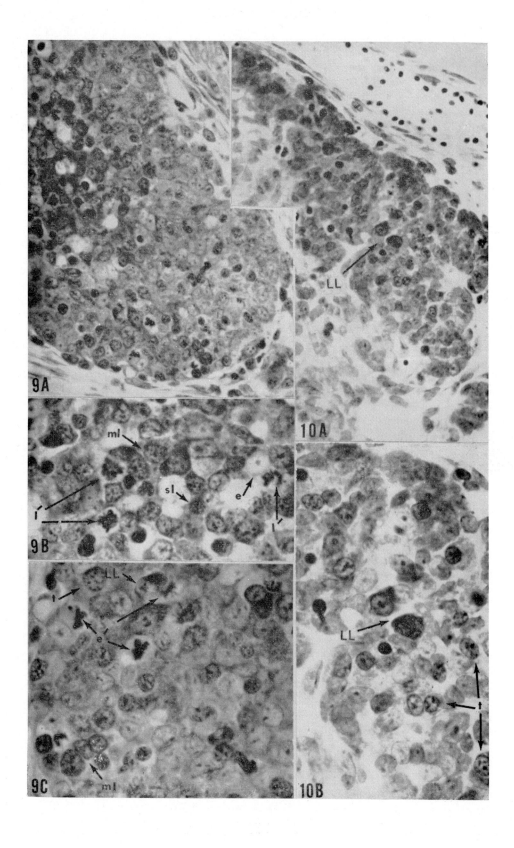

to investigate this phenomenon in immature eutherian embryos.

The opossum presents a unique opportunity to analyze development of specific antibodies and to assign origin of these antibodies to specific cells or tissues. For example, plasma cells are not found in opossums until 40 days after birth. Obviously antibodies formed prior to this time, provided the corresponding antigens did not stimulate plasma cell formation, must have been formed by cells other than plasma cells. Similarly, if antigenic stimulation at a time when only thymic but no extrathymic lymphatic tissue was present failed to induce antibody response, one could conclude that either the antigen did not reach the thymus or that thymic tissue was immunologically incompetent.

The opossum is able to form antibody to phage at a time when it lacks plasma cells and secondary nodules (11), although this investigation did not exclude the possibility that phage did not induce premature development of plasma cells and secondary nodules. Subsequently Rowlands showed that specific antibody in response to injection of flagellar antigen of *S. typhosa* was synthesized in opossums prior to development of plasma cells and secondary nodules but not prior to formation of extrathymic lymphatic tissue (20).

The role of the lymphocyte in inflammation.—The relationship of the circulating lymphocyte to mononuclear cells found in areas of inflammation has been bitterly disputed for over 100 years. One means to investigate this problem is to study inflammation in animals lacking lymphatic tissue and circulating lymphocytes. However, this condition cannot be produced experimentally in postnatal mammals without also inducing so many other abnormalities that the data obtained would be

difficult to interpret, and cannot be investigated in eutherian embryos immature enough to lack circulating lymphocytes and lymphatic tissues because of their inaccessibility. The opossum at birth, lacking circulating lymphocytes and lymphatic tissue and accessible by virtue of its position in the maternal pouch, is well suited for this type of experiment (1).

Fig. 11 is from the skin of a day-old animal that had been lightly burned on the 1st day of life, and Fig. 12 is from the skin of an animal that had been similarly burned on the 45th day of life. The younger animal lacked circulating lymphocytes and the older did not. Although both lesions show vasodilatation, very few mononuclear cells were found in the injured area in the younger animal, suggesting that extravascular mononuclear inflammatory cells are formed only in animals with circulating lymphocytes, and that these mononuclears are derived primarily from circulating lymphocytes rather than fixed connective tissue cells. This lack of inflammatory reaction to injury is similar to that found in the adult hagfish, which also lacks circulating lymphocytes (17, 18).

SUMMARY

The taxonomy, breeding habits, and postnatal development of hematopoietic tissues of the opossums have been described. At birth it is essentially a fetus in terms of development of its hematopoietic tissues. A series of experiments of interest to immunologists and embryologists have been described which would have been impossible in eutherian mammals but were feasible in the newborn opossum because of its accessibility in the maternal pouch.

Acknowledgment: This study was supported by USPHS Grant RG-4089.

FIG. 9. Thymus of a normal 4-day-old opossum: (A) Approximately 1/10 of the thymus is included on the illustration; the central area of the lobule composed primarily of small and medium lymphocytes; periphery of lobule composed primarily of epithelial (? mesenchymal) cells and a few large lymphocytes. x 425; (B) Central area of the lobule of (A) showing numerous medium (ml) and small lymphocytes (sl), numerous mitoses in lymphocytes (1′), and occasional epithelial (? mesenchymal) cells (e). x 900; (C) Peripheral area of the lobule of (A) showing numerous dividing epithelial (? mesenchymal) cells (e′); large lymphocytes (LL), occasional medium lymphocytes (ml) and transitions between epithelial (? mesenchymal) cells and lymphocytes (t). x 900

FIG. 10. Thymus of opossum exposed to 400 r total body radiation on the 1st day and sacrificed on the 4th day of life: (A) Section through entire length of thymus. Note small size, only 2 large lymphocytes (LL), and lack of differentiation *vs.* Fig. 9A of central and peripheral areas. x 400; (B) Central area of (A). Two large lymphocytes (LL), epithelial (? mesenchymal cells) and transitions between latter and former (t); note absence of mitoses. x 900

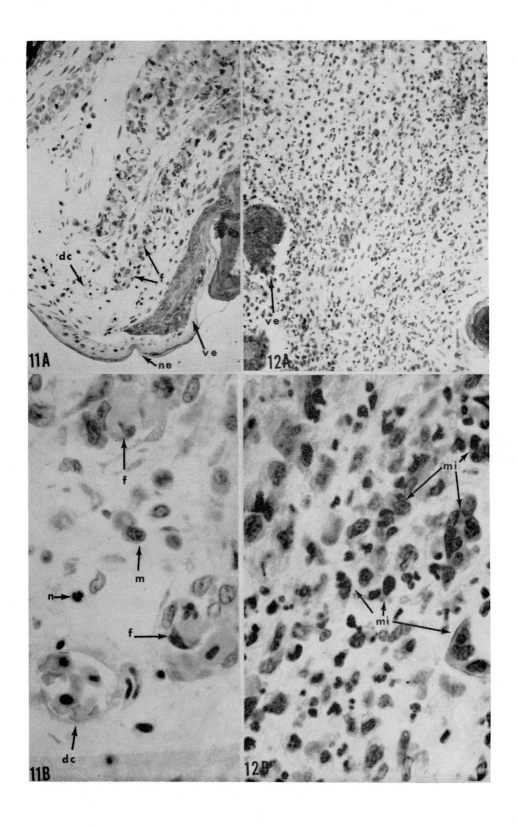

REFERENCES

1. Block, M. (1960): Wound healing in the new-born opossum (*Didelphis virginiana*); Nature *187*, 340.
2. Block, M. (1964): The blood forming tissues and blood of the newborn opossum (*Didelphis virginiana*). I. Normal development through about the one-hundredth day of life (in English). Ergebn. Anat. Entwicklungsgesch. *37*, 237.
3. Block, M.: Unpublished observations.
4. Bloom, W. (1938): Embryogenesis of mammalian blood. Chapter 13 in Handbook of Hematology, ed. Hal Downey, Paul B. Hoeber, New York, N. Y.
5. Dougherty, T., and White, A. (1945): Functional alterations in lymphoid tissue induced by adrenal cortical secretions. Amer. J. Anat. *77*, 81.
6. Fennestad, K. L., and Borg-Petersen, K. (1962): Antibody and plasma cells in bovine fetuses infected with *Leptospira saxkoebing*. J. Infect. Dis. *110*, 63.
7. Gross, L. (1960): Development of myeloid (chloro-) leukemia in thymectomized C₃H mice following inoculation of lymphatic leukemia virus. Proc. Soc. Exp. Biol. Med. 103, 509.
8. Hamilton, W., Jr. (1963): Success story of the opossum. Natural Hist. *72*, 17.
9. Hartman, C. G. (1921): Breeding Habits, Development and Birth of the Opossum; Report of Secretary of the Smithsonian Institution, Washington, p. 347.
10. Hartman, C. G. (1928): The breeding season of the opossum (*Didelphis virginiana*) and the rate of intrauterine and postnatal development. J. Morph. Physiol. *46*, 143.
11. Kalmutz, S. E. (1962): Antibody production in the opossum embryo. Nature *193*, 851.
12. Lende, R. A. (1963): Motor representation in the cerebral cortex of the opossum (*Didelphis virginiana*). J. Comp. Neur. *121*, 405.
13. Maximow, A. (1927): Bindegewebe and Blutbildende Gewebe; Vol. 2, part 1, in: W. von Möllendorf, ed.: Handbuch der Mikroskopischen Anatomie des Menschen. Berlin, Springer.
14. Miller, J. F. A. P. (1963): Role of the thymus in immunity. Brit. Med. J. 2, 459.
15. Miller, J. F. A. P., Block, M., Rowlands, D. R., Jr., and Kind, P. (1965): Effect of thymectomy on the hematopoietic organs of the opossum embryo. Proc. Soc. Exp. Biol. Med. *118*, 916.
16. Miller, J. F. A. P., Block, M., LaVia, M., and Kind, P. (1965): Unpublished observations.
17. Papermaster, B., Condie, R. M., and Good, R. A. (1962): Immune response in the California hagfish. Nature *196*, 355.
18. Papermaster, B. W., Condie, R. M., Finstad, J., and Good, R. A. (1964): Evolution of the immune response. J. Exp. Med. *119*, 105.
19. Reynolds, H. C. (1952): Studies on reproduction in the opossum (*Didelphis virginiana*). Univ. Calif. Publ. Zool. *52*, 223.
20. Rowlands, D. R., Jr., LaVia, M., and Block, M. (1964): Studies of the blood and blood-forming tissues of the newborn opossum. II. Observations of antibody formation to flagella of *S. typhi*. J. Immun. *93*, 157.
21. Schlesinger, M., and Mark, R. (1964): Wasting disease induced in young mice by administration of cortisol acetate. Science *143*, 965.
22. Silverstein, A. M. (1964): Ontogeny of the immune response. Science *144*, 1423.
23. Thrasher, J., and Block, M. (1966): Investigations in progress.
24. Uhr, J. (1964): The heterogeneity of the immune response. Science *145*, 457.
25. Waksman, B. H., Arnason, B. G., and Janković, B. D.: Role of the thymus in immune reactions in rats. III. Changes in the lymphoid organs of thymectomized rats. J. Exp. Med. *116*, 187.
26. Young, R., Ward, H., Hartshorn, D., and Block, M. (1963): The relationship between antibody formation and the appearance of plasma cells in newborn hamsters. J. Infect. Dis. *112*, 67.

DISCUSSION

PETERSON: Have you studied the effect of burns in older thymectomized animals?

BLOCK: No. We have studied only burns in animals of ages which have lymphocytes in their tissues and lymphocytes in circulating blood. As long as there are lymphocytes in the

FIG. 11. Skin of opossum burned during the 1st day of life and sacrificed 18 hours thereafter; (A) Viable epithelium (ve), necrotic epithelium overlying burn (ne), dilated capillary (dc). swollen muscle fibers (f). Note relatively acellular, edematous corium in comparison to Fig. 12A. x 200; (B) Corium of (A) showing dilated capillaries containing eosinophil megaloblasts (dc), swollen muscle fibers (f), occasional contracted mesenchymal cells (m), and rare neutrophils (n).

FIG. 12. Skin of opossum burned on the 45th day of life: (A) Viable epithelium (ve); corium contains many more inflammatory cells than in Fig. 11A. x 200; (B) Corium of (A); note numerous mononuclear inflammatory cells (mi) in comparison to Fig. 11B. x 900

tissues or in the circulating blood, they develop mononuclear inflammation. If they don't have lymphocytes, they do not show mononuclear inflammation.

SILVERSTEIN: When do histiocytes or phagocytic cells which mimic this inflammatory reaction in species without circulating lymphocytes appear?

BLOCK: The original papers show that rabbits at this stage of development, as well as opossums, mice, and rats, have histiocytic cells. Phagocytosis occurs in the connective tissues. It isn't a lack of potentially histiocytic cells that accounts for the lack of inflammation. The histiocytic cells would have had to divide in order to account for the increased number of cells.

GOOD: One of the aspects of the spleen of the neonatally thymectomized mice is not only the dearth of lymphoid development, but also the extraordinary persistence of erythropoiesis and myelopoiesis. It seems that one of the roles of the thymus revealed in the thymectomized mammal is inhibition of fetal type of erythropoiesis in this peripheral organ.

A certain type of human patient with aregenerative anemia shows enlargement of the thymus—actually a thymic tumor. In about half of these patients, removal of this tumor will result in the reinduction of effective erythropoiesis.

It is conceivable that the thymus is affecting fetal erythropoietic tissue at long range or through local effects of the ingressing lymphocyte. The effects of neonatal thymectomy on the lymphoid system of the mouse are very often delayed, we agree. In certain strains of mice, the circulating lymphocyte counts are maintained for about 3 weeks before they begin to drop to the low levels that characterize the neonatally thymectomized mouse at 6 or 8 weeks.

We thought that the mice had been under the influence of a mother with an adequate thymus. We removed the mother's thymus in adult life, and did neonatal thymectomies on her offspring. The lymphocyte levels were maintained for 3 weeks no differently from controls.

With respect to inflammation, we have a clinical observation to offer. In the Swiss type hypogammaglobulinemia, the mononuclear component of the inflammatory response is markedly depressed. These patients do have capacity for phagocytosis, but are lacking in bone marrow lymphocytes. The deficient cell type might ultimately be traced to the bone marrow or yolk sac or might derive from the thymus.

BLOCK: I would like to say a word about the clinical analogy you have just made. In the individual who has thymic hyperplasia and a lack of erythroblasts in his bone marrow, your analogy is not warranted. Such an individual shows an absence of erythroblasts in his bone marrow; he has no erythroblasts, granulocytes, or megakaryocytes in his spleen.

GOOD: What I am postulating is that the patient with thymic tumor may be producing abnormal amounts of something which under delicate balance in the normal embryo would suppress extramedullary erythropoiesis, but leave normal erythropoiesis in bone marrow unaffected. Removal of his thymus then might remove the pathological suppression.

BLOCK: You must realize that removing the thymus in opossums doesn't suppress erythropoiesis in the bone marrow. Apparently the thymus has no effect on intramedullary erythropoiesis.

GOOD: To produce the excessive amounts necessary to suppress the bone marrow might be achieved only by a tumor of the epithelial component of the thymus and not by normal thymus.

BLOCK: In these individuals, variation in the result of thymectomy is recognized. In our experience, removal of the thymus does not seem to help very much. Spleen removal seems to be essential.

We may be dealing with more than one disease. It is tenuous to draw analogies between such complicated, variable, and rare clinical situations and what we see at one stage of embryonic life in experimental animals.

GOOD: I must insist that the 47-50 instances of association of aregenerative anemia and this type of thymic tumor signal an important relationship that cannot be explained by chance alone.

19

W. H. ADLER, J. H. CURRY, and R. T. SMITH

Quantitative aspects of early postnatal immunoglobulin peptide chain synthesis in the rabbit

THE TIMING AND QUANTITATIVE ASPECTS of the immune response have been extensively studied in terms of classes of antibodies appearing in the serum (1-5). Interpreting such data with respect to timing and rate of synthesis of the various immunoglobulins and correlating these data with observable events at a cell level are compromised seriously by factors which vary independently for each class. These factors include rate of secretion by antibody-producing cells, distribution of immunoglobulins in the fluid spaces, rate of catabolism, epithelial secretion rate, and perhaps most significantly, the differing sensitivity of assay systems employed for their measurement.

Such considerations have led to various attempts to examine antibody-producing cells more directly. Jerne (6) and Ingraham and Bussard (7) have described techniques for determining sheep cell antibody secretion of individual cells *in vitro*. Sterzl and Riha (8), Borsos and Rapp (9), and Dresser and Wortis (10) have modified this approach in such a way as to differentiate γM- or γG-antibody secretion by such cells. Nossal *et al.* (11) examined single rat cell isolates *in vitro,* to determine the class of immunoglobulin antibody being produced.

It has not been possible to examine the intact mature lymphoreticular system by the fluorescent antibody technique to determine the class of immunoglobulins produced in response to a single stimulus, because of the multiple simultaneous immunologic events which are always in progress. The use of the newborn rabbit as an experimental model, however, offers an opportunity to examine peptide chain synthesis in an essentially virgin, but immunologically competent, lymphoreticular system.

In the studies to be described, goat anti-rabbit heavy chain specific fluorescent antibody reagents, as described by Cebra and Goldstein (12), were used to determine the natural background and induced order of appearance of immunoglobulins in the newborn rabbit responding to a bacterial antigen. The occurrence of γ or μ heavy chain production by cells in the spleen and lymph nodes was determined; the morphology of cells containing these heavy chains was observed; and indirect evidence for the identity of observed immunoglobulin formation with specific antibody synthesis was found.

Additional studies showing the ontogenetic sequence of α chain synthesis and the concurrent appearance of light chains in heavy chain producing cells are reported elsewhere (13).

MATERIALS AND METHODS

Preparation of the fluorescent reagents.— μ chain specific antibody was produced by immunizing goats with purified rabbit γM anti-*Salmonella* "O" antibody (14). The goat anti-rabbit γM was then absorbed with insoluble rabbit γG-globulin to remove non-μ chain antibody (15). Anti-rabbit γ chain was prepared by immunizing goats with Fc fragment (15).

50 ml aliquots of goat antisera to the rabbit heavy chains were precipitated by the addition of an equal volume of 3.2 M $(NH_4)_2SO_4$. The precipitate was then dissolved in 0.075 M NaCl and dialyzed against 0.01 M phosphate buffer at pH 7.5, and passed through a DEAE column (2.5 cm x 40 cm) equilibrated in .01 M phosphate buffer pH 7.5. The γG-containing peak was collected and concentrated to 10 to 20 mg of protein/ml by pressure dialysis. The goat γG anti-rabbit immunoglobulin reagents were then conjugated with either fluorescein isothiocyanate or tetraethylrhodamine isothiocyanate as described previously (12, 16, 17).

The two colors of fluorochrome conjugated goat antibodies were mixed in a proportion which by trial staining gave optimal staining by both (13). The final goat γG-immunoglobulin protein concentration of each reagent and the ratio of its optical densities at 280 mμ and 515 mμ (rhodamine) or 495 mμ (fluorescein) were as follows: rhodamine anti-γ chain (0.25 mg/ml) 2.1:1; fluorescein anti-μ chain (0.34 mg/ml) 7.3:1; rhodamine anti-μ chain (0.20 mg/ml) 2.9:1; and fluorescein anti-γ chain (0.32 mg/ml) 6.1:1.

Immunization and tissue preparation.—Litters of either New Zealand White or Dutch Black rabbits, born in the laboratory, were kept with the doe until sacrifice. After initial survey of a number of non-immunized and immunized animals during the first weeks of life, subsequent litters were divided into equal groups; one was immunized by a single i.p. injection of about 10^{10} flagellated *S. paratyphi B* (*4, 5, 12:b*), prepared as described by Bellanti *et al.* (3); the others were kept as controls. Spleen, mesenteric nodes, appendix, and popliteal lymphoid tissue were examined at varying intervals after birth. Touch prints were made of the spleen, mesenteric, and popliteal lymphoid tissue; cryostat sections of the appendix were prepared two to four microns thick. Tissues from the control groups of non-immunized rabbits were examined at birth, 5, 10, or 20 days of age. Tissue from immunized groups was examined at 1, 2, 3, 4, 5, or 10 days of age. Agglutinins of the flagellar antigen were titrated by a method described previously (3).

Fluorescent microscopy.—Imprints or cryostat sections were fixed in 95% ethyl alcohol for 20 minutes, air dried, flooded with appropriately diluted fluorescent antisera, and incubated at room temperature for one hour. Thereafter, they were rinsed with two changes of phosphate buffered saline, air dried, and mounted in buffered glycerol.

The stained tissues were examined with a Leitz microscope using an XB0-150-W light source and either a BG-13 or a 2x50 mm Corning #5840 glass filter. Barrier eyepiece filters used were Kodak Wratten celluloid filters; K2, 27A, and 57A. The K2 filter allows both red and green fluorescence to be seen, the 27A filter allows only red to be seen, and the 57A filter allows only green to be seen. Through the use of these filters it was possible to verify the color of fluorescence emitted by individual cells.

RESULTS

Spontaneously occurring immunoglobulin production.—The lymphoreticular tissues of the normal newborn unimmunized rabbit, as shown in Table 1, had no detectable heavy chain-producing cells. By the fifth day, however, very small numbers of both μ- and γ-containing cells were detectable in some animals. The number of heavy chain-containing cells seen through the 10th day of life was a very low percentage of the total lymphoid cells counted in each organ. For example, the number of lymphoid cells examined in the spleen prints of the 5-day-old rabbits was usually between $2x10^5$ and $3x10^5$. In the 5-day-old group, only two of six rabbits showed any γ- or μ-staining cells at all; four γ and two μ cells were seen in these three animals. This indicates that the normal occurrence of immunoglobulin-producing cells at five days is on the order of 0.5-1 per 10^5 lymphoid cells. By 20 days of age immunoglobulin-producing cells were found in all tissues of all normal animals examined. At this age the numbers were on the order of 3-4 per 10^5 lymphoreticular cells. Considerable variation in numbers of spontaneously occurring γ- and μ-containing cells was observed between litters, and even among littermates.

Of interest is the observation that γ-producing cells were the dominant type in the spleen and mesenteric nodes at 10 and 20 days of age in the normal rabbit. This represents a much lower relative prevalence of μ-contain-

TABLE 1.—OCCURRENCE OF HEAVY CHAIN CONTAINING CELLS OF THE UNIMMUNIZED
RABBIT AT VARIOUS AGES

Age of rabbits (days)	Tissue Examined*								
	Fraction having one or more fluorescent cells	Spleen		Mesenteric Lymph Node		Appendix		Popliteal Lymph Node	
		γ	μ	γ	μ	γ	μ	γ	μ
Day of birth	0/9†	0	0	0	0	0	0	0	0
4	2/5	10	4	7	0	0	0	0	0
5	2/6	4	2	0	0	0	0	0	0
6	1/6	0	1	0	0	0	0	0	0
10	3/5	24	3	10	0	40	0	2	2
20	5/5	34	3	60	1	30	10	6	0

*Number of cells in total imprints examined staining specifically for γ or μ heavy chains.

†Numerator of fraction: number of rabbits of the group showing at least one fluorescent staining cell; denominator: number in group.

ing cells than that found in the mature hyperimmunized rabbit (18). The appendix contained a somewhat higher proportion of μ cells but γ cells were also preponderant there. The proportions of γ and μ cells approach those found only in the mature rabbit intestine by Cebra *et al.* (18) where α chain-staining cells dominated. No spontaneous α chain synthesis was recognized in the newborn rabbit through 10 days of age in any organ studied.

Response to active immunization.—Upon this background of occasional spontaneously induced heavy chain production by the newborn lymphoreticular system, immunization at birth stimulated μ chain synthesis as early as 16 hours of age, and γ chain synthesis 20 hours later. Cell numbers in the immunized groups exceeded the numbers found in the unimmunized groups by a large factor (Table 2). The ratio of μ- to γ-containing cells ranged from 7.2 when γ cells first appeared at 2 days of age to .35 at 10 days of age. At 5 days, the number of μ-containing cells in the spleen were approximately equal in number to the γ-containing cells.

At the peaks of immunological activity as judged by cell counts, the proportion of lymphoid cells engaged in either γM or γG synthesis was approximately one in 10^3 to 10^4, or about 1,000-fold over background.

The response in the mesenteric nodes of the immunized rabbit lagged that observed in the spleen by about 24 hours, and the number of stained cells found was smaller. No immunofluorescent cells were found in some mesenteric nodes from animals which did have such cells present in their spleen, while the converse was never true. These nodes contained rare cells which apparently stained for both types heavy chains. These particular cells were of a single appearance — small mononuclear cells — and were found in no other tissue. No cells which stained with both reagents were observed in any spleen imprints.

Morphology of immunoglobulin-producing cells.—The range of cell morphology associated with heavy chain production in the spleen appeared to be identical regardless of which class was present (Fig. 1A, B, C, D). Namely, the earliest cell population evident in

TABLE 2.—OCCURRENCE OF HEAVY CHAIN CONTAINING CELLS IN THE LYMPHORETICULAR SYSTEM OF THE IMMUNIZED NEWBORN RABBIT*

Age of rabbits (days)	Number of animals in group‡	Spleen			Mesenteric Node		
		Cell Types			Cell Types		
		μ	γ	Ratio† $\mu:\gamma$	μ	γ	Ratio† $\mu:\gamma$
1	9	41	0	0	0	0	0
2	7	175	24	7.3	33	10	3.3
3	4	76	16	4.8	6	4	1.5
4	3	141	33	4.2	42	44	1.0
5	3	198	185	1	233	178	1.3
10	1	47	133	.35			

*Litters of rabbits in which the doe had a titer of *Salmonella paratyphi B* "H" agglutinins were 1:20 or lower were injected with 10^{10} of these organisms, and sacrificed at the indicated intervals.

†Ratio $\mu:\gamma$ indicates the average ratio of μ to γ staining cells observed.

‡All animals in these groups had at least 2 stained cells per 32 imprints.

each class after stimulation contained a high proportion of large, immature cells with narrow rims of fluorescent staining cytoplasm around large nuclei with open chromatin patterns. Intermediate and mature plasma cell morphology was observed later for each chain class. Although some clustering of stained cells of each type was observed, the imprint method does not permit any conclusions as to cloning of antibody-synthesizing cells.

Effect of passive antibody on active response.—A central question raised by these findings is whether, indeed, the clear evidence of heavy chain peptide synthesis can be equated to antibody produced in response to the specific antigenic stimulus. Although direct evidence on this point is not yet available, indirect evidence favors this conclusion.

Bellanti *et al.* (3) showed that newborn rabbits did not produce detectable flagellar antibody when transplacental antibody was present. Newborn humans (2, 19) who had titers of 1-20 or above of anti-d flagellar antibody had no active response to this antigen, but unaffected responses to other flagellar antigens. This phenomenon has been extended to show that passively administered γG-immunoglobulin antibodies inhibit specifically the active immune response (20, 21,

22). Thus, γG-antibody derived either transplacentally or by injection has an effective and specific suppressive effect on the active immune response.

It was therefore of considerable interest that the newborn animals in this study in which the mother had an antibody titer of 1:20 or more developed no cell response to the antigenic stimulus beyond the background level (Table 3). Conversely, a cellular response to the antigen occurred in all those litters in which the mothers had serum antiflagellar antibody titers of less than 1:20. These data, then, provide indirect evidence that the immunoglobulin-producing cells found in response to an antigenic stimulus are involved in specific antibody synthesis.

TABLE 3.—EFFECT OF MATERNAL ANTIBODY TITER ON OCCURRENCE OF FLUORESCENT STAINING IN THE SPLEEN OF IMMUNIZED NEWBORN RABBITS

Titer of flagellar agglutinin in serum of does	Proportion of immunized litters with fluorescent positive cells at 5 days of age
1:5 - 1:20	6/6
1:40 - 1:80	0/5

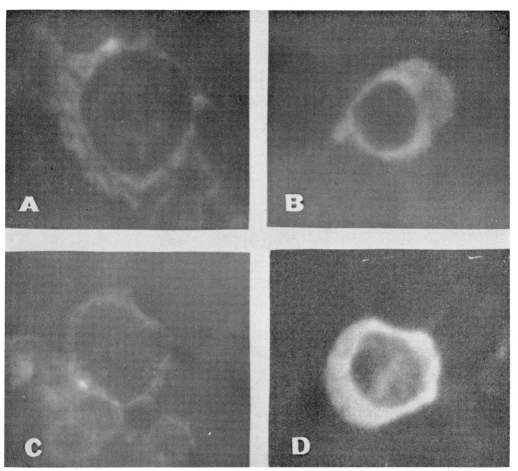

FIG. 1. (A) Spleen cell from 1-day-old rabbit showing specific μ chain fluorescence; (B) Spleen cell from 3-day-old rabbit showing specific μ chain fluorescence; (C) Spleen cell from 3-day-old rabbit showing specific γ chain fluorescence; (D) Spleen cell from 5-day-old rabbit showing specific γ chain fluorescence.

DISCUSSION

The studies described here extend those of Cebra *et al.* (18) to evaluation of the sequential appearance of cells producing γM- and γG-immunoglobulins during the active immune response. Goat anti-rabbit γM and γG heavy chain fluorescent reagents of two colors were employed simultaneously to examine the earliest evidence of heavy chain synthesis in the newborn rabbit, both as it occurs spontaneously, and in active response to an injection of *S. paratyphi B*. Normal newborn rabbits through the tenth day of life were found to have a very low level of immunological ac-

tivity of spontaneous origin by these criteria. However, following immunization at birth, γM-producing cells appeared as early as 16 hours later and γG cells were first found 20 hours after that. Five days after birth the numbers of each type of cell were approximately equal.

An apparent discrepancy exists between these findings and those of Bellanti *et al.* (3), who used an identical technique of immunization. Bellanti *et al.* found peak serum antibody titers at 10 days of age as high as 1:320, and that the serum activity was limited to γM as characterized by susceptibility to 2-ME reduction and sucrose density gradient ultracentrifugation. Antibody of the γG class was not detected until the fourth or fifth week of life. The interval between γM and γG appearance in that model could be shortened somewhat by more intensive immunization. The data reported here, in contrast, suggest that activity in cells producing both classes is nearly equal. Several possible explanations of the differences in serum antibody class and events at a cellular level deserve consideration.

Recent data (5) show that when assays of known sensitivity for γG and γM classes of antibody are employed, a γG element of the primary response to the "O" antigen is unmasked which cannot be detected by simple agglutination. Differential assay sensitivity could therefore explain the occurrence of γ chain-producing cells in the absence of detectable γG-antibody, providing such a differential sensitivity applies to detection of flagellar agglutinins.

A related explanation depends upon the relative avidity of the two classes of antibody in a primary response. Eisen has shown that binding affinity of antibodies changes up to 10,000-fold during a primary immune response to haptens; i.e., early antibody has an intrinsic association constant which is much lower than that found in antibody pools sampled late after primary immunization or after repeated antigenic challenges (23). Early γG- and γM-antibodies both have low apparent affinity for specific somatic antigen as compared to later antibodies in the primary response (5). However, the rate of increase of the capacity to effect agglutination of somatic antigen was much more rapid in the case of γM. Thus, apparent γG-antibody detectable in serum could conceivably lag γM-agglutinins on this basis.

Evidence is available in other contexts to confirm that γG-synthesis occurs in the newborn period (24, 25). For example, Wainer et al. (25) showed that the newborn rabbit incorporated S^{35} methionine and C^{14} leucine into γ-globulin as early as 12 hours after birth. Altemeier (unpublished data) found that γG-agglutinins of the somatic antigen were detectable after immunization of the newborn rabbit, providing a sufficiently sensitive assay was used. Studies of the normal human fetus (26 and this volume) have apparently demonstrated γG-containing plasma cells at the 27th

week of gestation. Similar findings in antenatal infections have also been reported (27).

The conclusion that heavy chain-synthesizing cells are making complete specific antibody depends upon three lines of indirect evidence. First, the chain-containing cells in immunized newborn rabbits numbered over 1,000 times those found in the unimmunized normal control animals. Secondly, the response to antigenic challenge was specifically inhibited by the presence of transplacental antibody. Thirdly, these cells appear to produce complete antibodies in that light chain production was found in every cell in which heavy chains were detected, regardless of antibody class or phase of cell differentiation (13). However, data provide no direct evidence that the demonstrated chain synthesis represents actual antibody production. In fact, the number of cells involved in an active immune response exceeds that producing antibody by a large factor, and all cell response is inhibited by passive antibody.

Direct proof would depend upon demonstration of specific antigen binding by cells shown also to be synthesizing the heavy chains. This is technically within the capability of the two-color fluorescent technique, if the concentration of bound antigen adhering to the cell were sufficient to be visualized unmistakably. However, the probability of a very low antigen-binding capacity of early antibody to bacterial antigens (5) suggests that the prospects of such a demonstration are not good.

These studies also appear to shed some light on the question of whether (a) the sequence of γM—γG synthesis depends upon differentiation of a single cell line through two types of heavy chains in sequence, or (b) the differentiation which determines the heavy chain precedes that of morphologic differentiation.

Nossal et al. (11) and Mellors and Korngold (28) have described findings considered consistent with a mechanism whereby a single cell line differentiates to produce two types of heavy peptide chains during its antibody-synthesizing life. For example, Nossal found nearly 10% of cells producing both γM and γG antiflagellar antibodies at a time when the transition from γM to γG was occurring in the serum of his animals.

Cebra et al., in contrast, have shown that populations of lymphoreticular cells in humans

(15) and hyperimmune rabbits (18) studied by the use of peptide chain-specific fluorescent antibody reagents contained essentially no cells which produced two heavy peptides simultaneously. The recent observation that germinal centers may contain cells which apparently absorb immunoglobulins from the circulation rather than synthesize them (29) may explain the differences in the results of past studies on this point. This may explain also the rare cells in the mesenteric lymph nodes which were found in this study to contain both classes of heavy chain.

The earliest cells seen in our studies, regardless of chain produced, shared similar morphology—a large cell with a narrow rim of fluorescent cytoplasm and a large immature appearing nucleus. Although single cells were not followed through the various stages of differentiation, the timed population sampling technique used here yielded an array of morphological types for both chain classes ranging from the earliest immature cells to mature plasmacytes. No double staining cells, indicating simultaneous production of both classes, were observed in the spleen at any stage of cell differentiation. These data are therefore consistent with the hypothesis that morphological differentiation is independent of the heavy chain class produced. It suggests that the step in differentiation which determines heavy chain synthesis occurs prior to morphologically distinctive plasma cell differentiation.

In summary, these studies appear to provide a model for examining the sequences, morphologic and distributional aspects of immunoglobulin synthesis by cells of an intact virgin lymphoreticular system. Such studies should be useful in complementing those which depend upon *in vitro* phases and upon responses to antigens of broad specificity such as sheep erythrocytes.

Acknowledgments.—The authors acknowledge with gratitude the advice and assistance of Dr. John Cebra in these studies.

Supported in part by a training grant in Developmental Physiology (HD-0054), and grants from the National Institute of Child Health and Human Development (HD-00384), the American Heart Association (64G158), and the American Cancer Society (Institutional Grant IN-62-E).

Dr. Adler was a Research Fellow in Immunology (NIAID Training Grant #5T1-A1-128-06).

REFERENCES

1. Smith, R. T., Eitzman, D. V., Miller, B. (1960): Qualitative differences in the immune response of infants and adults receiving *Salmonella* vaccine. J. Clin. Invest. *39*, 1029.
2. Smith, R. T. (1960): Response to active immunization of human infants during the neonatal period. Ciba Foundation Symposium on Cellular Aspects of Immunity *23*, 348.
3. Bellanti, J., Eitzman, D. V., Robbins, J. B., Smith, R. T. (1963): The development of the immune response. J. Exp. Med. *117*, 479.
4. Bauer, D. C., and Stavitsky, A. B. (1961): On the different molecular forms of antibody synthesized by rabbits during the early response to a single injection of protein and cellular antigens. Proc. Nat. Acad. Sci. *47*, 1667.
5. Altemeier, W. A., Robbins, J. B., and Smith, R. T. (1966): Quantitative studies of the immunoglobulin sequence in the response of the rabbit to a somatic antigen. J. Exp. Med. *124*, 443.
6. Jerne, N. K., and Nordin, A. A. (1963): The agar plate technique for recognizing antibody producing cells in cell bound antibodies. Edited by Amos, B., and Kopronski, H. Philadelphia, Wistar Institute Press, p. 109. Science *140*, 405.
7. Ingraham, J., and Bussard, A. (1964): Application of a localized hemolysin reaction for specific detection of individual antibody forming cells. J. Exp. Med. *119*, 667.
8. Sterzl, J., and Riha, I. (1966): Detection of cells producing 7S antibodies by the plaque technique. Nature (London) *208*, 858.
9. Borsos, T., and Rapp, H. J. (1965): Complement fixation on cell surfaces by 19S and 7S antibodies. Science *150*, 505.
10. Dresser, D. W., and Wortis, H. H. (1966): Use of an antiglobulin serum to detect antibody with low hemolytic efficiency. Nature (London) *208*, 859.
11. Nossal, G. J. V., Szenberg, A., Ada, G. L., and Austin, G. M. (1964): Single cell studies on 19S antibody production. J. Exp. Med. *119*, 485.
12. Cebra, J. J., and Goldstein, G. (1965): Chromatographic purification of tetramethylrhodamine-immune globulin conjugates and their use in the cellular localization of rabbit γ globulin polypeptide chains. J. Immun. *95*, 230.
13. Adler, W. H., Curry, J. H., and Smith, R. T. (1966): Submitted for publication.
14. Robbins, J. B., Kenny, K., and Suter, E.

(1965): The isolation and biological activities of rabbit γM and γG anti-*Salmonella typhimurium* antibodies. J. Exp. Med. *122*, 385.

15. Bernier, G., and Cebra, J. J. (1965): Frequency distribution of α, γ, κ, and λ and polypeptide chains in human lymphoid tissues. J. Immun. *95*, 246.

16. Jaquet, H., Bloom, B., and Cebra, J. J. (1964): The reductive dissociation of rabbit immune globulin in sodium dodecylsulfate. J. Immun. *92*, 991.

17. Wood, B. T., Thompson, S. H., and Goldstein, G. (1965): Fluorescent antibody staining. III. Preparation of fluorescein isothiocyanate labeled antibodies. J. Immun. *95*, 225.

18. Cebra, J. J., Colberg, J. E., and Dray, S. (1966): Rabbit lymphoid cells differentiated with respect to α, γ, and μ heavy polypeptide chains and to allotypic markers Aa1 Aa2. J. Exp. Med. *123* (3), 547.

19. Smith, R. T., and Eitzman, D. V. (1964): The development of the immune response: Characterization of the response of the human infant and adult to immunization with *Salmonella* vaccine. Pediatrics *33*, 163.

20. Möller, G., and Wigzell, H. (1965): Antibody synthesis at the cellular level: Antibody-induced suppression of 19S and 7S antibody response. J. Exp. Med. *121*, 969.

21. Neiders, M. E., Rowley, D. A., and Fitch, F. W. (1962): The sustained suppression of hemolysin response in passively immunized rats. J. Immun. *88*, 718.

22. Finklestein, M. S., and Uhr, J. W. (1964): Specific inhibition of antibody formation by passively administered 19S and 7S antibody. Science *146*, 67.

23. Eisen, H. N., and Suskind, G. W. (1964): Variations in affinities of antibodies during the immune response. Biochemistry *3*, 7.

24. Thorbecke, G. J. (1960): Gamma globulin and antibody formation *in vitro*. I. Gamma globulin formation in tissues from immature and normal adult rabbits. J. Exp. Med. *112*, 279.

25. Wainer, A., Robbins, J., Bellanti, J., Eitzman, D., and Smith, R. T. (1963): Synthesis of gamma globulin in the newborn rabbit. Nature *198* (4879), 487.

26. Van Furth, R., Schuit, H. R. E., and Hijmans, W. (1965): The immunological development of the human fetus. J. Exp. Med. *122*, 1173.

27. Silverstein, A. M., and Luker, R. J. (1962): Fetal response to antigenic stimulus. I. Plasmacellular and lymphoid reactions in the human fetus to intrauterine infection. Lab. Invest. *11*, 918.

28. Mellors, R. C., and Korngold, L. (1963): The cellular origin of human immunoglobulins (γ2, γ1M, γ1A). J. Exp. Med. *118*, 387.

29. Humphrey, J. H. (1966): Personal communication to the authors.

DISCUSSION

SILVERSTEIN: Have you done radioactive amino acid incorporation studies in the rabbit to find out whether immunoglobulins are formed?

SMITH: Wainer *et al.* (25) have shown that the newborn rabbit incorporates C^{14} and S^{35} labelled amino acids into immunoglobulins given on the day of birth.

VAN FURTH: Thorbecke did this with a different technique in newborn rabbits and found early postnatal immunoglobulin synthesis.

BLOCK: Was there any correlation between when the rabbit is weaned and the appearance of heavy chains in the appendix?

ADLER: We found γ chains in the 10-day-old rabbit, but they were still suckling.

20

G. J. THORBECKE and R. VAN FURTH

Ontogeny of immunoglobulin synthesis in various mammalian species

UNTIL RECENTLY the normal fetus and new-born were considered not to be engaged in the production of immunoglobulins. These proteins, when present in the serum of the fetus, were regarded to be of maternal origin only, and plasma cells were not observed in the lymphoid tissues of the normal fetus and newborn.

The study of C^{14}-labelled amino acid incorporation into immunoglobulins by tissues *in vitro* provides a sensitive method to detect the synthesis of small amounts of these proteins. With this method it has been shown that various mammalian species synthesize immunoglobulins during the gestation period. The present review summarizes the data obtained so far. The method used in obtaining the results, represented in Table 1, was the

TABLE 1.—INITIATION OF IMMUNOGLOBULIN SYNTHESIS IN VARIOUS MAMMALIAN SPECIES

Species	Gestation Period* (days)	Synthesis by spleen tissue†		
		First day observed	γG	γM
Human	280	140 (before birth)	+	+
Sheep	150	60 (before birth)	—	+
Guinea pig	68	10 (before birth)	—	+
Rabbit	31	at birth‡	—	+
Mouse	21	at birth	—	—
		3 (after birth)	—	+
Rat	21	at birth	—	—
		7 (after birth)	—	+

*Reference 1.
†γA was always negative.
‡Not studied during fetal period.

incubation of spleen tissue in the presence of C^{14}-amino acid for 24 to 48 hours, and subsequent analysis of labelled proteins in the dialyzed and concentrated culture fluids. The method of analysis of the proteins employed a combination of autoradiography and immunoelectrophoresis; immunoelectrophoretic patterns were prepared with the use of appropriate carrier sera and antisera. These methods were described in detail in previous publications (2, 3).

Human.—Production of γG and γM is regularly found in the spleen of the human fetus after the 20th week of gestation (4). No production of γA has been demonstrated even as late as the 31st week (4). This observation was substantiated by studies employing immunofluorescent staining of fetal tissues (4). Fluorescein-labelled specific antisera to γG, γA, and γM were used (5). γG and γM positive plasma cells, even with Russell bodies, and immunoglobulin-containing large and medium-sized lymphoid cells were found in the spleens of fetuses aged 20 weeks and older. Some small lymphocytes were found to contain γM (Fig. 1) (4).

Sheep.—Approximately at the 90th day of gestation the spleen of the normal sheep embryo starts to produce γM (6). Induction of other immunoglobulins is usually not observed before birth, except for, occasionally, a little γ_1 globulin. Intrauterine immunization, however, may result in production of all immunoglobulins, including γM, γ_1 and γ_2, and what appears to be γA, as early as the 90th day of the gestation period (6).

Guinea pig.—Production of γM by the spleen in this species can already be detected by the 58th day of the gestation period, and remains the only immunoglobulin produced by the spleen for 1 to 2 weeks after birth (7). In autoradiographs of immunoelectrophoretic patterns performed with such culture fluids there is also some labelling of the fast-moving γ-globulin, which always accompanies γM production, but this was shown to be due to formation of free light chains (7, 8). Around 2 weeks after birth the production of γ_2 globulin can be shown in both spleen and lymph nodes, whereas production of the specific γ_1 determinant normally develops at 3 to 4 weeks after birth (7, 8). Immunization at birth results in detectable production of all these immunoglobulins in lymph node or spleen of 1- to 2-week-old guinea pigs (Fig. 2) (8).

Rabbit.—Spleen cultures never showed synthesis of γG at birth, but some γM production was detected (8). However, Wainer *et al.* (9) showed, with autoradiography of immunoelectrophoretic patterns of sera from animals given labelled amino acid *in vivo,* some production of γG at birth. Under normal conditions, the production of immunoglobulins by rabbit spleen increases rather suddenly around the 3d week of life (10), whereas appropriate immunization at birth may result in γG production by regional lymph nodes as early as 1 week after birth (11).

Mouse.—Newborn mouse spleen tissue from mice does not produce immunoglobulins, but spleen tissue from 3-day-old animals synthesizes γM (8, 12). This is soon followed by the production of γ_1, and the formation of γA and γ_2 appears several weeks later (12).

Rats.—γM production could not be shown with spleen tissue from newborn rats but became detectable within approximately 1 week after birth (8).

The time of appearance of immunoglobulin formation in relation to the time of birth depends on the length of the gestation. In mice and rats, animals with a short gestation period, γM production begins only after birth. In all other species examined the production of γM is detectable in the fetus or newborn. In the human even the formation of γG could be demonstrated during fetal life. In those species in which the earliest time of immune responsiveness for certain antigens has been established, a similar relationship appears to hold. In bovine embryos (13) the earliest responsiveness is found at approximately 140 days before birth (gestation period 280 days), in sheep (14) at approximately 80 days before birth, and in pigs (15) at approximately 30 days before birth (gestation period 90 days). In the opossum, which has a gestation period of only 12.5 days, antibody production can be induced at about 8 days after birth (16).

It cannot be ascertained whether the "spontaneous" immunoglobulin production seen in fetal or newborn animals represents maturation of *normal* globulin production, or the production of proteins with antibody specificity induced by intrauterine antigenic stimulation. The sequence of immunoglobulin

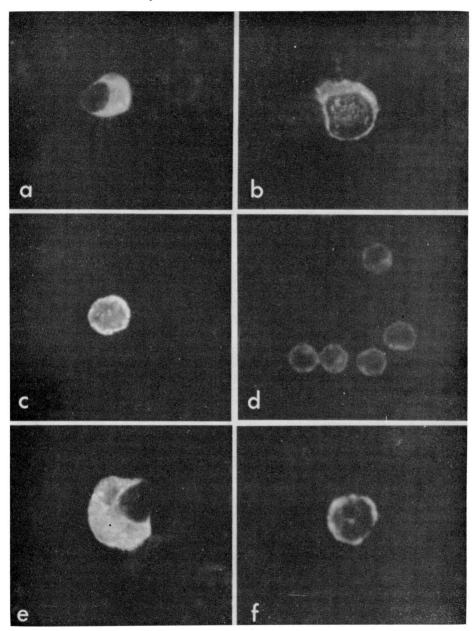

Fig. 1. Immunofluorescent staining of human fetal spleen cells. (a) γM-positive plasma cell; (b) γM-positive large lymphocyte; (c) γM-positive medium-sized lymphocyte; (d) γM-positive small lymphocytes; (e) γG-positive plasma cell; (f) γG-positive large lymphocyte. x 500

production, γM before γG, which develops spontaneously, is similar to the one seen after active immunization. At no time has immunoglobulin formation been observed before a stage at which immunization was also feasible.

If exposure to antigen occurred *in utero*, it would be expected that antigens enter via the circulation and have easy access to the spleen. In fact, the spleen has been shown to have the earliest and most active production of γM in fetal and neonatal humans, sheep (6), and guinea pigs (8).

175

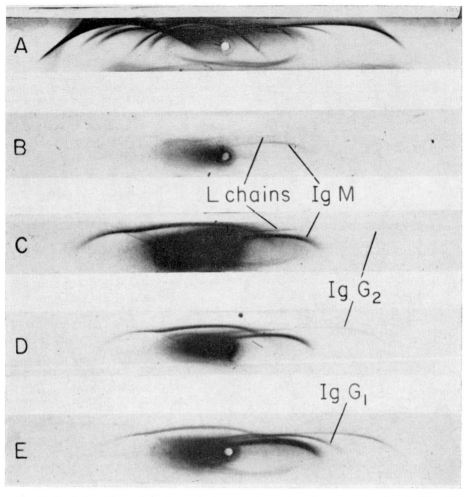

Fig. 2. Typical carrier guinea pig serum immunoelectrophoretic pattern developed with rabbit anti-whole guinea pig serum (A). The accompanying autoradiographs are of spleen culture fluids from fetal (B), normal 15-day-old (C) and 22-day-old (D), and immunized 16-day-old (E) guinea pigs.

Acknowledgments.—Dr. G. J. Thorbecke is the recipient of a Career Development Award (#GM-K3-15,522). Dr. R. van Furth is a recipient of a fellowship from the Netherlands Organization for Pure Research (ZWO). These studies were supported by a grant from the U.S.P.H.S. No. AI-3076.

REFERENCES

1. Altman, P. L., and Dittmar, D. S., eds. (1964): Biology Data Handbook, Fed. of Am. Soc. for Exp. Biol., p. 57.
2. Hochwald, G. M., Thorbecke, G. J., and Asofsky, R. (1961): Sites of formation of immune globulins and of a component of C'3. I. A new technique for the demonstration of the synthesis of individual serum proteins by tissues *in vitro*. J. Exp. Med., *114*, 549.
3. Williams, C. A., Jr., Asofsky, R., and Thorbecke, G. J. (1963): Plasma protein formation *in vitro* by tissues from mice infected with staphylococci. J. Exp. Med. *118*, 315.
4. Van Furth, R., Schuit, H. R. E., and Hijmans,

W. (1965): The immunological development of the human fetus. J. Exp. Med. *122,* 1173.

5. Van Furth, R., Schuit, H. R. E., and Hijmans, W. (1966): The formation of immunoglobulins by human tissues *in vitro.* I. The methods and their specificity. Immunology *11,* 1.

6. Silverstein, A. M., Thorbecke, G. J., Kraner, K. L., and Lukes, R. J. (1963): Fetal response to antigenic stimulus. III. Gamma-globulin production in normal and immunized fetal lambs. J. Immun. *91,* 384.

7. Thorbecke, G. J. (1964): Development of immune globulin formation in fetal, newborn, and immature guinea pigs. Fed. Proc. *23,* 346.

8. Stecher, V. J., and Thorbecke, G. J.: Sites of formation of immune globulins and of a component of C′3. III. B$_{1c}$ and immune globulin formation by tissues from germfree and normal animals of various ages. Immunology, in press 1967.

9. Wainer, A., Robbins, J., Bellanti, J., Eitzman, O., and Smith, R. T. (1963): Synthesis of gamma-globulin in the newborn rabbit. Nature *198.* 487.

10. Thorbecke, G. J. (1960): Gamma-globulin formation and antibody production *in vitro.* I. Gamma-globulin formation in tissues from immature and normal adult rabbits. J. Exp. Med. *112,* 279.

11. Pernis, B., Cohen, M. W., and Thorbecke, G. J. (1963): Specificity of reactions to antigenic stimulation in lymph nodes of immature rabbits. I. Morphological changes and gamma-globulin production following stimulation with diphtheria toxoid and silica. J. Immun. *91,* 541.

12. Asofsky, R. (1965): Immunoglobulin formation by lymphoid tissues from germfree mice. Fed. Proc. *24,* 502.

13. Fennestad, K. L., and Borg-Petersen, C. (1962): Antibody and plasma cells in bovine fetuses infected with *Leptospira saxkoebing.* J. Infect. Dis. *110,* 63.

14. Silverstein, A. M., Uhr, J. W., Kraner, K. L., and Lukes, R. J. (1963): Fetal response to antigenic stimulus. II. Antibody production by the fetal lamb. J. Exp. Med. *117,* 799.

15. Sterzl, J., Vesely, J., Jilek, M., and Mandel, L. (1965): The inductive phase of antibody formation studied with isolated cells, in: Sterzl, J., ed.: Molecular and Cellular Basis of Antibody Formation. Czech. Acad. Sci., Prague, p. 463.

16. Rowlands, D. T., Jr., La Via, M. F., and Block, M. H. (1964): The blood forming tissues and blood of the newborn opossum (*Didelphis virginiana*). J. Immun. *93,* 157.

DISCUSSION

Good: Dr. van Furth, I know it is hazardous to extrapolate from species to species, but I think the specific pathogen-free piglet raised under germ-free conditions provides especially pertinent information concerning at least one of the questions raised. Kim and Watson have with great care shown that newborn piglets, whose mothers have been minimally exposed to antigens, are free of all traces of immunoglobulins in their circulation. Nonetheless they can respond within 48 hours to primary stimulation with bacteriophage. One would think that if nonsense γ-globulin were formed *in utero* without antigenic stimulation, such piglets would have small amounts of immunoglobulins. Further, when antigenic stimulation occurs in human fetuses *in utero,* significant increases in γM components can be demonstrated at birth. It seems reasonable that the few immunoglobulin-producing cells you demonstrate in human fetuses reflect antigenic stimulation from some source.

One possible source is the histocompatibility antigens. A case recently reported by Zuelzer is of interest. He described what appears to be a type of immunological deficiency disease in which the child was a male but all the lymphoid cells present were of female karyotype. Thus, Zuelzer's patient was a lymphocytic chimera. Maternal white blood cells had entered the circulation of the baby. If this occurs on a less massive basis in the normal child, it would surely evoke an immunological response, one component of which might be immunoglobulin synthesis.

I would like to know what you found in the centrally located lymph nodes, those of the mediastinal, mesenteric, and cervical locations. In Florence Sabin's classical study of the development of lymphoid tissue, she pointed out that long before the spleen became lymphoid, and almost immediately after the thymus became lymphoid, the centrally located lymph nodes developed a lymphoid structure.

Smith: It would be quite interesting to examine preparations of human fetal tissue, like those described here, stained with fluorescent anti-light chain (κ or λ) reagents. This might provide more direct confirmation of the data of Epstein and co-workers, showing that a high proportion of human cord bloods have macroglobulin anti-λ chain antibody, higher in titer than the mother, while few have anti-κ chain antibodies.

It is reasonable to conceive that the fetus can undergo antigenic stimulation from his mother's histocompatibility antigens. It has been demonstrated in many different circumstances that maternal polymorphonuclear leucocytes as well as other white cells do pass the placenta, and certainly are histoincompatible with respect to the fetus. A second possible source might be the virus infections that the mother has during pregnancy which, although they don't produce teratological changes in the fetus, could also infect the fetus.

Our own data (Ciba Foundation Symposium, *The Cellular Basis of Immunity*, 1959) contained several premature infants of 23-26 weeks of gestation who were immunized on the day of birth, and produced detectable specific γM-antibodies in the circulation by the 4th day of age. Thus it is quite probable that the heavy chain synthesis in the fetus demonstrated by Dr. van Furth indeed indicates active antibody formation.

In summary, the known sources of stimuli for active antibody formation in the infant *in utero* are:

(a) Isoantigens from the mother including λ light chain allotypes, Gm allotypes, haptoglobin allotypes, etc.

(b) Maternal histocompatibility antigens in maternal WBC which are known to pass the placenta into the fetal circulation.

(c) Asymptomatic or symptomatic viral infections of the mother—and fetus.

(d) Prenatal infections such as syphilis, toxoplasmosis, and cytomegalovirus infections as have been described by Silverstein and others.

SILVERSTEIN: I am sure that we cannot extropolate across species lines. However, in the normal lamb we found γM, no γA, and no adult γG, but a peculiar fetal γG, perhaps analogous to 5S γG in the piglet, as reported by the group in Prague.

AUERBACH: Could Dr. Silverstein comment on the results he has obtained with the fetal monkey? How does the timing of immunoglobulin production compare? Is it correlated with white pulp development in the spleen?

SILVERSTEIN: While the data are less complete for the fetal monkey compared to the fetal lamb, both appear to form antibodies before any organized white pulp appears in the spleen.

HILDEMANN: Despite the absence of an antigen-free fetal test system, can you consider the possibility that the immunoglobulins you detect in the fetus are naturally occurring products rather than specific antibodies? Secondly, how good is the evidence that γM-antibodies fail to traverse the placenta—how about commonly observed A-B-0 hemolytic disease of the newborn?

VAN FURTH: It is very difficult to argue against the suggestion of non-antibody γ-globulins. We don't have any test in the human model to determine whether these immunoglobulins are really antibodies.

SMITH: The antibodies that normally pass the human placenta are limited to the γG-immunoglobulins. But we have seen circumstances under which we could feel reasonably certain that γM-antibodies pass from the mother to the fetus through placental leaks. The circumstances under which this might occur include those in which other cells also leak, such as red cells and white cells that are identifiable by their different cell type. Under these circumstances, we have found antibodies of the γM type in the fetus which we feel were of maternal origin.

SILVERSTEIN: I would like to assure Dr. Hildemann that not everyone here makes the assumption that these fetal globulins are antibody globulins. But those of us who do not make the assumption are very much on the defensive. I happen to be one of those who believe in "nonsense" globulins. I dislike the term "immunoglobulin" because I don't really believe it is a proper term to use for all of these proteins.

SMITH: That's nonsense indeed, unless you can show such a entity exists.

HILDEMANN: You can't do so without an antigen-free system. And where are you going to find it? That's the dilemma. It was reported at a workshop about a year ago that γM-globulin was produced by chick fibroblasts in culture. Even the investigators were very defensive about the notion that such a cell as a fibroblast could possibly be making γM. But from what Dr. van Furth has said, I sort of wonder how far out this notion really was.

VAN FURTH: The immunoglobulin production in the human fetus is by lymphoid cells and plasma cells in the spleen; 15 out of 17 thymus cultures were negative and the appendix is negative in the human fetus at 25 and 27 weeks. We haven't looked at other organs.

CEBRA: Are complete immunoglobulin molecules being synthesized by the early human fetuses? Do those cells which are stained for heavy chain also stain positively for light chain? Do you find positive radio-labelled precipitin arcs upon development of the electrophoresed fetal proteins with anti-light chain? Dr. Fraňek reported the presence of an "incomplete" γG-immunoglobulin related to the γ chain in germ-free piglets taken by Caesarean section. Such proteins may be one form of "nonsense" immunoglobulin.

VAN FURTH: Yes, I think there is evidence for the synthesis of complete γG and γM. We found positive autoradiographic lines with specific anti-γG and anti-γM sera as well as with anti-κ or anti-λ sera. Also in the immunofluorescent test we found positive cells when stained with anti-κ or anti-λ conjugates.

CEBRA: It would be interesting to carry out a quantitative analysis to see if more than a very few per cent of cells that one finds in an adult stain only for one of these heavy chains, but don't stain for, say, light chains. That's probably a kind of nonsense. So if you want to defend a nonsense level, that's what we want.

SMITH: It would be quite interesting to do that because it would appear that the capacity for κ chain synthesis is developed in the human fetus before that of λ chain synthesis.

M. COOPER: Has Dr. Hirschhorn looked at cultured lymphocytes' responsiveness to PHA on an ontogenetic basis?

HIRSCHHORN: The earliest I know of is a blood from a 30-week fetus which did respond.

21

ARTHUR J. L. STRAUSS, PIERSON G. KEMP, and
STEVEN D. DOUGLAS

An immunohistological delineation of striated muscle cells in the thymus

IMMUNOGLOBULINS WHICH REACT *in vitro* with portions of the A-Band in striated muscle and with large cells of the thymic medulla (Fig. 1) are found in sera from 30% of randomly studied patients with myasthenia gravis (5). Virtually all patients with myasthenia gravis who have associated thymomas possess this serological reactivity; and approximately 25% of patients with thymomas not associated with myasthenia gravis have reactive sera (6).

Reciprocal absorption studies using striated muscle and thymic homogenates indicate that this concurrent reactivity is due to reactants shared by striated muscle and thymus, but otherwise unique (8). The reactive cells in thymus were first observed by van der Geld *et al.* (7) in postnatal calf, and were subsequently identified in late human fetal material (5). Upon restaining with hematoxylin and eosin, following fluorescent antibody studies, such cells appeared to conform to the criteria for thymic epithelial cells-round cells several times larger than the predominating lymphoid elements seen mostly in thymic medulla, possessing abundant eosinophilic cytoplasm, and often eccentric nuclei. Recently, however, new findings and some nearly 80 years old have come to light which prompt some change in these views concerning the identity of these reactive cells.

The very interesting and possibly pertinent studies of Van de Velde and Friedman (9) and Raviola and Raviola (4) dealing with myoid cells in thymus have come to our attention. These investigators have studied the ultrastructural features of thymic cells, which have been repeatedly described in German anatomical reports from 1888 to 1952 (but not, it appears, elsewhere). As originally viewed by light microscopy (Fig. 2) and now by electron microscopy these cells have the appearance of variously modified striated muscle. Although most numerous in reptilian thymuses, they also have been seen in amphibian, avian, and now even in human material (3). The subject of myoid cells in thymus was extensively and authoritatively reviewed by W. Bargmann in 1943 (1). It is curious that no major reference to such cells has appeared since; these cells are not described in current standard histology texts.

We have studied the fine structural features of the thymus of the red-eared turtle, *Pseudemys scripta elegans,* three months posthatching and have confirmed the findings of Van de Velde *et al.* (9) and Raviola and Raviola (4) that there are indeed present thymic cells with the sarcomeric and myofilamentous structure of striated muscle (Figs. 3A, B, and 4).

In addition, we have studied the thymus of the same species for reactivity with serum immunoglobulins of patients with myasthenia gravis, etc. The indirect immunofluorescence technique for detection of immunoglobulin binding was employed. Prior to quick-freezing for sectioning, thymuses were fixed in 10% formalin buffered with 2% calcium acetate

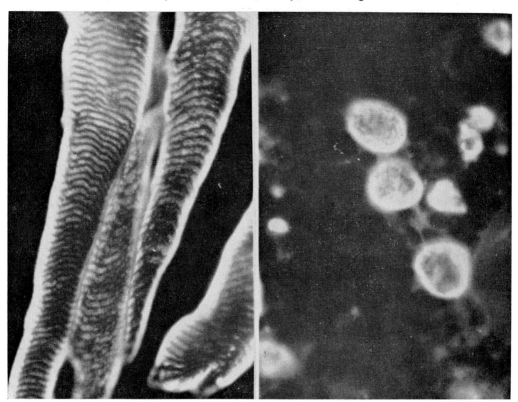

Fig. 1. Characteristic pattern of "myasthenic" serum immunoglobulin reactivity seen versus skeletal muscle and thymic cells *in vitro* by means of the indirect immunofluorescence technique. Bovine tissues were the substrates in this instance. x 900

(pH 7.3) for one-half hour at 3°C, and then washed in chilled 0.9% saline buffered at pH 7.2 with 0.01 molar phosphate. This procedure has been found greatly to enhance the delineation of striations (2). Immunofluorescent striated cells were present in impressive numbers, primarily in medullary regions. Such cells appeared generally elongated, with "head and tail" configurations often with prominent single nuclei. The pleomorphism seen in cells, as illustrated in composite Fig. 5, is at least in part due to differing orientations in relation to the plane of section. Various control serums from both normal and disease states failed to delineate these cells; nor were these cells seen in other organs of the turtle.

In a recent preliminary communication, Henry (3) has described striated muscle cells in the thymus of a human 38-week fetus. We

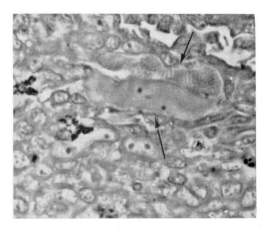

Fig. 2. Positive phase contrast photomicrograph of the thymus of the red-eared turtle, *Pseudemys scripta elegans*. Arrows point to myoid cells which are surrounded by the predominant thymocyte population. x 1800

181

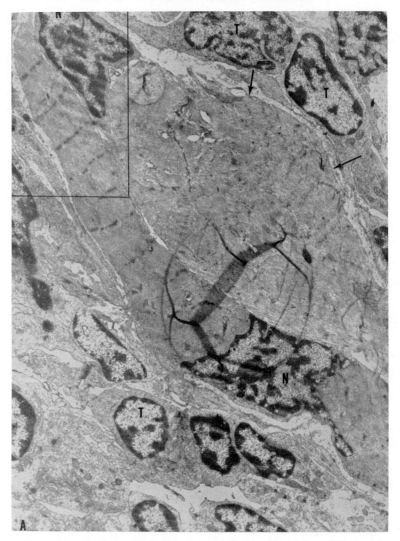

FIG. 3(A). Electron micrograph of turtle thymus. Thymocytes (T), muscle cell nuclei (N). Note oblique striated muscle (arrows). x 10,000

have found in fetal calf thymuses of comparable gestation, reactive cells possessing the "head and tail" shape of myoid cells of the turtle thymus (Fig. 6), but striations within these remain to be demonstrated. In view of these findings, it is entirely possible that with the aid of reactive myasthenia gravis serums we will ultimately be able to reaffirm the presence of striated muscle cells in mammalian thymus.

Thymic cells of mammals, postnatal calf, and man in particular, which had earlier been described by Van der Geld *et al.* (7) as reactive with serums from patients with myasthenia gravis, though clearly sharing an antigenic reactant with striated muscle did not display the obvious appearance of striated muscle. At present, however, in the light of Bargmann's 1943 review (1) and on the basis of Van de Velde's (9) and Raviola and Raviola's (4) recent electron microscopic studies, and Henry's (3) observation it is possible that cells which Van der Geld described and had interpreted as epithelial cells were, in fact, atrophic rounded up striated muscle cells which had lost their morphologic identifying

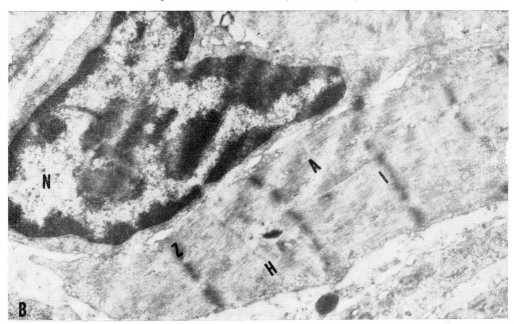

FIG. 3(B). Higher power electron micrograph of blocked area shown in Fig. 3(A). Muscle nucleus (N); Z, A, I, H zones are labelled. x 25,000

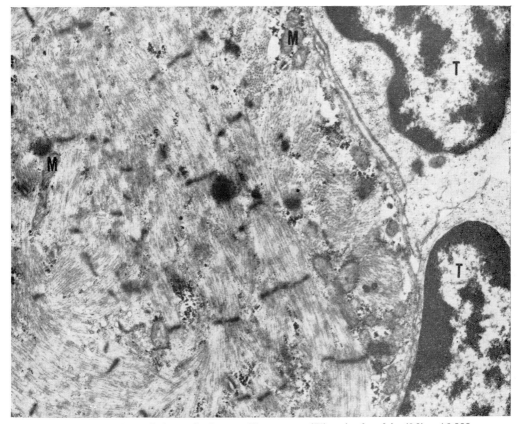

FIG. 4. Striated muscle in turtle thymus. Thymocytes (T), mitochondria (M). x 16,000

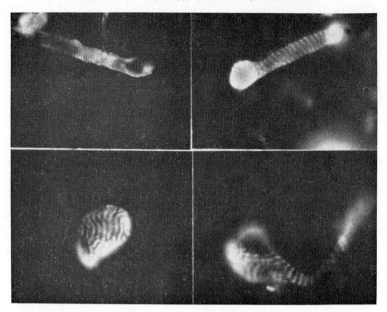

Fig. 5. Several examples of myoid cells of turtle thymus delineated with myasthenia gravis sera using immunofluorescence technique. x 1800

features save for antigenic determinants which could be detected with serum immunoglobulins from patients with myasthenia gravis and/or thymomas.

At this time we can only speculate as to the biological significance of striated muscle cells in thymus and further as to the implications of these cells in relation to thymic pathology and autoimmune phenomena associated with myasthenia gravis. At present, there is no convincing information pertinent to either issue. Though it has been suggested that these cells are more or less fortuitously derived from mesenchyme surrounding the thymic primordium, it may be significant that similar cells have not been identified in either thyroid or parathyroid which similarly take origin from pharyngeal pouches. Presumably these organs might also incorporate adjacent mesenchyme in the course of embryogenesis. It is conceivable that the thymus could exert special inductive influences toward myogenesis by entrapped mesenchyme. The fact that such cells occur even in distantly related species constitutes a kind of biological significance for these cells, and is against their mere accidental presence. Serum immunoglobulins from patients with myasthenia gravis constitute a versatile immunohistological reagent for the

study of the origin and possible significance of such cells.

The fact that serums from patients with myasthenia gravis, especially those with thymomas, and from patients with thymomas not associated with myasthenia gravis react with striated muscle may have no direct relevance to the occurrence of thymic myoid cells. This serological reactivity can be demonstrated *in vitro* with striated muscle from a variety of vertebrate and non-vertebrate sources, and in this context the thymus may be an additional,

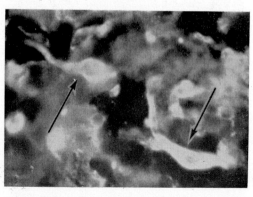

Fig. 6. Reactive cells in fetal calf thymus. Note "head and tail" appearance of some cells but no evident striations. x 1800

184

albeit unconventional, substrate for striated muscle. On the other hand the occurrence of serologic reactivity in individuals with manifest thymic lesions is a compelling argument for further study of these cells. If the occurrence of autoantibodies to striated muscle can be viewed as a break in immune tolerance to self constituents and the thymus can be assigned a crucial role in the establishment, maturation, and possible maintenance of immunocompetence, then in such a context it is possible that thymic myoid cells may have some special role in the development of tolerance to muscle constituents.

REFERENCES

1. Bargmann, W. (1943). Der Thymus, in: von Möllendorf, W., ed.: Handbuch der mikroskopischen Anatomie des Menschen, Vol. 6 Part 4.1, Berlin, Springer-Verlag.
2. Douglas, S. D., Gottlieb, A. J., Strauss, A. J. L., and Spicer, S. S. (1966): Selectivity of ferritin-protein conjugates for sites on skeletal muscle. Exp. Molec. Path. Suppl. 3, 5.
3. Henry, K. (1966): Mucin secretion and striated muscle in the human thymus. Lancet 1, 183.
4. Raviola, E., and Raviola, G. (1966): Fine structure of the myoid cells of the reptilian and avian thymus. Anat. Rec. 154, 483.
5. Strauss, A. J. L., Van der Geld, H. W. R., Kemp, P. G. Jr., Exum, E. D., and Goodman, H. C. (1965): Immunological concomitants of myasthenia gravis. Ann. N. Y. Acad. Sci. 124, 744.
6. Strauss, A. J. L., Smith, C. W., Cage, G. W., Van der Geld, H. W. R., McFarlin, D. E., and Barlow, M. (1966): Further studies on the specificity of presumed immune associations of myasthenia gravis and consideration of possible pathogenic implications. Ann. N. Y. Acad. Sci. 135, 557.
7. Van der Geld, H. W. R., and Strauss, A. J. L. (1966): Myasthenia gravis, immunological relationship between striated muscle and thymus. Lancet 1, 57.
8. Van der Geld, H., Feltkamp, T. E. W., and Oosterhuis, H. J. G. H. (1964): Reactivity of myasthenia gravis serum γ-globulin with skeletal muscle and thymus demonstrated by immunofluorescence. Proc. Soc. Exp. Biol. Med. 115, 782.
9. Van de Velde, R. L., and Friedman, N. B. (1966): Muscular elements of the thymus. Fed. Proc. 25, 661.

DISCUSSION

FELDMAN: Dr. Strauss, you said that your active sera gave positive reactions with myoblasts of 3-day-old embryos, similarly to the anti-myosin of Holtzer which react with 3-day-old myoblasts. Did you test the activity of your sera against pure preparations of myosin? If the reaction is directed against myosin, did you try to absorb the sera with thymus cells, and test whether some reactivity is retained against the muscle and if so, is this reactivity directed against myosin?

STRAUSS: Hale has been attempting to purify the reactive material in muscle, and indicates that this material is, if not myosin, intimately associated with it in initial preparative ultracentrifugation. We have been unable to absorb out this reactivity with purified myosin; crude whole striated muscle is an effective absorbent however. Other tissues do not absorb this reactivity save for some preparations of crude thymus.

BLOCK: Myasthenia gravis is a disease of the motor end plate (myoneural junction). Were you able to show fixation of fluorescent antibody on the motor end plate rather than on striations? I note that the immunofluorescent stain ran transversely. If the motor end plate were stained, I would expect the immunofluorescence to run parallel to the muscle fiber.

STRAUSS: McFarlin, who has worked with us, has studied just this issue. He has done immunofluorescent staining with serums that are reactive against striations and with nonreactive sera. He has then restained the motor end plate areas enzymatically and fails to find any localization of immunofluorescence in these latter areas.

BLOCK: The reason I didn't think they were staining the motor end plates is because the plates run parallel to the length of the fiber.

AUERBACH: Although you may be marking muscle with your antibody, there is some question of whether, in fact, an antibody made against muscle would react against the thymus. I think this is the key question.

STRAUSS: One might predict they would react against reptilian myoid cells.

AUERBACH: Just because the reptilian has myoid cells which are quite apparent, and possibly the 12-day thymus has a few cells that might be myoid cells, you are asking us to believe that those nice cells you showed in the adult thymus are muscle cells. I don't believe it.

STRAUSS: I am merely suggesting a homology; Henry (3) has in fact seen striated cells in human fetal thymus.

AUERBACH: They are not muscle cells; they are particularly good, self-respecting thymus cells with nice nuclei.

VAN FURTH: Have you stained thymus cell suspensions? What is the distribution of the fluorescent cells in the thymus sections?

STRAUSS: Hugo Van der Geld has stained thymic cell cultures. In the first few hours following dispersion of these cells, one can find substantial numbers of reactive cells. But continued growth of the culture involves disappearance of reactivity, not disappearance of epithelial cells, but disappearance of reactivity.

22

ARTHUR G. JOHNSON and GIOVANNA HOEKSTRA

Acceleration of the primary antibody response

OUR LABORATORY has been exploring the changes in the antibody-forming apparatus when endotoxins markedly increase the synthesis of antibody to protein antigens (8). How does the first cell seen with antibody, which possesses relatively little of the cell apparatus associated with protein synthesis and secretion, become a plasma cell fully equipped for this task? This differentiation or maturation is accompanied by division of the cell and acquisition of greater amounts of endoplasmic reticulum and ribosomes. Our findings suggest the hypothesis that early cells normally possess suboptimal amounts of nutritive materials required for differentiation, and that their responsiveness can be accelerated by oligonucleotides supplied either exogenously by injection or endogenously by cytotoxic agents (including endotoxin) which liberate cellular nucleic acids *in vivo*. The evidence supporting this hypothesis is as follows.

The general question asked was why inclusion of microgram amounts of endotoxin with the first injection of any of a number of protein antigens results in a decrease in the time necessary for antibody to appear in the circulation and enhancement of the early γM-antibody as well as an early and late appearing γG-antibody.

One of the first clues to an answer to this question was from the experiments of Taliaferro and Jaroslow (14). Animals rendered incapable of synthesizing antibody by x-irradiation were induced to do so when sources high in nucleic acids, or nucleic acids and their breakdown products, were injected with antigen. Data were obtained establishing that endotoxin overcame inhibition of antibody formation in x-irradiated rabbits (10). It was then postulated that such a restorative effect, as well as the enhancing action of endotoxin in normal rabbits, was mediated through damage to cells by endotoxin with release of nucleic acids or their breakdown products. Evidence that the latter possess the property of increasing cell division and the activity of enzymes during DNA synthesis has been accumulated by several investigators (1, 2, 4, 5, 9).

Support for this hypothesis was gained by histologic examination of the rabbit spleen following injection of endotoxin. Within hours small lymphocytes were seen to be damaged in the white pulp in the immediate vicinity of antibody-forming cells (16). Cytotoxic effects of endotoxin on spleen cells *in vitro* had also been reported by Heilman and Bernton (7), and on macrophages by Braun and Kessel (1). Endotoxin was found capable of inciting antibody formation in mice treated with 5-fluoro-2-deoxyuridine (FUDR), a specific inhibitor of DNA synthesis. The capability of this and many similar drugs to enhance early antibody formation when given as a single large cytotoxic dose was also in accord with this hypothesis (3, 12).

It was reasoned that if oligonucleotides mediated the enhancing action of endotoxin, they must also elevate antibody titers and shorten the induction period, similar to endotoxin and drugs. This proved to be the case

(13). The appearance time of circulating antibody was shortened and antibody levels were raised when DNA or RNA was injected with antigen. These characteristics were associated with a dialyzable fraction of nuclease-treated nucleic acids (13).

An *in vitro* system for study of antibody formation in organ culture has been under study in our laboratory (11). However, addition of nucleic acids not only failed to enhance the meager synthesis of such organs, but inhibited all antibody synthesis (6).

Isolation of the smaller dialyzable fragments, active as adjuvants, was attempted. The procedure of Tomlinson and Tener was adopted employing DEAE cellulose and urea-NaC1 mixtures as eluant (15). Under these conditions, the oligonucleotides are fractionated according to their net charge, and thus the number of linked bases. The flow sheet (Fig. 1) depicts the handling of the DNA-DNAse digest. The resultant chromatogram (Fig. 2) indicated the presence of at least 6-7 distinct entities. The effect of each of these peaks on the antibody response of Balb/c mice to a single injection of 3 mg of bovine γ-globulin is shown in Table 1. All fractions except peak 4 substantially increased the immune response. Analysis of their base composition and their activity in organ culture is under study.

It is apparent that adjuvant activity was not a function of any particular size of oligonucleotide. Rather, this adjuvant effect appears to be due to a property of oligonucleotides independent of base composition.

SUMMARY

Evidence is presented favoring the hypothesis that cells responding early after primary antigenic stimulation may not possess optimal amounts of nucleic acid building blocks when called upon for the burst of nucleic acid synthesis prior to antibody formation. If oligonucleotides are supplied from exogenous sources (or endogenously following cytotoxic agents) the primary antibody response is accelerated with respect to the time of appearance of antibody and higher antibody levels. Fractionation of DNA-DNAse digest mixtures by gradient elution with urea on DEAE-cellulose ion exchange resin revealed adjuvant activity associated with all but one oligonucleotide fraction.

DNA

↓ Hydrated in 0.015M $MgC_2H_3O_2$ overnight at room temp. in presence of chloroform

DNA + DNAse

↓ Incubated 3 hr at room temp.

DNA DIGEST

↓ Heated at 100°C for 5 min

Cooled to room temp.; filtered

Stored at -20°C until needed

DEAE—CELLULOSE (CHLORIDE) COLUMN

↓ Eluted with a linear gradient formed by 1 L 7M urea + 25 ml $NaC_2H_3O_2$ buffer, pH 4.8 and 1 L (7M urea + 0.3M NaCl) + 25 ml $NaC_2H_3O_2$ buffer, pH 4.8

FRACTIONS

↓ Molecular extinction measured at 271 mμ
Pooled; concentrated by pervaporation

SEPARATION OF NaCl—UREA FROM OLIGONUCLEOTIDES

↓ Pooled fractions desalted by molecular sieving on a BioGel P-2, 100-200 mesh column

LYOPHILIZATION

FIG. 1. Flow sheet diagram separating oligonucleotides following treatment of DNA with DNAse.

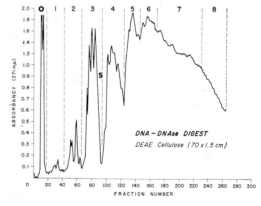

FIG. 2. Fractionation of DNA-DNAse digest on DEAE cellulose column. Elution was accomplished with a linear gradient formed by 1 L 7M urea + 25 ml $NaC_2H_3O_2$ buffer and 1 L (7M urea + 0.3M NaCl) + 25 ml $NaC_2H_3O_2$ buffer. Numbers indicate peaks pooled and injected into mice.

TABLE 1.—ADJUVANT ACTION OF OLIGONUCLEOTIDES SEPARATED FROM DNA-DNASE MIXTURE BY DEAE CELLULOSE CHROMATOGRAPHY

BGG* (3 mg) +	Amount Injected	Probable Size of Oligodeoxyribonucleotide†	Antibody Titer (Day 9)
——	——	None	80
Endotoxin	10 μg	None	2560
Peak 0	2 mg	?	2560
" 1	0.2 mg	Mononucleotides	320
" 1	2.0 mg	"	1280
" 2	0.2 mg	Dinucleotides	320
" 2	1.0 mg	"	2560
" 2	2.0 mg	"	1280
" 3	1.0 mg	Trinucleotides	1280
" 3	2.0 mg	"	5120
" 4	2.0 mg	Tetranucleotides	80
" 5	0.1 mg	Pentanucleotides	640
" 5	2.0 mg	"	2560
" 6	2.0 mg	Hexanucleotides	1280
" 7	2.0 mg	Higher nucleotides	1280
" 8	——	" "	Not tested

*Inbred mice, Balb/c strain, 8-week-old males, injected ip in groups of 3 with 3 mg bovine γ-globulin in 0.5 ml saline. Oligonucleotides injected ip separately in 0.5 ml saline at same time as antigen. Antibody titers determined by passive hemagglutination.
†Size inferred from data of Tomlinson and Tener (15).

REFERENCES

1. Braun, W., and Kessel, R. W. I. (1964): Cytotoxicity of endotoxins in relation to their effects on host resistance. Chapt. 36, p. 397. Landy, M. and Braun, W., eds.: Bacterial Endotoxins. Rutgers Univ. Press.
2. Bryant, B. J. (1963): Reutilization of lymphocyte DNA by cells of intestinal crypts and regenerating liver. J. Cell Biol. 18, 515.
3. Buskirk, H. H., Crim, J. A., Petering, H. G., Merritt, K., and Johnson A. G. (1965): Effect of uracil mustard and several antitumor drugs on the primary antibody response in rats and mice. J. Nat. Cancer Inst. 34, 747.
4. Eidam, C. R., and Merchant, D. J. (1965): The plateau phase of growth of the L-M strain mouse cell in a protein-free medium. Exp. Cell Res. 37, 147.
5. Firshein, W. (1965): Influence of deoxyribonucleic acid degradation products and orthophosphate on deoxynucleotide kinase activity and deoxyribonucleic acid synthesis in pneumococcus type III. J. Bact. 90, 327.
6. Han, I., and Johnson, A. G. (1964): Unpublished observations.
7. Heilman, D. H., and Bernton, H. W. (1961): The effect of endotoxin on tissue cultures of spleen of normal and tuberculin-sensitive animals. Amer. Rev. Resp. Dis. 84, 862.
8. Johnson, A. G. (1964): Adjuvant action of bacterial endotoxins on the primary antibody response; Chapt. 24; p. 252, in: Landy, M. and Braun, W., eds.: Bacterial Endotoxins; Rutgers Univ. Press.
9. Keir, H. M. (1962): Stimulation and inhibition

of DNA nucleotidyltransferase by oligodeoxyribonucleotides. Biochem. J. *85,* 265.

10. Kind, P., and Johnson, A. G. (1959): Studies on the adjuvant action of bacterial endotoxins on antibody formation in x-irradiated rabbits. J. Immun. *82,* 415.

11. Kong, Y. M., and Johnson, A. G. (1963): Factors affecting primary and secondary antibody production by splenic tissues. J. Immun. *90,* 672.

12. Merritt, K., and Johnson, A. G. (1963): Studies on the adjuvant action of bacterial endotoxins on antibody formation. V. The influence of endotoxin and 5-fluoro-2-deoxyuridine on the primary antibody response of the Balb mouse to a purified protein antigen. J. Immun. *91,* 266.

13. Merritt, K., and Johnson, A. G. (1965): Studies on the adjuvant action of bacterial endotoxins on antibody formation. VI. Enhancement of antibody formation by nucleic acids. J. Immunol. *94,* 416.

14. Taliaferro, W. H., and Jaroslow, B. N. (1960): The restoration of hemolysin formation in x-rayed rabbits by nucleic acid derivatives and antagonists of nucleic acid synthesis. J. Infect. Dis. *107,* 341.

15. Tomlinson, R. V., and Tener, G. M. (1963): The effect of urea, formamide, and glycols on the secondary binding forces in the ion-exchange chromatography of polynucleotides on DEAE-cellulose. Biochemistry *2,* 697.

16. Ward, P. A., Johnson, A. G., and Abell, M. R. (1959): Studies on the adjuvant action of bacterial endotoxins on antibody formation. III. Histologic response of the rabbit spleen to a single injection of a purified protein antigen. J. Exp. Med. *109,* 463.

23

WERNER BRAUN and MASAYASU NAKANO

The reinforcement of immunological stimuli by oligodeoxyribonucleotides

It has been known for some time that cell breakdown products, specifically oligodeoxyribonucleotides (cf. 1, 5) and also oligoribonucleotides (21) can enhance the immune response. On the basis of such findings it has been suggested that at least part of the action of cytotoxic adjuvants, such as bacterial endotoxins and Freund's adjuvant, may be attributable to the release of stimulatory oligonucleotides. In this communication we shall review some previously published, as well as some new and unpublished, evidence regarding the nature and probable causes of such reinforcement of immunological stimuli. We shall also cover the apparent contribution of these effects to the natural course of immune responses, and their role in antibody formation in newborn as compared with adult animals. We shall put particular emphasis on the nature and effects of the active materials in enzymatic digests of calf thymus DNA (DNA digests = DD) since we have found these materials to be far more active than the oligoribonucleotides that result from the enzymatic digestion of RNA (5).

Oligodeoxyribonucleotide effects on bacteria, DNA synthesis, and mammalian cells. The effects of DD were first discovered in studies with gram-positive bacteria (cf. 1 for a more complete review). The rate of multiplication of the virulent (S) forms of these bacteria was found to be greatly enhanced by oligodeoxyribonucleotides (di- to pentanucleotides) but not by mononucleotides and -sides.

This stimulation of growth was subsequently shown to be associated with a selective stimulation of DNA synthesis (9), and more recent evidence (10) revealed that, at least in pneumococci, such stimulation is the consequence of an oligodeoxyribonucleotide-induced elevation of nucleotide kinase levels. In other words, in cells exposed to oligodeoxyribonucleotides, enzymes concerned with the formation of DNA precursors are present in much higher concentrations.

It has not yet been established that the stimulatory effects of oligodeoxyribonucleotides on the rate of multiplication of mammalian cells, especially on antibody-forming cells and on tumor cells (4), are also due to enhanced nucleotide kinase activity. However, in view of the striking parallelism of modifying and inhibitory effects which are produced by the same agents in both the bacterial and the mammalian cell systems, one can suspect that the mode of action of DD is identical in both systems. It is interesting to note that in the bacterial test systems, large DNA fragments interfere with the activity of the small DNA fragments (1), whereas in the mammalian cell system even large DNA fragments are active. It has been concluded that this difference is apparent rather than real. The animal possesses nucleases which can rapidly degrade large DNA fragments to small ones, thus assuring arrival of the stimulator in the form of oligodeoxyribonucleotides at sites of target cells.

The effects of DD on antibody formation was first indicated by their ability to restimulate impaired antibody-forming systems (8, 25, 26). These effects were difficult to discern in studies with normal animals in which circulating antibodies were assayed (cf. 1 for a detailed review). However, techniques capable of measuring the number of antibody-forming cells in spleen and lymph nodes (19, 24) revealed the effects of DD on increases in antibody-forming cell populations.

The oldest and most widely used of the techniques for scoring numbers of antibody-forming cells employs the well-known phenomenon of lysis of red blood cells in the presence of specific antibodies and complement (19). The spleen of a mouse immunized with sheep red blood cells (sRBC) is removed 2, 3, or 4 days following immunization, broken up into a single cell suspension, and mixed with sRBC in agar. The agar is flooded with fresh serum (as a source of complement) with the result that red blood cells are lysed, and plaques are formed in the neighborhood of spleen cells which formed specific hemolysins.

Influence of oligodeoxyribonucleotides on early events in antibody formation. It was demonstrated that DD, given in conjunction with sRBC, affects principally the early period of increase in antibody-forming spleen cell populations (5). Thus, the number of hemolysin-forming cells, 48 hours after immunization with heterologous red cells, is significantly higher if antigen is administered with an enzymatic digest of calf thymus DNA (Table 1). Stimulation by oligodeoxyribonucleotides is

TABLE 1.—INFLUENCE OF DNA DIGEST ON THE NUMBER OF HEMOLYSIN-PRODUCING SPLEEN CELLS 48 HOURS AFTER IMMUNIZATION OF AKR MICE

Treatment of spleen donors	Number of hemolysin-producing cells ($\pm$ S. E.) per 1/5 spleen after 48 hrs.
None	2.6 ± 0.9
Sheep red blood cells (10^8/mouse)	27.0 ± 4.2
Sheep red blood cells + DNA digest	73.2 ± 16.1
DNA digest	2.6 ± 0.8

not matched by comparable effects of oligoribonucleotides; mixtures of monodeoxyribonucleotides or -sides are inactive. Stimulation appears to involve a stimulated multiplication of early appearing, or early activated, antibody-forming clones, and is more difficult to detect as the interval between time of immunization and time of assay of spleen cell populations increases (Table 2).

Data similar to those just reviewed have been collected when *E. coli*, instead of sRBC, served as immunizing agent and the number of bactericidin-forming spleen cells was assayed by the technique of Schwartz and Braun (24).

Both dosage and route of administration influence the magnitude of the DD effect (cf. 5). An enhanced rate of increase of hemolysin-forming cells occurs in the presence of oligodeoxyribonucleotides in the primary response as well as in the secondary response. Actinomycin

TABLE 2.—EXTENT OF THE DNA DIGEST EFFECTS AT VARIOUS TIMES FOLLOWING IMMUNIZATION OF AKR MICE WITH SHEEP OR HORSE RED BLOOD CELLS. ITALICIZED FIGURES REPRESENT VALUES THAT IN T TESTS PROVED TO BE SIGNIFICANTLY DIFFERENT FROM CORRESPONDING VALUES OBTAINED IN THE ABSENCE OF DD. FROM (5)

Treatment of spleen donors	Average number of hemolysin-producing cells per 1/5 spleen after			
	24 hr.	48 hr.	72 hr.	96 hr.
Sheep red blood cells (10^8/mouse)	4.2	16.0	234.8	4,580
Sheep red blood cells + DNA digest	4.0	*44.8*	328.0	4,560
Horse red blood cells (10^9/mouse)	-	3.6	13.8	80.4
Horse red blood cells + DNA digest	-	7.8	19.8	*161.0*

D has been shown to interfere with the primary response in the absence as well as in the presence of oligodeoxyribonucleotides. However, in the secondary response, which ordinarily is insensitive to actinomycin D, the antibiotic will inhibit all of the DD-stimulated response, an indication that part of the secondary response is a repetition of the primary response.

Kinetin riboside, the riboside of 6-furfuryl amino purine, was found to inhibit the stimulatory effects of DD in the bacterial system (11) as well as in the antibody-forming cell system.

It has been determined recently that stimulatory levels of oligodeoxyribonucleotides are maintained in the circulation for relatively long periods of time (23). Table 3 shows that following the passive transfer of serum (0.4 ml i. v.) from mice injected with DD (1.0 ml i. p., 0.5 ml i. v.) to mice injected with sRBC, an enhanced rate of increase in antibody-forming cells can be achieved as late as 48 hours following the injection of DD into the serum donor.

Stimulation of antibody formation by DD requires the concurrent administration of antigen (5). In contrast, endotoxin can produce such stimulation in the absence of antigen, causing a rapid increase in pre-existing hemolysin- or bactericidin-forming spleen cells, for example. Endotoxin may stimulate because it can cause the release of DD-like materials from intracellular sites (3); thus, the difference in antigen requirements between endotoxin and DD stimulation was puzzling. The possibility was considered that a stimulated increase in antibody-forming cell populations may require two factors: the stimulator *and* an agent permitting the entrance of the stimulator into the cells to be stimulated. In this case endotoxin may possess both attributes: release of stimulator and the capability to alter the permeability of the target cells. In contrast, antigen may be required in the case of DD because by reacting with antibody on the surface of the antibody-forming cell it may alter the permeability of the cell membrane, thus permitting the entrance of oligodeoxyribonucleotides. If such considerations were correct, it should be possible to replace the requirement for antigen, in the DD-elicited stimulations, by factors that can alter the permeability of target cells in a non-specific manner.

This was found to be the case. Chlorpromazine, cortisone, and also phenoxybenzamine, agents that are known to alter, or suspected of

TABLE 3.—EFFECTS OF PASSIVE TRANSFER OF SERUM (0.4 ML I. V.) FROM CF-1 MICE, INJECTED 3 TO 72 HOURS EARLIER WITH DNA DIGEST, ON THE NUMBER OF HEMOLYSIN-PRODUCING SPLEEN CELLS IN CF-1 MICE INJECTED I. V. WITH 10^8 SHEEP RED BLOOD CELLS (sRBC) 48 HOURS EARLIER

Treatment of spleen donors	Average number (± S. E.) of hemolysin-producing cells per 1/5 spleen
None	4.8 ± 0.7
sRBC	34.6 ± 6.2
″ + DNA digest	83.6 ± 9.9
″ + normal serum	33.4 ± 4.8
″ + serum from a mouse that received DNA digest 3 hrs. earlier	60.2 ± 4.4
″ + serum from a mouse that received DNA digest 24 hrs. earlier	72.4 ± 6.5
″ + serum from a mouse that received DNA digest 48 hrs. earlier	59.8 ± 14.8
″ + serum from a mouse that received DNA digest 72 hrs. earlier	39.6 ± 10.4

TABLE 4.—THE EFFECT OF CHLORPROMAZINE ON HEMOLYSIN-
FORMING SPLEEN CELLS OF CF-1 MICE TREATED WITH
DNA DIGEST.

Treatment of spleen donors	Average number (± S. E.) of hemolysin-producing cells per 1/5 spleen after 48 hrs.
None	3.0 ± 1.2 ←
sRBC	66.7 ± 14.5
DNA digest	4.7 ± 1.9 ←
DNA digest + chlorpromazine*	24.0 ± 4.7 ←
Chlorpromazine*	3.4 ± 1.3
sRBC + DNA digest	131.7 ± 7.9

*100 γ/mouse at 0 and 24 hrs.

altering, cell permeability are capable of mediating an increase in the number of hemolysin-forming spleen cells when given with DD, in the absence of specific antigen. Table 4 presents an example of such effects. We, therefore, conclude that the enhancement of the rate of increase in antibody-forming cell populations requires both a stimulator and an agent permitting its entrance into the cells to be stimulated.*

Oligodeoxyribonucleotides also can enhance the rate of phagocytosis (13) and such stimulation occurs without a requirement for anti-

*Since these studies showed that antibody-forming cells can be "opened up" by chlorpromazine, we employed this compound to determine whether macrophages, presumably involved in an early step in antibody formation (12), may produce a "turning-on" RNA that can activate all the plasma cell precursors that it can enter. We made the assumption that macrophages, having phagocytosed an antigen, will process it and complex it with a "turning-on" RNA. The processed antigen, through its reaction with a specific antibody-like recognition site on, or in, a stem-cell of antibody-forming cell populations, may then guide this RNA into the proper stem-cell. It was suspected that chlorpromazine, through its ability to cause general changes in the permeability of antibody-forming cells might open up all available stem-cells to the "turning-on" RNA. Evidence for this was found in the recent observation that a specific antigen (sRBC) when given to mice with chlorpromazine will cause an increase in spleen cells that form heterologous antibodies (anti-cRBC, anti-E. coli) while decreasing the specific response (anti-sRBC). These and related experiments on the possible significance of RNA-antigen complexes will be reviewed in a separate communication (2).

gen. Like the DD effect on antibody formation, the effect of DD on phagocytosis can be reversed by kinetin riboside.

Clonal distribution of antibody-forming cells. The normal and the stimulated increases in cells forming a specific antibody have a clonal pattern in the spleen. Recent studies (22) have shown that hemolysin-forming cells in the spleens of mice immunized with heterologous red blood cells are non-randomly distributed throughout the spleen. This non-random distribution has a different pattern for cells that form antibodies to one antigen compared to those forming antibodies to another one. Thus, in spleens of mice immunized with both sheep red blood cells (sRBC) and chicken red blood cells (cRBC) the non-random distribution of cells forming antibodies to sRBC is quite different from that occurring in the same spleen for cells forming anti-cRBC. These data were obtained by assaying, with the plaque technique, 20 different fragments of one spleen against both sRBC and cRBC.

It should be noted that the normal and stimulated increases in the antibody-forming spleen cell populations are not necessarily due to a clonal multiplication of antibody-forming cells. It is possible that these increases are due to the spread of an activator, or possibly even of information, in an exponential fashion through neighboring cells. The end result could be the same, i. e., a production, within lymphoid tissues, of separate micropopulations of cells forming a given type of antibody protein. We shall come back to this point once more when we discuss stimulated antibody formation in newborn animals.

Relationships between oligodeoxyribonucleotides and naturally released stimulators. We suggested previously (1, 3) that the stimulatory effects of adjuvants with cytotoxic activity can be attributed to their ability to release oligodeoxyribonucleotides from intracellular sites, either by cell leakage or by cell destruction. This suggestion has found support through the finding that a known inhibitor of DD effects, namely kinetin riboside, can also reverse the stimulatory effects of adjuvants such as endotoxin (20) and FUDR (7). Also, if endotoxin is regarded as the trigger for the release of stimulatory intracellular materials, rather than as the stimulator itself, it should be possible to provoke stimulatory effects of DD in endotoxin-tolerant animals that can no longer be stimulated by endotoxin. This was shown to be the case in recent experimental tests (14). In addition, prior studies have shown that crystalline silica and CCl_4—agents with preferential cytotoxicity for macrophages—can cause the release of intracellular materials with stimulatory capacities for antibody-forming cells (cf. 1).

More recently, it has been demonstrated that reactions *in vitro* between antibody-forming cells and specific antigen can release intracellular materials capable of producing striking enhancing effects on antibody synthesis (23). These experiments were performed as follows. Mice were immunized with cRBC (which do not cross-react with sRBC). Five days later, when the spleen has a maximum number of cells forming anti-cRBC, the animals were sacrificed and their spleens broken up in Eagle's medium into a suspension of single cells. Chicken red blood cells (approx. 4×10^8/ml) were then added and the mixed suspension of spleen and cRBC was incubated for 6 hours. The suspension was then centrifuged and 1.0 ml of the supernatant, corresponding roughly to the supernate obtained from cells of one spleen, was then injected, partially i. v. (0.5 ml) and partially i. p. (0.5 ml) into mice that simultaneously received 1×10^8 sRBC i. v. As illustrated in Table 5 such treatment resulted in a significant elevation of the number of sRBC hemolysin-forming cells in the recipient mouse 48 hours later, when compared to the number of such hemolysin-forming spleen cells in animals that had received only antigen. Preliminary tests on the stimulatory supernatants,

TABLE 5.—STIMULATORY EFFECTS OF THE SUPERNATANT OBTAINED FOLLOWING A 6-HOUR INCUBATION OF CHICKEN RED BLOOD CELLS (cRBC) WITH SPLEEN CELLS FROM CF-1 MICE IMMUNIZED 5 DAYS EARLIER WITH cRBC*

Treatment of spleen donors	Average number ($\pm$ S. E.) of hemolysin-producing cells per 1/5 spleen
None	5.4 $\pm$ 1.8
sRBC	74.8 $\pm$ 6.0
" + DNA digest	112.0 $\pm$ 14.2
" + supernatant from immune cells	221.2 $\pm$ 27.2
" + " " normal cells	77.8 $\pm$ 12.4
" + culture medium	78.0 $\pm$ 11.8
Supernatant from immune cells	24.4 $\pm$ 8.8

*One ml of the supernatant was injected i.v./i.p. into each of several CF-1 mice which simultaneously received 10^8 sRBC i.v. The animals were then sacrificed 48 hours later. The table shows the number of spleen cells forming anti-sRBC hemolysins in these supernatant-treated mice. One ml of supernatant corresponds approximately to the yield obtained from the incubation of one spleen + 4 x 10^8 cRBC.

obtained following reactions between anti-body-forming cells and antigen, indicate that the active materials could be oligodeoxyribonucleotides. However, a great deal more work remains to be done before this conclusion can be regarded as definite. In any event, these observations suggest that stimulators of rates of increases in antibody-forming clones may be released naturally, some time after the initiation of an immune response, as the consequence of interactions between antibody-forming cells and antigen. This may account for the fact that the artificial introduction of such stimulators can influence only the very early period of immune responses, i. e., a period during which the natural release of similar stimulators may be deficient. This may also account for the increased capacity of stimulators to exert effects in newborn animals, i. e., in an environment where the background level of cell-breakdown products, and of cell-released materials, may be much lower than in adult animals. The following section will deal with data on events in newborn animals.

Oligodeoxyribonucleotide effects in new-born animals. In comparison with adult animals, the stimulatory effects of DD on increases in numbers of antibody-forming cells are even more pronounced in newborn animals (16, 17). The administration of sRBC in conjunction with DD to newborn AKR and Ha/ICR mice not only enhances the rate of increase in antibody-forming cells in mesenteric and pancreatic lymph nodes, but can even advance the detectable onset of cellular immune responses by 48 to 72 hours (Fig. 1). This speed-up, however, occurs only after the animal has reached the age where it can show any response to a given antigen. In other words, oligodeoxyribonucleotides can stimulate increases in antibody-forming cell populations once immunological competence has been attained, but they cannot advance the maturation of immunological competence. We may assume that oligodeoxyribonucleotides do not advance the point at which stem-cells with specific recognition sites occur in lymphoid tissues. However, these stimulators can greatly increase the rate at which the number of cells increase in such activated clones.

In studies with AKR, $C_{57}B1$, and Ha/ICR mice it was found that newborn AKR mice

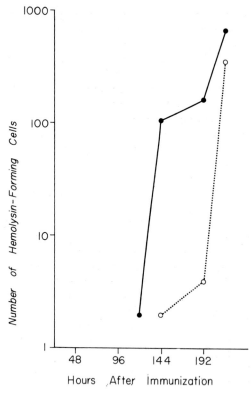

Fig. 1. Graphic representation of the average number of hemolysin-forming mesenteric lymph node cells in AKR mice immunized at 5 days of age with 10^8 sRBC (———— DNA digest-treated, ... saline-injected).

attain the ability to respond to sRBC at 5 days of age, Ha/ICR at 7 days of age, and $C_{57}B1$ not until 10 days of age (18). Once competence for response to sRBC has been attained, the actual degree of responsiveness does not parallel the sequence with which competence developed in different strains (Table 6). Thus, as far as circulating hemolysins are concerned, AKR, the earliest responding strain, shows only low titers for at least 2 weeks after immunization, whereas responding Ha/ICR and $C_{57}B1$ mice show high titers. AKR and Ha/ICR show a large number of antibody-forming cells, $C_{57}B1$ a small one. This discrepancy between titers of circulating hemolysin and numbers of hemolysin-forming spleen- and lymph-node cells suggests that cellular efficiency (number of antibody molecules formed per cell per unit time) is not equal in different strains. Newborn strain differences determined by Hechtel and those of adult animals studied by Friedman (15) might be explained on this basis. Regardless of strain, the order of appearance of hemolysin-forming cells in the newborn animals was spleen → pancreatic lymph nodes → mesenteric lymph nodes.

The ability of oligonucleotides to stimulate immune responses in newborn mice appears to be roughly inverse to the intensity of the normal response. It is noteworthy that oligonucleotide effects are discernible in the level of circulating antibodies of several strains. It has been very difficult to detect such stimulatory effects by studying the sera of adult animals although the effects are clearly apparent when numbers of antibody-forming cells are assayed (1). This difference in oligonucleotide effects on cellular responses and levels of circulating antibodies in adult mice has been ascribed to the fact that the effects of injected stimulators are principally on early responses. Consequently, stimulated responses are no longer discernible by the time that circulating hemolysins are detectable; as discussed above, by that time normally released stimulators probably hide the effects of artificially introduced stimulators.

In newborns, however, the intensity of the stimulation by nucleotides is greater and appears to persist longer. This difference between young and adult animals may be attributable to the higher background level in the adult of oligodeoxyribonucleotides and of other naturally released cell-breakdown products which can act as stimulators for immune responses. Such materials may become available from a variety of postnatal environmental stimuli. It should be possible to obtain further support for this concept through studies in which newborns are purposely exposed to a series of simultaneous or consecutive heterologous immunological responses. From the existing evidence it would be expected that such early multiple exposures may increase the rate at which specific antibody-forming cells increase in numbers.

In newborn animals a rapid increase in detectable hemolysin-forming cells was found to occur in lymph nodes and spleen of sRBC-exposed animals. This increase appeared to involve principally those cells that are able to form the specific antibody under study, since no corresponding over-all increases in cell numbers could be noted in the organs of DD-treated or untreated mice (16). If one

TABLE 6.—SUMMARY OF THE IMMUNE RESPONSES OF NEWBORN MICE OF DIFFERENT STRAINS TO sRBC AND THE EFFECT OF DNA DIGEST ON THIS RESPONSE. FROM (16)

Strain	*	Antibody levels in the circulation	Spleen	Numbers of antibody-forming cells in	
				Pancreatic lymph nodes	Mesenteric lymph nodes
AKR	1	intermediate	early	intermediate	late
	2	low	high	high	high
	3	no	no	yes	yes
	4	early	early	early	early
Ha/ICR	1	intermediate	early	intermediate	late
	2	high	high	high	low
	3	yes	no	yes	no
	4	intermediate	intermediate	intermediate	late
$C_{57}B1$	1	late	early	late	late
	2	high	low	low	low
	3	yes	yes	yes	yes
	4	late	late	late	late

*1 = Detectable response: early to late after immunization.

2 = Intensity of response: high or low.

3 = Influence of DNA digest at any time: yes or no.

4 = Comparative time after birth of the development of responsiveness by mouse strain.

accepts that the generation time of 12-14 hours for lymphoid cells of adult mice (6) is also applicable to newborn mice, then the results obtained with newborn immunized mice indicate the occurrence of both functional differentiation (activation of pre-existing specific competence?) as well as multiplication. Thus, for example in the spleen of mice, immunized at 10 days of age with 10^8 sRBC, the number of detectable hemolysin-forming cells increased from an average of 2 at 48 hours to an average of 209 at 72 hours after immunization, an increase that would require about seven generations within 24 hours if all of the increase were due to multiplication. Similarly,

the number of hemolysin-forming cells in DD-treated mice increased during the same period from 9 to 1,274, again equivalent to seven generations. It remains to be established whether the rates of multiplication of antibody-forming cells in newborn animals are much higher than anticipated from the results on adult animals, or increases in antibody-forming cell populations may, under certain conditions, involve both functional differentiation and multiplication.

Acknowledgment: Current studies reported herein are being supported by Grant AM-08742 of the U.S.P.H.S.

REFERENCES

1. Braun, W. (1965): Influence of nucleic acid degradation products on antibody synthesis, in: Molecular and Cellular Basis of Antibody Formation. Czech. Acad. Sci. p. 525.
2. Braun, W., and Cohen, E. P. (1966): On the role of nucleic acids in antibody formation, in: Regulation of the Antibody Response, B. Cinader, ed. [In press]
3. Braun, W., and Kessel, R. W. I. (1964): Cytotoxity of endotoxins in relation to their effects on host resistance, in: Bacterial Endotoxins. Rutgers Univ. Press, p. 397.
4. Braun, W., Lampen, J. O., Plescia, O. J., and Pugh, Leonora (1963): Effects of nucleic acid digests on spontaneous and implanted tumors of C3H mice, in: Conceptual Advances in Immunology and Oncology, New York, Hoeber, p. 540.
5. Braun, W., and Nakano, M. (1965): Influence of oligodeoxyribonucleotides on early events in antibody formation. Proc. Soc. Exp. Biol. Med. *119*, 701.
6. Capalbo, E. E., Makinodan, T., and Gude, W. D. (1962): Fate of H3-thymidine-labeled spleen cells in *in vivo* cultures during secondary antibody response. J. Immun. *89*, 1.
7. Cohen, E. P. (1966): Unpublished data.
8. Feldman, M., Globerson, A., and Nachtigel, D. (1963): The reactivation of the immune response in immunologically suppressed animals, in: Conceptual Advances in Immunology and Oncology. New York, Hoeber.
9. Firshein, W. (1963): The induction of deoxycytidylic acid kinase activity by a dinucleotide fraction derived from an enzymatic DNA digest in pneumococci. Biochem. Biophys. Res. Commun. *11*, 187.
10. Firshein, W. (1965): Influence of deoxyribonucleic acid degradation products and orthophosphate of deoxynucleotide kinase activity and deoxyribonucleic acid synthesis in pneumococcus Type III. J. Bact. *90*(2), 327.
11. Firshein, W., and Braun, W. (1964): Inhibitors of preferentially stimulated deoxyribonucleic acid

synthesis in pneumococci. J. Bact. *87*, 1245.
12. Fishman, M., van Rood, J. J., and Adler, F. L. (1965): The initiation of antibody formation by ribonucleic acid from specifically stimulated macrophages, in: Molecular and Cellular Basis of Antibody Formation. Czech. Acad. Sci. p. 491.
13. Freedman, H. H., and Braun, W. (1965): Influence of oligodeoxyribonucleotides on phagocytic activity of the reticuloendothelial system. Proc. Soc. Exp. Biol. Med. *120*, 222.
14. Freedman, H. H., Nakano, M., and Braun, W. (1966): Antibody formation in endotoxin-tolerant mice. Proc. Soc. Exp. Biol. Med. *121*, 1228.
15. Friedman, H. (1964): Distribution of antibody plaque forming cells in various tissues of several strains of mice injected with sheep erythrocytes. Proc. Soc. Exp. Biol. Med. *117*, 526.
16. Hechtel, M. A. (1965): Influence of Oligodeoxyribonucleotides on Immune Responses in Newborn and Thymectomized Mice. Dissertation, Rutgers University.
17. Hechtel, M., Dishon, T., and Braun, W. (1965a): Influence of oligodeoxyribonucleotides on the immune response of newborn AKR mice. Proc. Soc. Exp. Biol. Med. *119*, 991.
18. Hechtel, M., Dishon, T., and Braun, W. (1965b): Hemolysin formation in newborn mice of different strains. Proc. Soc. Exp. Biol. Med. *120*, 728.
19. Jerne, N. K., Nordin, A. A., and Henry, Claudia (1963): The agar plaque technique for recognizing antibody-producing cells, in: Cell-Bound Antibodies. Philadelphia, Wistar Institute Press, p. 109.
20. Kessel, R. W. I., and Braun, W. (1966): Endotoxin-enhanced host resistance: Reversal by kinetin riboside. Nature *211*, 1001.
21. Merritt, Katharine, and Johnson, A. G. (1965): Studies on the adjuvant action of bacterial endotoxins on antibody formation. VI. Enhancement of antibody formation by nucleic acids. J. Immun. *94*, 416.

22. Nakano, M., and Braun, W. (1966): Fluctuation tests with antibody-forming spleen cell populations. Science 151, 338.
23. Nakano, M., and Braun, W. (1966): unpublished data.
24. Schwartz, S., and Braun, W. (1965): Bacteria as an indicator of formation of antibodies by single spleen cells in agar. Science 149, 200.
25. Simić, M. M., Petkovic, M. Z., and Mancic, D. (1959): Partial restoration of hemolysin-forming capacity in x-irradiated rats by homologous spleen deoxyribonucleic acid. Bull. Inst. Nucl. Sci. "Boris Kidrich" (Belgrade) 9, 155.
26. Taliaferro, W. H., and Jaroslow, B. N. (1960): The restoration of hemolysin formation in x-rayed rabbits by nucleic acid derivatives and antagonists of nucleic acid synthesis. J. Infect. Dis. 107, 341.

DISCUSSION

HIRSCHHORN: Dr. Johnson, with reference to your experiment showing an abolition of antibody response by FUDR given 1 to 2 days after the antigen, you mentioned Elion and Hitchings' experiment. They showed that a second injection of antigen at this time and up to one week later also abolished the antibody response. They also stated that this inhibition can be avoided if phytohemagglutinin is given with the first injection of antigen. Have you tried phytohemagglutinin with the later injection of FUDR?

JOHNSON: No.

HIRSCHHORN: Dr. Braun, with reference to your experiment using the supernate from immune cells, there were two recent reports from Canada showing a factor in the supernate of mixed lymphocyte cultures (and, in lower dose, from cultures of lymphocytes from single donors) which can stimulate other lymphocytes to enlarge and divide. This could be the same factor as you describe.

The results you describe are very similar to the effect of phytohemagglutinin. That is, more cells make antibody than with antigen alone, and they respond earlier with morphological change, immunoglobulin production, and the ability to destroy allogeneic fibroblasts. The cells also seem to be derepressed for whatever they can make, as they do in your misdirected system. Have you tried phytohemagglutinin in your system?

BRAUN: I have long been intrigued with the possible relationship of some of your observations and our results. We are attempting to see whether spleen cell mixtures from two different strains can give us supernatants of similar action. I immediately thought when I saw the Canadian paper that they may be dealing with the same stimulator, but I would suggest that these people as well as you determine whether kinetin riboside can depress your effects. If it does, we then would have some very suggestive experimental evidence for a relationship. We find that the effects which we can achieve with phytohemagglutinin are very much dependent on the time of administration. We can get it in certain dosages if given at certain times.

FELDMAN: Dr. Braun, you described the effect of the oligodeoxyribonucleotides as increasing the numbers of plaque-forming cells and decreasing the latent period. This could result either from the increase in incidence of clones of plaque-forming cells or from the increase in rate of replication within each clone. This could be studied by testing fragments of spleens, similarly to tests applied by Papermaster and Playfair (Science, 1965). Have you done any experiments along these lines?

A second question: Dr. Johnson claimed that RNA affected the immune response similarly to DNA. Since you, Dr. Braun, confined yourself to the effect of DNA and DNA digests, would you care to comment on the possible effect of RNA as compared to DNA in your experimental system?

Finally, a question to Dr. Johnson: You demonstrated the effect of ATP in activating an immune response. Since I have been taught that ATP does not penetrate living cells (at least there is no evidence that it does), do you have any notion as to whether in your experimental system the ATP does get into any of the cells associated with the phenomenon which you have described?

BRAUN: We immunized mice with red blood cells; took the spleen and sectioned it into 24 equal parts, then assayed each part ten times. The same numbers of plaques was found in each sample from individual fragments. But different fragments varied greatly in the number of plaques.

The question here is, is this non-random distribution an anatomical feature or a reflection of clonal distribution of antibody-forming cells? We then immunized the spleen donor with two different antigens which do not cross-react. Each fragment was similarly assayed against each one of the antigens. If the explanation was purely anatomical, then all of the fragments having few plaques with one antigen should have few with the other; all high responders for one should be high to the other.

This was not the case. A completely independent, non-random distribution of response to the antigens was found. Stimulation did not increase the number of these clones per spleen but increased the rate at which clones increased in size.

FELDMAN: You have confined yourself to the effect of oligodeoxyribonucleotides, and we learned from Dr. Johnson that RNA does the same. Do you have a comment?

BRAUN: Except for poly-A, poly-U mixtures, which work well, our few attempts to use RNAse digest of a variety of RNA preparations have not given us comparable effects to those of oligoribonucleotides in our test system. But I don't see any *a priori* reason that the oligodeoxyribonucleotides shouldn't be active as well, if these are inducers of nucleotide kinase.

JOHNSON: In response to Dr. Feldman's question, I know nothing about the entry of ATP into cells. The ATP experiment was a shot in the dark which yielded this weird effect that I can't explain.

BLOCK: Dr. Braun, you infer that the number of antibody-containing cells in each clone increases rather than the number of clones. This means that the feed-in mechanism from stem cells is not altered. Therefore, the time between mitosis must be decreased and/or the time each antibody-containing cell remains in the clone is increased. Which is the mechanism you postulate? The situation is similar to that which occurs in erythroblasts where the number of erythroblasts is dependent on the rate of feed-in from stem cells, the number of divisions in erythroblasts, the number of dying erythroblasts, and the rate at which they become red cells or leave the area.

BRAUN: Dr. Hechtel, in working with newborns, observed that the detectable increase in numbers of antibody-forming cells during a 24-hour period is of such a nature that if it were due to division, you would have to assume seven generations. The same is true in some of the stimulated adult animals, but it is much more remarkable in the newborns. So either you can have in the newborn a much more rapid multiplication of antibody-forming cells, or it is multiplication plus something else. Perhaps we are not really measuring just multiplying cells, but something which involves also functional differentiation at the same time. I don't know.

BLOCK: You have to take into account also that the number of cells in any clone depends not only on division after the first cell of a clone is formed, but also in part on whether the cells in the clone are disappearing and leaving the clone.

MITCHISON: Dr. Braun, does the non-antigen-dependent effect that you observe (chlorpromazine + DNA digest) increase if the cells are left longer than 48 hours to assay?

BRAUN: It increases to 72 hours, but then it levels off.

MITCHISON: Dr. Johnson, does the bovine test you used detect the γM-antibody?

JOHNSON: I have no evidence that the Farr technique does not pick up γM-antibody. I would expect it to detect any antibody combining with antigen. However, even if it did not, it doesn't detract from our main point, that an early γG-antibody was enhanced by endotoxin.

MITCHISON: The effects observed by Dr. Johnson with FUDR injected shortly after antigen seems to be analogous to the effect described by Taliaferro and by Dixon, which they interpret as selection in favor of antigen-stimulated cells, rather than cell stimulation.

·········· Synthesis and speculation ··········

Editors:

R. T. SMITH

R. A. GOOD

and

P. A. MIESCHER

EBERT EMPHASIZED that for a number of years we have recognized two phases in the development of immunologically competent cells: that which we consider as independent of antigenic stimulus and which is part of the normal development of the cell system, and that which is antigen-dependent.

Block has raised the question whether this distinction is, in fact, a proper one; whether the evolution of all immune cells is in some way or other antigen-dependent.

To Ebert the great bulk of indirect evidence would indicate that differentiation proceeds up to a certain point independent of antigen. We need to re-examine in as many ways as possible the basis upon which we have made the assumption of two phases in the past. Experiments which are needed to clarify this issue involve those which might establish whether the stem cells in the yolk sac or even in the thymus are, in fact, capable of any degree of differentiation in the *absence* of an antigenic stimulus. Experiments are also needed to establish whether there are any cells in the absence of antigenic stimulus which are capable of producing γM-globulins.

A second series of questions which Ebert felt needed answers emerged from the discussion

of the function of the lowly macrophage. It has become quite evident that a need for critical understanding exists of the timing of macrophage function in the embryo. A large battery of old evidence with respect to clearance of various antigens yields practically no information on the precise fate of any given antigen or families of antigens.

He was impressed with Silverstein's data on the ontogeny of capacity for producing several different antibodies in the sheep fetus. Here the antibodies against bacterial products, against particulate materials such as ferritin, appeared much earlier than the antibodies to more soluble and more highly purified antigens.

It is important to carry these studies further using, say, three different antigens of three different sizes of particle to determine antigen-processing at different stages of embryonic life. Until such information is available, we cannot understand whether processing of antigen is a meaningful aspect of differentiation of the lymphocytic series independently or dependently.

We need to know whether a primordial type of stem cell exists in the embryo from which the several lymphocytic series arise. Using laser beams, one can now eliminate very specific parts of embryos cleanly. With such a technique one ought to be able to examine the capacities of various lines of embryonic cells both *in vivo* and *in vitro* with a great deal more precision and elegance than has heretofore been possible.

Several other issues need more study from the standpoint of the embryologist and immunobiologist.

First is the transfer of messages between cells. Accumulating evidence infers that messages are transferred from cell to cell. Does this really occur? And if so, just how does it occur?

Another important question is the relationship of tolerance to the phenomena of general biology. Experiments with induction of the tryptophan pyrrolase enzyme system show that inhibition is achieved at a time when the enzyme was not inducible by the administration of substrate. Is this a general phenome-

201

non? Are there really truly tolerant cells or is tolerance a question of interference with communication between cells?

Another important area covered is the nature of the preparation of antigen and the significance of the macrophage function. The phylogenetic perspective may assist materially in providing further relevant data.

The last issue raised implicit in many of our remarks is the question of recognition. We have talked about recognition, and we have assumed that lymphocytes have recognition sites. What is recognition? Even when starving amoeba do not eat other amoeba. Is this, therefore, due to a recognition phenomenon—a function dependent on membrane characteristics?

The reaggregation of cells, both in embryos and in tissue cultures, although controversial at the moment, implies a recognition process that may involve a surface language. A form of this language may be the language of receptors, for example, for virus particles.

Joshua Lederberg has shown for bacteria and Thomas Block for yeasts that exchange of nuclear material in conjugation involves first surface recognition mechanisms involving the surface proteins and carbohydrates—veritable sexes as well as sexuality seem to exist in these primitive forms.

Gessner's work on the circulation of lymphocytes through the postcapillary venules in the lymphoid organs, then on to recirculate, possibly also involves a recognition language between cells of the same genotype. Gessner showed that disaccharidase treatment of lymphocytes inhibits recirculation. It has also been shown that contact inhibition in tissue culture with T_3 fibroblasts involves an enzyme-sensitive saccharide structure.

Surface recognition processes, then, probably involve surface polysaccharides, and represent a complex but general biological language.

Among unanswered questions are: Can host proliferation in the graft-versus-host reaction be attributed to a recognition phenomenon? Does allogeneic inhibition initiating cytoplasmic and nuclear destruction start at the cell surface as a recognition phenomenon?

We should surely comment on a parallelism which can be developed between those conditions under which tolerance can be induced and those in which the activation of the immune response is characteristically incomplete; i.e., γM-antibody synthesis is evoked but the γG-component is either delayed or inhibited.

In the newborn rabbit, the parallelism appears complete. In this situation, the bacterial antigen elicits γM-globulin synthesis qualitatively and quantitatively mature in character. This is consonant with Adler's report here that μ chain synthesis is elicited as early as 24 hours postnatally in the rabbit spleen. The γG-globulin component of the sequence, however, is delayed in the serum after a variety of antigenic stimuli. Further, γ chain synthesis in the spleen lags μ chains by several days. This pattern persists through the first two weeks of life. Tolerance induction with a level dose of antigens such as BSA has a similar timing.

The effect of adjuvants, whether water-in-oil emulsions, endotoxins, or oligonucleotides, interferes with the induction of tolerance at this age as well as accentuating the immune response, and giving the mature sequence timing. 6-mercaptopurine renders the adult animal susceptible to induction of tolerance by protein antigens, and also delays the appearance of the γG-antibody formation when bacterial antigens are employed.

Braun's data suggest that at least one difference between the newborn and the more mature animal with respect to the induction of tolerance and the full expression of the immunological response might be the difference in the availability of a pool of oligodeoxyribonucleotides upon which to draw for the "tooling up" process anticipating a full immune response.

A working hypothesis, then, would hold that an excess pool of nucleotides is required to prevent tolerance and to activate the full range of the immunologic response.

Such an effect of oligonucleotides could be completely unrelated to specific immunological function. It is well established that newborns have the high rates of DNA and RNA turnover by any measurement. Apparently this reflects synthesis of cytochromes and other enzyme systems required to utilize molecular oxygen efficiently and produce liver and intestinal enzymes required for conjugation and nutrition.

These circumstances might conspire to give a rate-limiting effect on the pool of nucleotide precursors available for active immunological responses. This hypothesis could be tested by experiments such as giving RNA coupled antigens; or providing excess nucleotides to newborns and testing for the sequence of γM and γG response to a bacterial antigen or susceptibility to tolerance induction. If oligonucleotides restore responsiveness as Braun has stated, do they restore a full response?

Dr. Braun felt that preliminary experiments on ability of oligodeoxyribonucleotides to modify the response of the newborn are not in conflict with the hypothesis presented by Smith.

A secondary hypothesis would be that nucleotides are necessary to activate fragments of antigen rather than to have the general function of providing precursors for all of the processes necessary to protein antibody synthesis. Perhaps they act by specific attachment to certain peptides related to the antigenic determinant and yielding "superantigen" which has the new property of intrusion into otherwise privileged portions of the cell.

Experiments testing this could be devised, such as determining the rate of access to cells of nucleotide-antigen complexes compared to uncomplexed antigen. This type experiment might best employ the type of nucleotide-antigen complex which Garvey and Smith found in the liver of the tolerant rabbit, since no antibody would be concurrently present.

The question has been raised of the importance of macrophages in initiation of immunization. This question should perhaps be rephrased—can macrophages recognize foreignness? Are macrophages capable of recognition?

Fishman feels there is evidence for recognition by macrophages in that the ability of an animal to respond to an antigen is governed by the carrier portion of the antigen rather than the antigenic site.

The inability to form antibody may be due to several reasons. Either the cell lacks genetic information to give rise to a specific antibody or it was not made competent via the thymus or the antigen was or was not processed properly.

We should suggest, speculatively, that there may be dual roles for antigen. One, of course, is to "instruct" cells in a way which results in the specific response.

A second role of antigen may be to stimulate division by initiating cell mitosis and differentiation sequences now familiar to everyone. This second function could simply represent the effect of an antigenic determinant of broader specificity on a complex antigen. On the other hand, in the intact system this stimulatory effect may conceivably be related to the combination of antigen and nucleic acid. The stimulatory but not the instructive role of antigen may be the missing element allowing induction of tolerance. If this were correct, the tolerant animal would be expected to have a small, finite number of cells instructed and available for antibody production if stimulated to divide and initiate the process. It requires, of course, that Mitchison is wrong regarding the fate of cells which recognize antigen in the animal which becomes tolerant.

If the putative stimulating element were provided, perhaps by injecting the animal with PHA or providing a small amount of nucleotide-associated antigen, the tolerant state would be broken. Or if the hypothetically tolerant cells were in explant *in vitro*, perhaps clonal development of specific antibody-producing cells could be elicited by stimulation with PHA, inferring that tolerant cells *were* present.

We should like to close this symposium by introducing subject material to be considered at our conference in developmental immunobiology next year. In this conference we plan to deal in detail with diseases of man associated with developmental abnormalities of the lymphoreticular system. We shall deal with these abnormalities in a framework that considers not only the bases for the defective development of the processes, but in a perspective which we anticipate will feed back from the clinical and immunological-pathological observations in man focus and insight into the basic operations of the lymphoid system.

As an example one current clinical and pathological orientation is based upon the model in chickens being studied at Minnesota. The chicken which has been thymectomized and irradiated at hatching exhibits a reduction of small lymphocytes in the circulating blood and tissues, together with depletion of the white pulp of the spleen. However, germinal centers and plasma cells in these animals are normally present and the chickens have normal immunoglobulins. The striking observations are that such chickens show significantly reduced total antibody production, reduced graft-versus-host reactions, reduced capacity to reject homografts, and reduced ability to develop delayed allergic reactions.

By contrast, chickens which have been bursectomized and irradiated at hatching show delayed formation of germinal centers and plasma cells. Lymphocyte levels in their circulation and in their tissues are normal. No γM- or γG-immunoglobulins are demonstrable by immunoelectrophoresis. They do not form significant antibody in response to stimulation. They have normal graft-versus-host reactions and only a very slight impairment of homograft immunity.

Chicks bursectomized at hatching *without* irradiation show no consistent abnormality in the structure of the lymphoid apparatus; however, they have low γG-globulin, excessive amounts of γM, reduced ability to form circulating antibody, but normal delayed hypersensitivity.

The functional and anatomic analogies between these chicken models and examples of the spectrum of immunological deficiency disorders studied over the past ten years are striking.

With the analogy to the chicken in mind, we have made an attempt now to classify more than 200 cases of immunological deficiency and lymphoreticular malignancies of our own together with approximately 150 available in the literature.

The "Swiss-type" agammaglobulinemia is a simple Mendelian recessive by best evidence in which all parameters of immunity are absent —delayed sensitivity, homograft immunity, and antibody synthesis.

Such patients show striking reduction in small lymphocytes in the circulating blood and lymph nodes, and plasma cells are absent. The thymus often cannot be found, and appears entirely epithelial with no lymphocytes.

We visualize this condition as being analogous to the bursectomized and thymectomized irradiated chick in that immunological function of both immunoglobulin and cellular immune systems is defective. This disease must either represent deficiency of the stem cell in its response to differentiation, or failure to develop, in association with the gut, epithelial components that can differentiate to lymphoid cells.

A variation of this type patient has been described by Nessloff in which lymphoid elements were absent but germinal centers, plasma cells, and immunoglobulin production were intact. Perhaps this functional combination parallels the thymectomy and irradiation model.

The Bruton type hypogammaglobulinemia shows normal lymphocytes in the circulation and lymphatic tissues. These patients are capable of developing a normal delayed sensitivity response. They can reject a homograft, and their thymus is morphologically normal. They completely lack plasma cells, however, and do not form secondary follicles. They are deficient in intestinal epithelium-associated lymphoid tissue including tonsils and Peyer's patches. They make at most small quantities of each of the immunoglobulins.

This clinical condition seems to parallel the bursectomized irradiated chicken both morphologically and functionally. Perhaps the defect is an absence of some genetically determined key step, which, in mammals, fulfills bursal function in the chicken.

Certain patients with so-called acquired hypogammaglobulinemia have a disease analogous to visceral lymphomatosis of chickens in which proliferation in the germinal center components of the lymphoid apparatus is striking, resembling giant follicular lymphoma.

Ataxia telangiectasia syndrome is a progressive cerebellar ataxia in which γA-globulins are absent in the circulation and in the secretions; in addition, however, these patients have abnormalities of delayed sensitivity. Delayed sensitivity develops slowly or not at all and homografts are not rejected normally. If they live long enough they develop malignancy of the lymphoreticular system, particularly lymphosarcoma. Peterson biopsied the thymus of such patients and found an incompletely developed thymus without Hassall's corpuscles or normal medullary development, and minimal lymphoid cell production.

Another group of patients show hypoparathyroidism, with failure of parathyroid development, absence of the thymus, and reduction of circulating and tissue lymphocytes. In such patients both epithelial derivatives of the third- and fourth-pharyngeal pouch do not develop; however, these patients show germinal centers, normal plasma cells, and normal immunoglobulin levels.

We believe that examination of these experimental models in the chicken assists in understanding the various aberrant structural defects and abnormal functions, seen in what otherwise appears to be an amorphous clinical group of disorders of the lymphoreticular system. In the long run we expect that development of such animal models will assist materially in developing an understanding which will subtend rational therapy in humans. In the conference to be held next winter we shall try to bring together those who have contributed the great bulk of this clinical experience and try to gain from past experience understanding of the clinical diseases associated with immunological deficiency. From this study it is hoped that improved directions of analyses and study as well as improvement of approaches to therapy will be forthcoming. Perhaps of greatest moment will be the focus of important questions concerning differentiation and development of the lymphoid apparatus by the experiments of nature represented in these diseases of immunologic deficiency.

Index